AN ATLAS

OF

HUMAN ANATOMY

FOR STUDENTS AND PHYSICIANS

BY

CARL TOLDT, M.D.

ASSISTED BY

PROFESSOR ALOIS DALLA ROSA, M.D.

Adapted to English and American and International Terminology

BY

M. EDEN PAUL, M.D. Brux., M.R.C.S., L.R.C.P.

FIRST SECTION

A. THE REGIONS OF THE HUMAN BODY

B. OSTEOLOGY

(FIGURES 1 TO 377 AND INDEX)

REVISED EDITION

NEW YORK

REBMAN COMPANY

141, 143 AND 145 WEST 36TH STREET

ILLUSTRATED &

PUBLISHED BY

E-KİTAP PROJESİ & CHEAPEST BOOKS

www.facebook.com/EKitapProjesi

www.cheapestboooks.com

ISBN:

978-625-6629-60-8

Cover Image: Henry Vandyke Carter - Henry Gray (1918) Anatomy of the Human Body

TRANSLATOR'S PREFACE

THE science of human anatomy is purely descriptive in its methods, the field it covers is not very extensive, and its boundaries are sharply limited; it is, therefore, one of the few sciences in which something closely verging on finality and completeness has been attained. Even, however, if no new anatomical data are likely to be forthcoming, there is yet scope for originality in the method of presentation of those data of which the science now consists; and originality of this kind Professor Toldt's "Atlas of Human Anatomy" exhibits in a high degree. In the many admirable manuals of human anatomy now extant in English, the illustrations, even when numerous, as they are often, and when good, as they are occasionally, form a mere supplement—usually a very imperfect supplement—to the text. Atlases of anatomy, and useful atlases, also exist in English, but all are quite fragmentary. Some, like the well-known and valuable, but somewhat antiquated, "Illustrations of Dissections," consist of a series of pictures of selected regions carefully prepared on the cadaver: these are models for the imitation of the student in his own dissecting work, but are not of much value for private study. Others, like Bellamy's English edition of Braune's atlas of frozen sections of the human body, present a small number of anatomical facts from a striking and unfamiliar point of view. But among English works, an accurate pictorial representation of *all* the data of human anatomy, carefully drawn to scale from actual specimens, and arranged suitably for systematic study, has hitherto been lacking.

Whilst a true knowledge of anatomy, a knowledge that will through life supply the needs of the physician and the surgeon in their practical work, can be obtained only in the dissecting-room, the student's labours with scalpel and forceps must be preceded and supplemented by systematic private study. Now, for this purpose, the textual descriptive treatise is not alone sufficient; or, if sufficient, it is so at an excessive expenditure of time and labour. Both in his work preparatory to dissection and in his revision of his anatomical knowledge subsequent to dissection, the energy of the student will be enormously economized if he has at hand a graphic representation of every structure named and described in his systematic treatise. An increased use of the visual or graphic method, both in the acquirement and in the revivification of knowledge, is a feature of the age in all educational departments; but this English translation of Professor Toldt's work is, as far as the English-speaking races are concerned, the first adequate application of the method to the study of human anatomy.

In speaking of the finality and completeness of anatomical science, one exception must be made, and this exception relates to anatomical terminology, which, though nearly completed, has not yet attained finality. Had there been a universal anatomical nomenclature—a nomenclature, that is, adopted by, or even fully intelligible to, anatomists of all nationalities—an English edition of this work would have been superfluous. Anatomy, however, like all other sciences, has suffered from the dispersion of tongues that ensued on the Renascence, when the good and the evil of mediævalism became inextricably confounded, and were cast away together, and the inestimable gift of a language common to the learned of all lands was lost for ever. The German-speaking peoples have a fairly complete and fairly pure Latin anatomical nomenclature, needing, however, to be eked out here and there by the vernacular; whilst in England, as in France, a strange and bastard dialect, half Latin and half vernacular, has come into use. Uncouth jargon as it is, being current and familiar, it is not likely in England and America ever to be replaced by the more consistent terminology in use in the anatomical schools of Germany and Austria; I have, however, in this English edition of the "Atlas of Anatomy" retained the terminology of the original side by side with the English translation, distinguishing between the two by a difference of type.

In some cases, in the nomenclature used by the author, terms are met with which have no counterpart in English anatomical terminology: either because the author regards as normal a structure which English anatomists regard as a variety; or, and far more commonly, because the structure in question, though normal, is unimportant, and English anatomists have therefore neglected to name it. Sometimes, in such cases, I have given a literal English translation of the Latin name used by the author; sometimes, however, a periphrasis has been required to explain what the structure is, or to account for the absence of an English name, and this periphrasis, when lengthy, has been printed as a foot-note. In all such cases, *an asterisk* is prefixed both to the Latin name and to its English equivalent, to indicate to the reader that there is something unusual in the terms employed.

I must further point out that in a few instances the author's nomenclature actually conflicts with that commonly used in England, so that the literal translation of the author's name for a certain structure is applied in England to a structure totally different. For instance, what the author calls *canalis pterygopalatinus* is in England called the *posterior palatine* or *palatomaxillary canal*, while the *pterygopalatine canal* of English anatomists is called by the author *canalis pharyngeus*. But for this warning, beginners might imagine such divergencies to be due to carelessness on the part of the translator or to errors of the press.

A further difficulty has arisen from the fact that English anatomical nomenclature is itself not yet finally settled, nor even wholly consistent. Not merely is the same structure often known by several names; but, which is worse, the same name is sometimes applied to two different structures. Reform is therefore needed, but it is not the part of a translator to undertake it, and I have perforce been content to follow the authorities. My leading authority has been the tenth edition of Quain's "Elements of Anatomy," but I have also had Macalister's "Text-book of Human Anatomy" in constant requisition. From these works I have, when more than one name is used to denote any structure, taken all those in common use, the order in which the alternative names have been printed showing most often the relative frequency of employment; in a few cases, however, where a name less commonly used has appeared to me distinctly preferable for any reason to an alternative name more commonly used, I have given the less usual but preferable name the precedence. To this small extent only have I been influenced by my own views in the matter of anatomical terminology; and, with the exception of those names which for the reason already furnished are preceded by an asterisk, all the terms in the English nomenclature are in use by one or more of the leading English authorities.

As regards the terminology employed in the United States of America, the contributions of the scientific investigators of that country to anatomy have, owing to the early perfection of this branch of study, been far less extensive than in the case of the other sciences ancillary to medicine; and the science of anatomy was for the most part taken bodily over, text-books, terminology, and all complete. A few differences, however, exist, and I have therefore collated my manuscript with that useful little work, Young's "Synopsis of Human Anatomy," and any divergent terms in use in America only have been inserted in my translation, and distinguished by the addition of the letters "U.S."

A considerable number of the references to the figures will be found to be in the English nomenclature only. These are either cases in which the English and the International descriptive terms were identical, and the printing of both was therefore superfluous; or else cases in which in the original the reference was wholly in German.

Measurements given in the original in centimetres have in all cases been reduced to inches. In illustrations of fœtal parts the age of the fœtus is given in months from the date of fertilization of the ovum. On the Continent, however, the period of utero-gestation is usually reckoned as ten "months" of four weeks each; not, as with us, as nine calendar months. To avoid mistake, I have in all such cases after the word "month" or "months" added in parentheses the words "months of four weeks each."

I cannot dismiss mention of the works of reference I have employed without alluding to the German-English "Dictionary of Medical Terms," by Treves and Lang—a book invaluable to all those engaged in the translation of German medical works.

Since this Atlas is intended for the use of beginners, as well as for that of advanced students of human anatomy and of practitioners of medicine, I may fitly conclude this preface with a few words on the general principles of anatomical nomenclature. For descriptive purposes the body is regarded as being in the upright posture, with the arms extended by the sides, and the hands fully supinated, so that the palms look forward. With this attitude kept in mind, the meaning of the terms *superior* and *inferior*, *anterior* and *posterior*, *external* and *internal*, is obvious. Sometimes, however, descriptive terms of another kind are used, to remove the confusion liable to arise from the adoption by man of an attitude different from that of all the other vertebrata, and to homologize the nomenclature of human with that of comparative anatomy. Thus, *cephalic* and *caudal* in comparative anatomy correspond respectively with *superior* and *inferior* in human anatomy; *ventral* and *dorsal*, with *anterior* and *posterior*. Dividing the body into right and left halves by a vertical *median plane*, which cuts the surface of the body at the *median line*, *medial* or *mesial* and *lateral* correspond respectively with *internal* and *external* in denoting position respectively nearer to, or more remote from, the median plane. Other terms in frequent use are *superficial* and *deep*, *central* and *peripheral*, *proximal* and *distal*; these are self-explanatory.

In some cases descriptive terms applied to portions of certain structures denote the relation of these portions to other structures, as when we speak of the *vertebral* and the *sternal* extremities of the ribs, or the *acromial* and the *sternal* extremities of the clavicle. Terms of similar import are *radial* and *ulnar* applied to structures of the forearm; *tibial* and *fibular* (or *peroneal*) of the leg; *palmar* and *dorsal* of the hand; *plantar* and *dorsal* of the foot; *flexor* and *extensor* of any of the extremities. It is to be noted that *internal* and *external* are sometimes used in a sense different from that previously explained, being employed to denote the interior and exterior positions respectively, either in relation to the general axis of the body or to the axis of one of its cavities. In this sense, for instance, we may speak of the *internal* and the *external* tables of the cranial vault, or of the *internal* and the *external* oblique muscles of the abdomen; but it is, as a rule, better to use the words *inner* and *outer* to denote this relation, and to reserve *internal* and *external* for position in respect to the median plane.

Finally we have to explain the terms used to denote certain directions, more especially the direction of certain sections: these are *horizontal* and *vertical*, requiring no definition; *sagittal*, denoting a dorso-ventral direction either in or parallel to the median plane; and *frontal* or *coronal*, which are synonymous terms, denoting direction in a transverse vertical plane.

The definition of many of the terms used in descriptive anatomy, such as *condyle* and *tuberosity*, *process* and *tubercle*, *sinus* and *cavity*, *ligament*, *tendon*, and *aponeurosis*, would be superfluous, since the student will best gain an accurate notion of their meaning by an examination of the structures to which they are respectively applied.

M. EDEN PAUL.

ALDERNEY, *August*, 1903.

REGIONES CORPORIS HUMANI

THE REGIONS OF THE HUMAN BODY

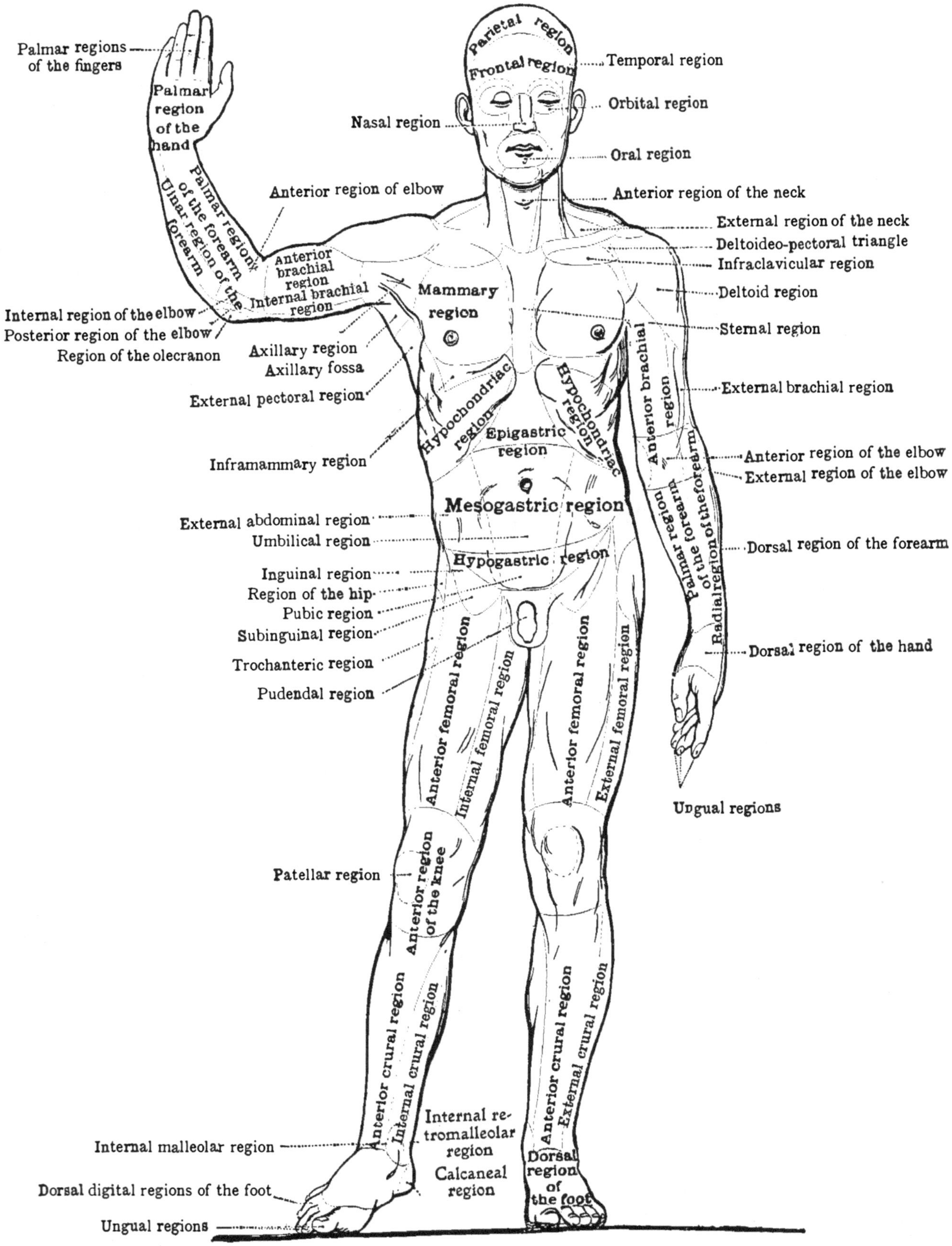

FIG. 1.—ANTERIOR SURFACE OF THE BODY.

Regions of the Human Body.

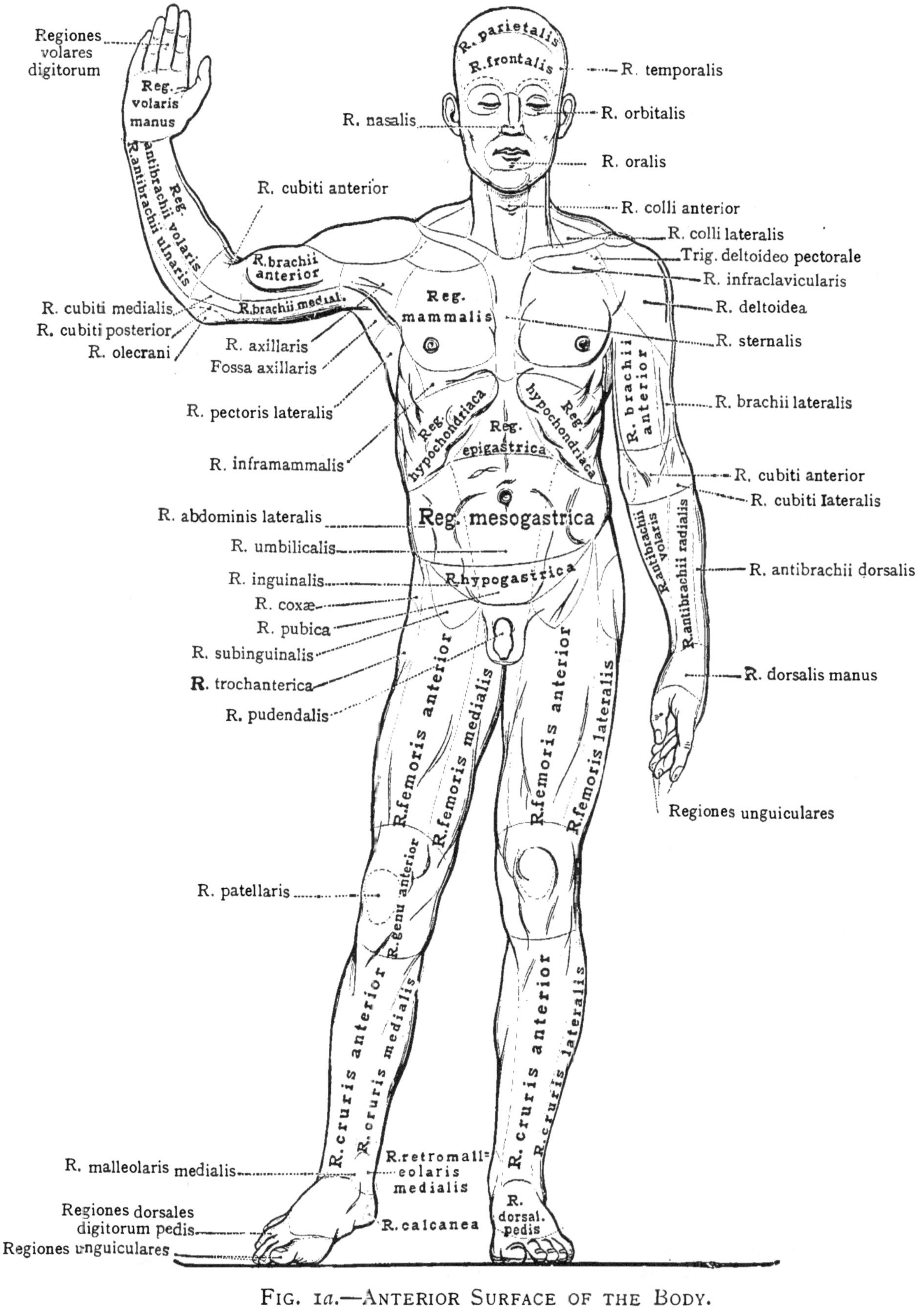

FIG. 1a.—ANTERIOR SURFACE OF THE BODY.

Regiones Corporis Humani.

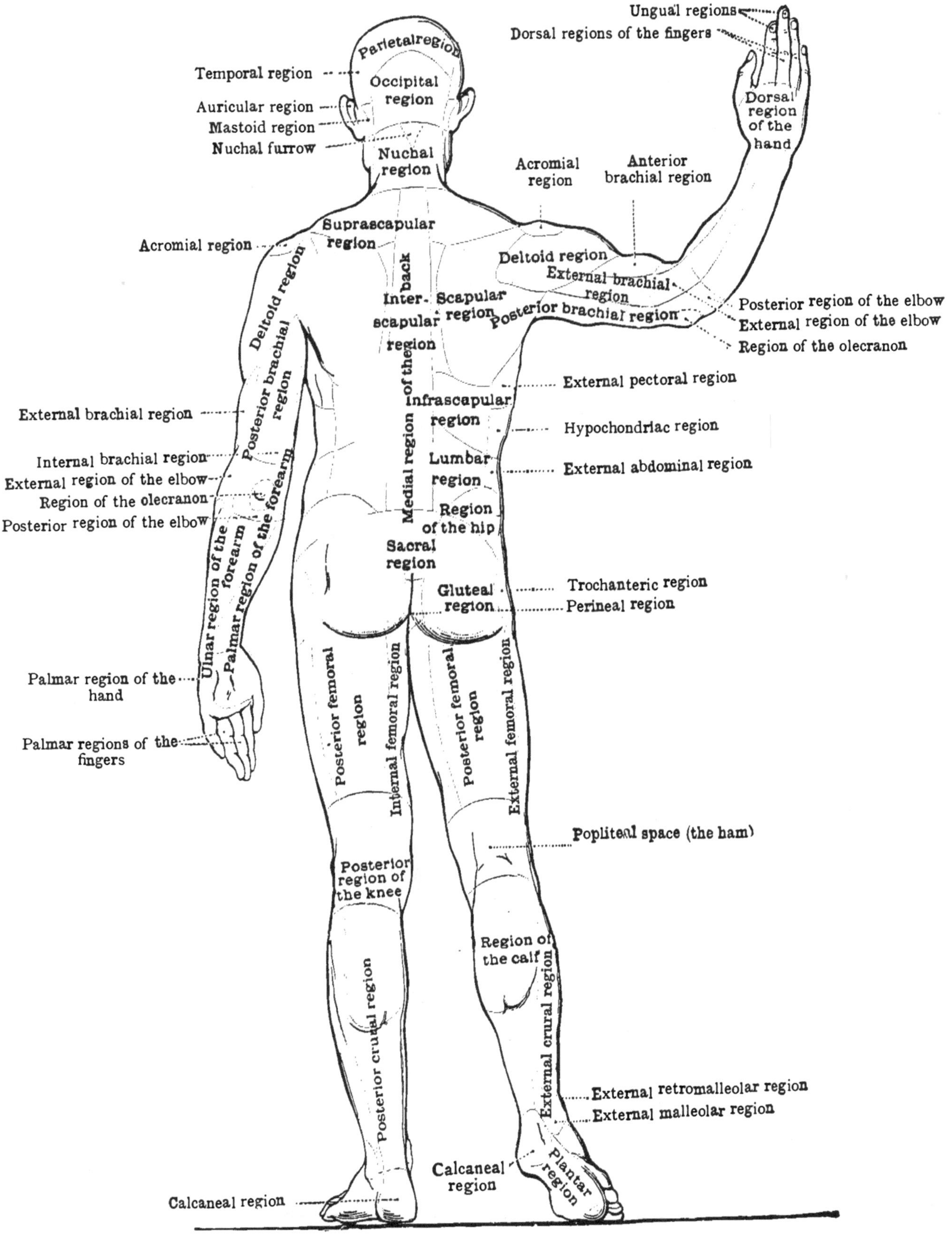

FIG. 2.—POSTERIOR SURFACE OF THE BODY.

Regions of the Human Body.

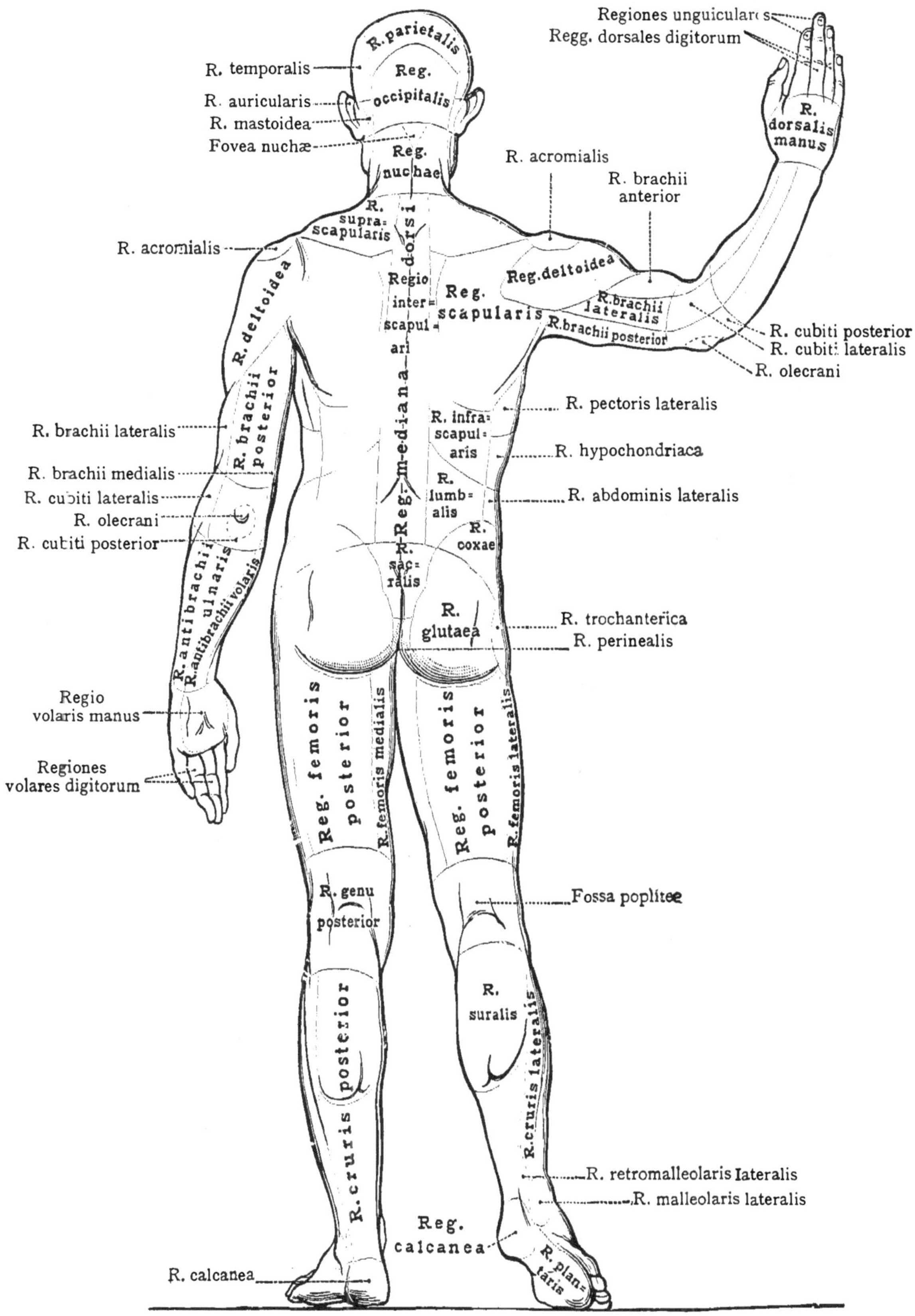

FIG. 2a.—POSTERIOR SURFACE OF THE BODY.

Regiones Corporis Humani.

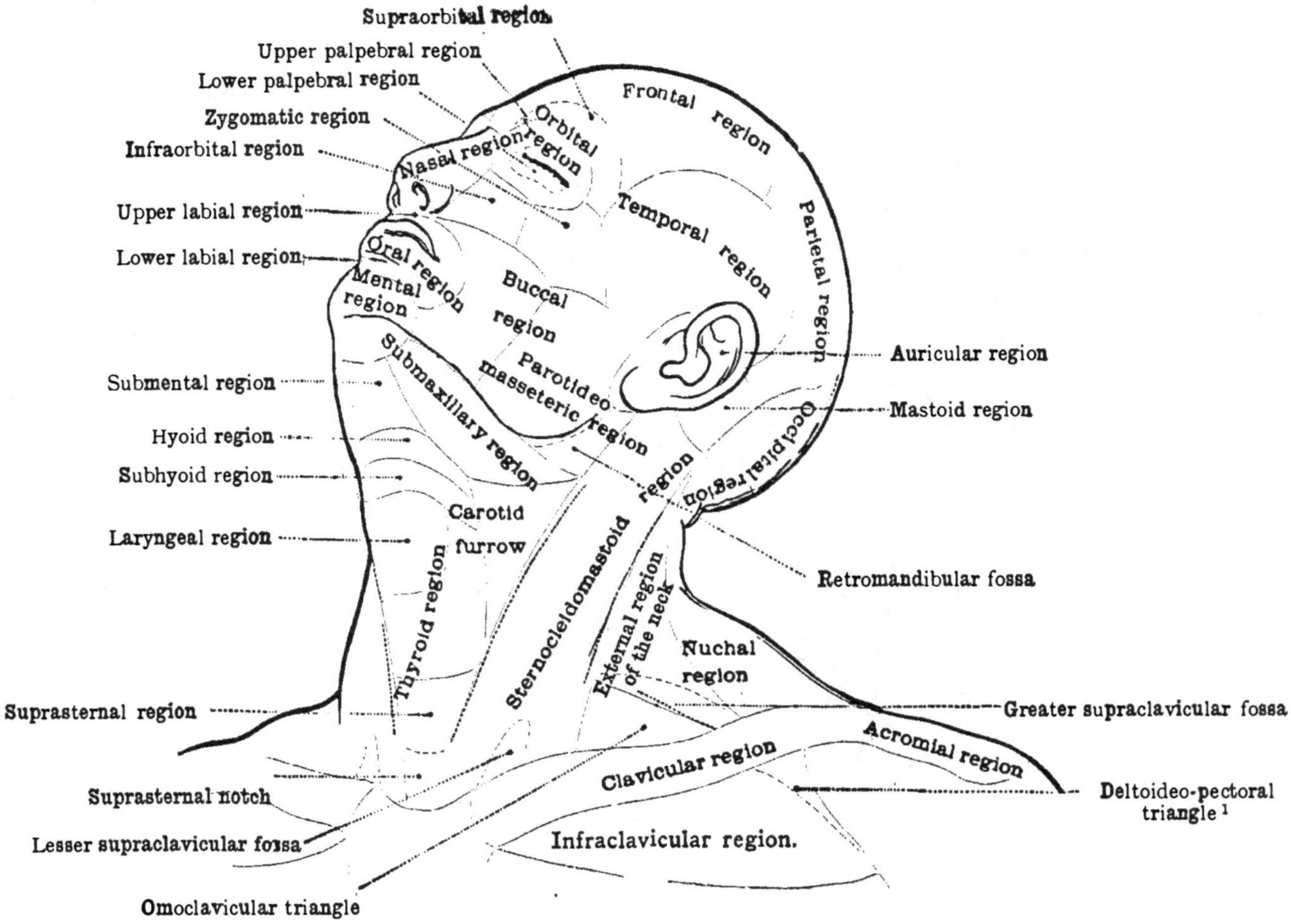

[1] Known also as the *infraclavicular triangle* or *infraclavicular fossa*, and sometimes called *Mohrenheimer's space.*

FIG. 3.—HEAD AND NECK.

Regions of the Head and Neck.

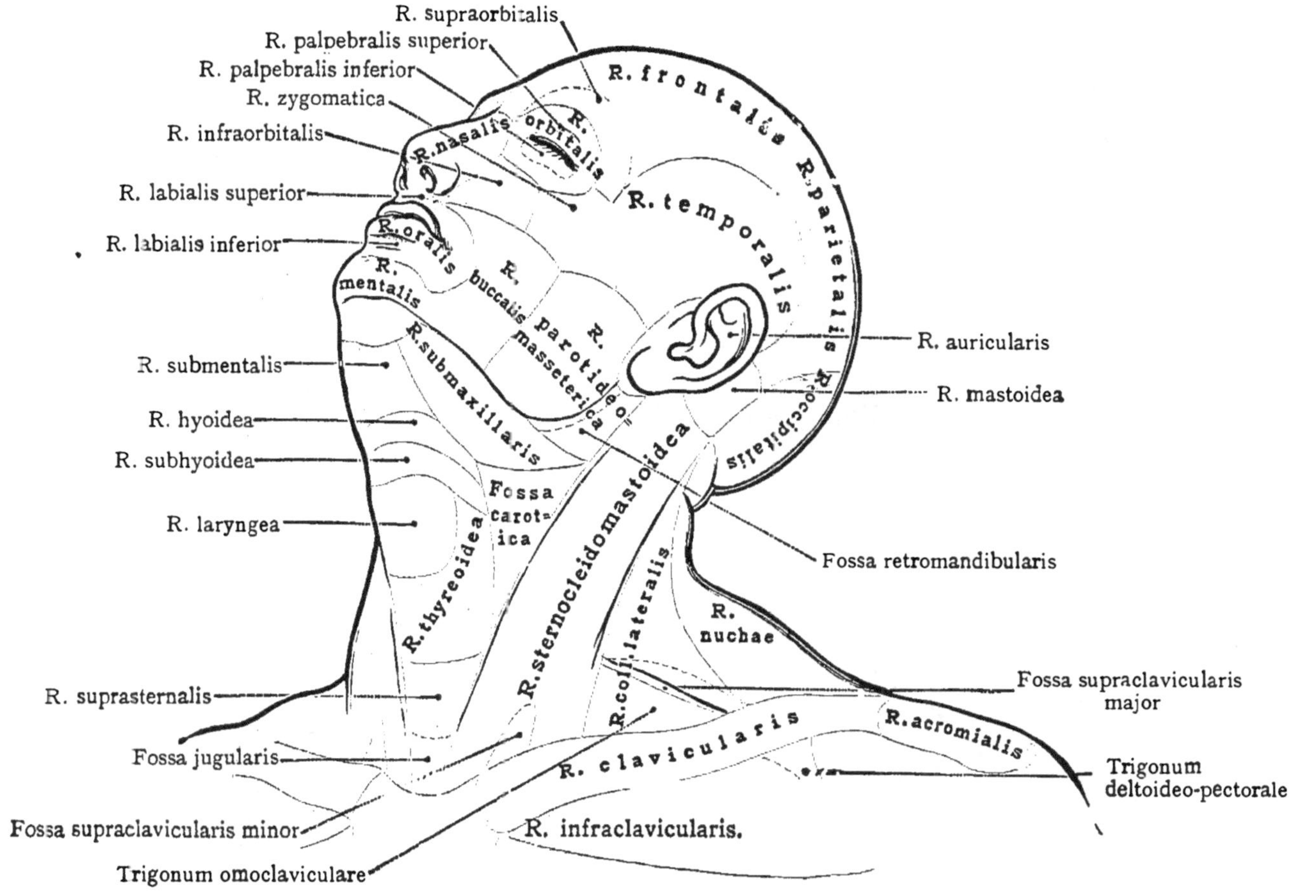

FIG. 3a.—HEAD AND NECK.

Regiones Capitis et Colli.

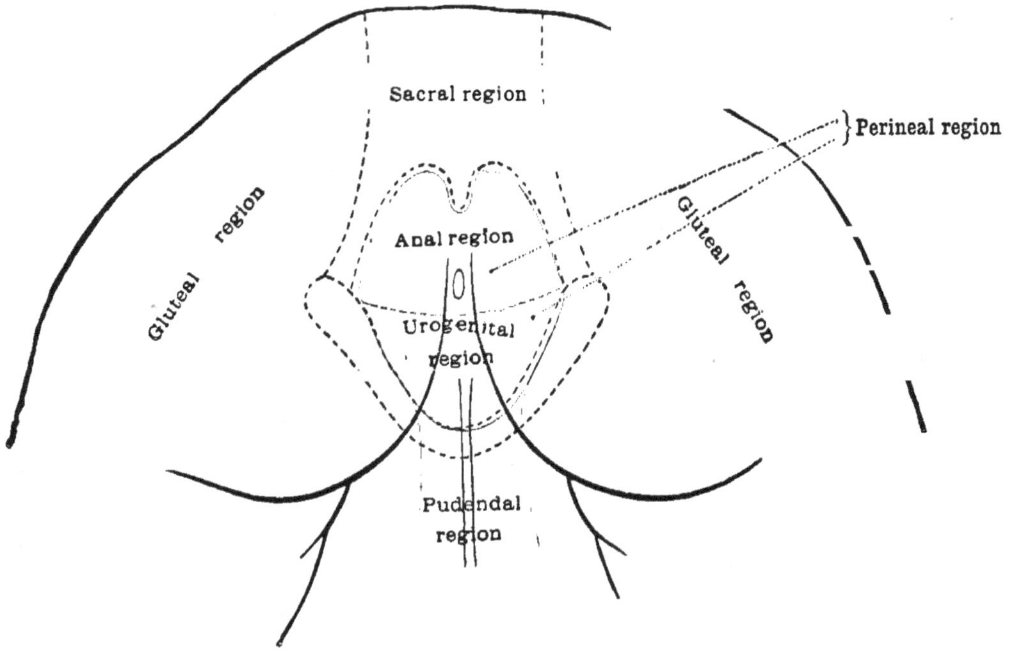

FIG. 4.—MALE PERINEAL REGION.

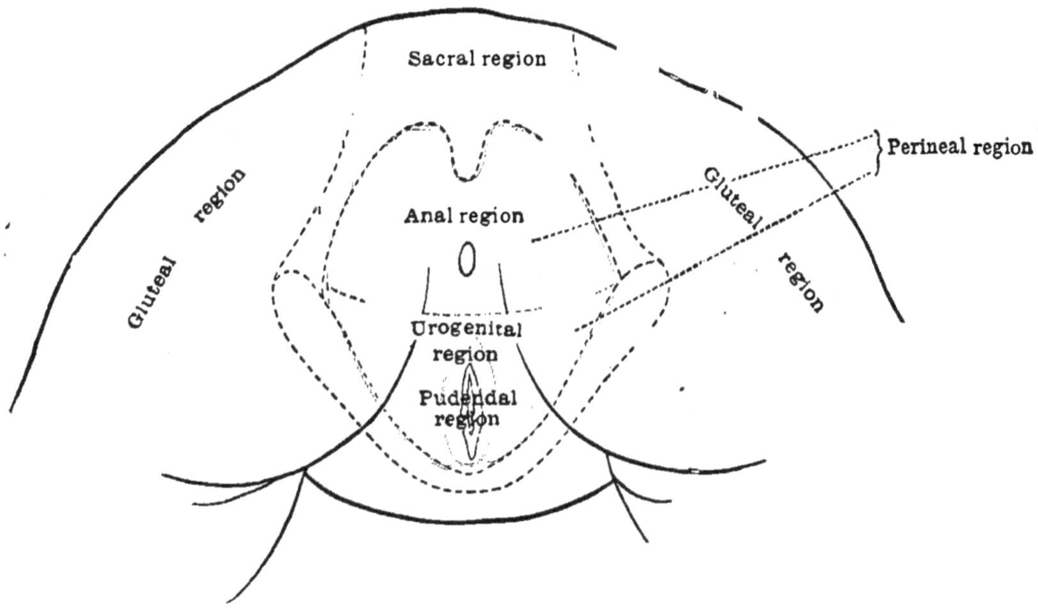

FIG. 5.—FEMALE PERINEAL REGION.

Perineal Region.

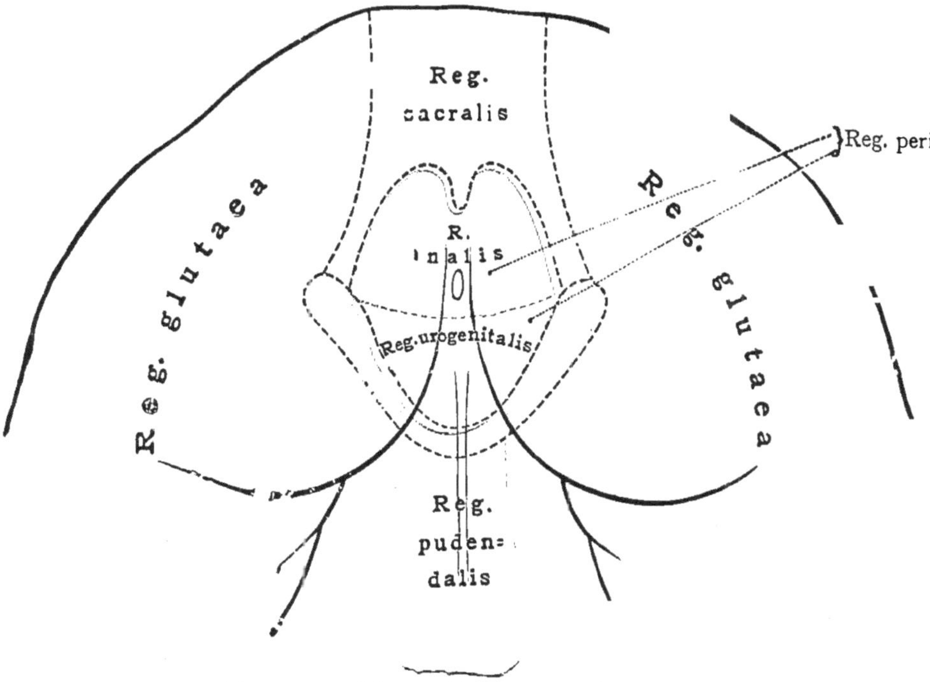

FIG. 4a.—MALE PERINEAL REGION.

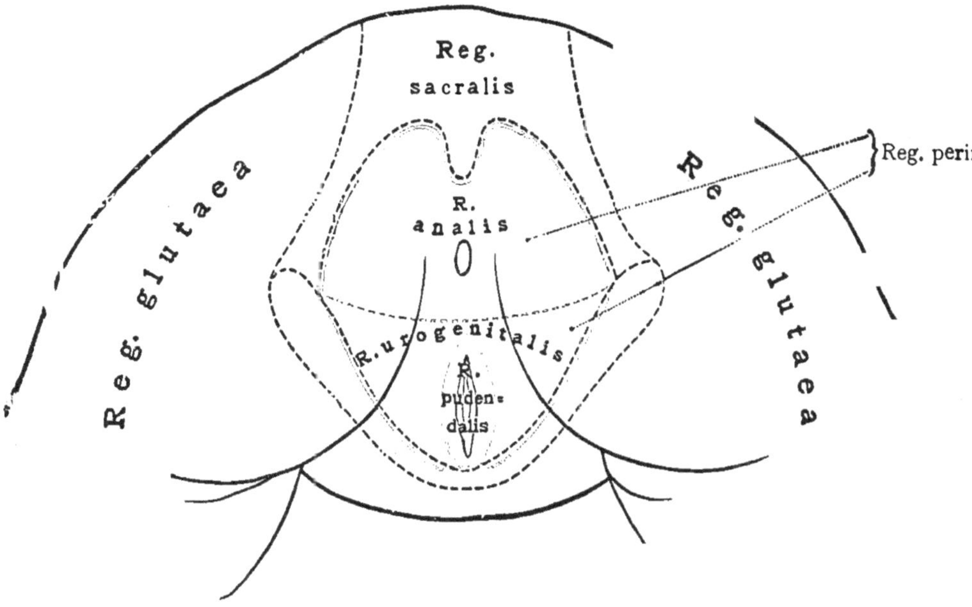

FIG. 5a.—FEMALE PERINEAL REGION.

Regio Perinealis.

OSTEOLOGIA

OSTEOLOGY

THE STRUCTURE OF THE BONES

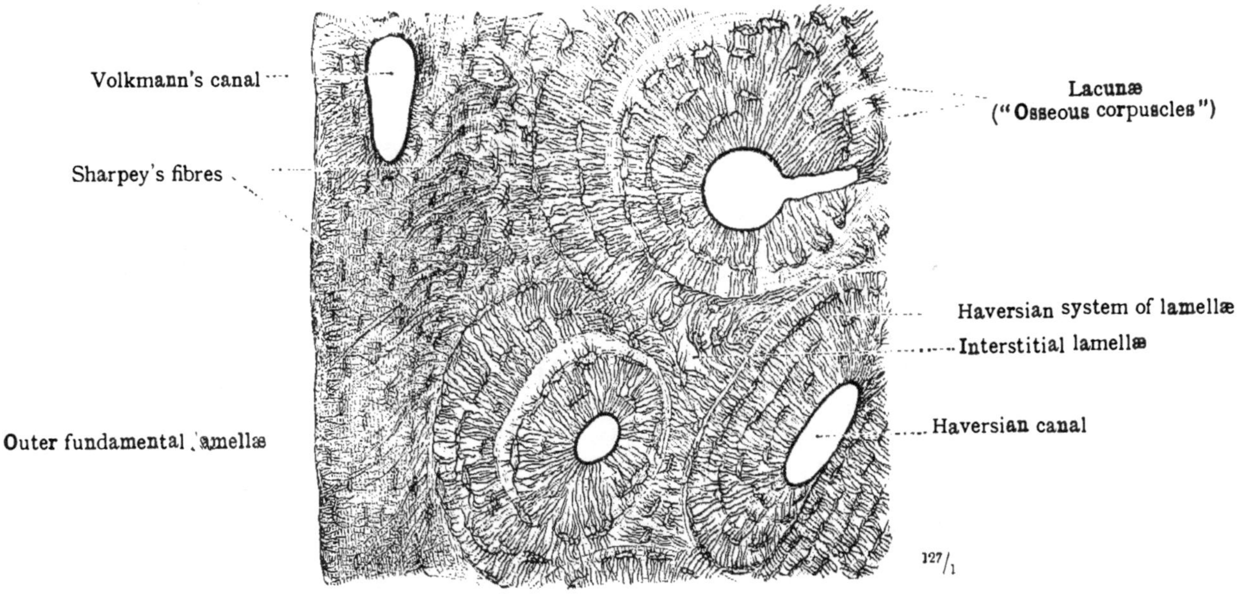

FIG. 6.—PORTION OF A CROSS-SECTION THROUGH THE COMPACT TISSUE OF LONG BONE.

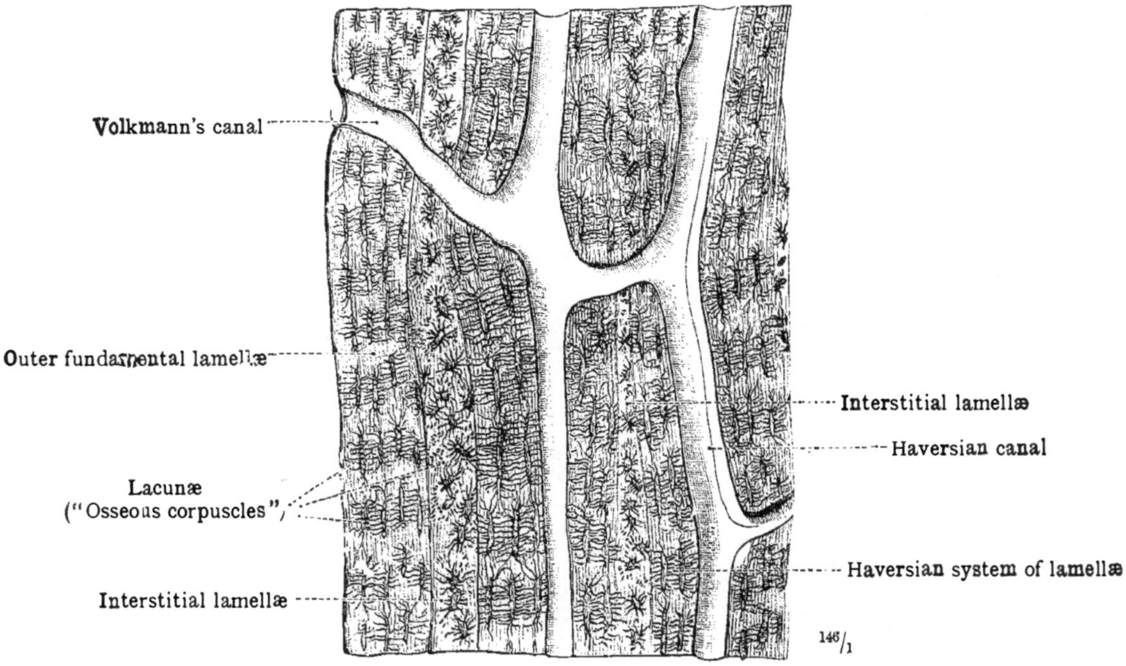

FIG. 7.—PORTION OF A LONGITUDINAL SECTION THROUGH THE COMPACT TISSUE OF A LONG BONE.

Microscopical Structure of Bone.

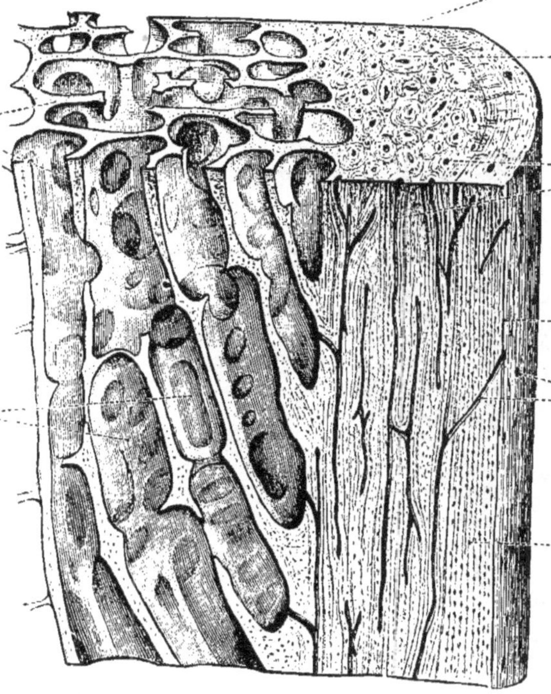

FIG. 8.—DIAGRAM OF THE STRUCTURE OF BONE.

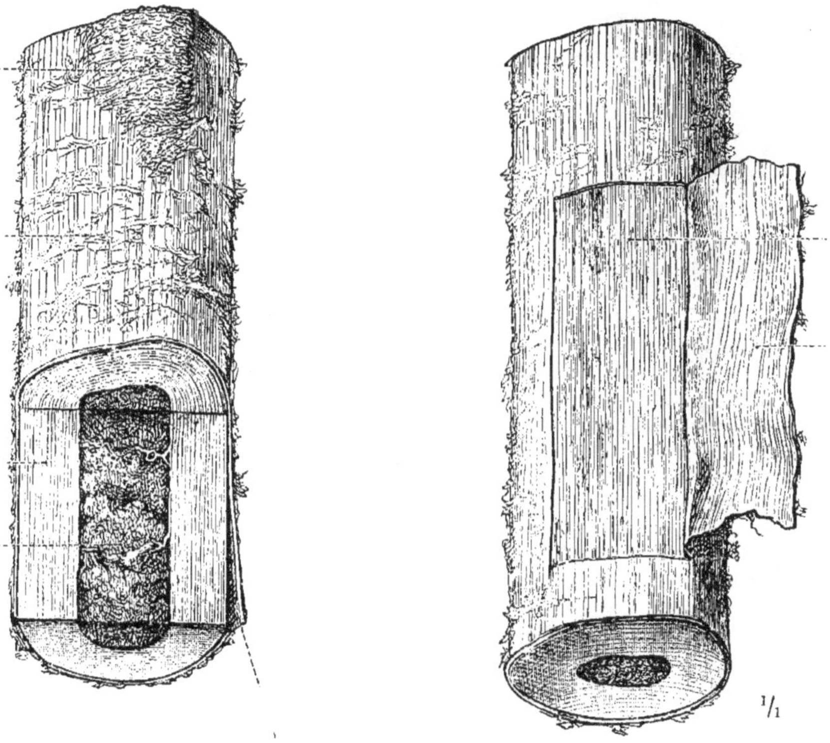

FIG. 9.—PART OF THE MIDDLE SEGMENT OF THE FEMUR FROM WHICH THE PERIOSTEUM HAS BEEN PARTIALLY REMOVED.

The medullary canal (cavum medullare) has been opened, and the bone-marrow (medulla ossis) is seen.

Periosteum and Bone-Marrow (Medulla Ossium).

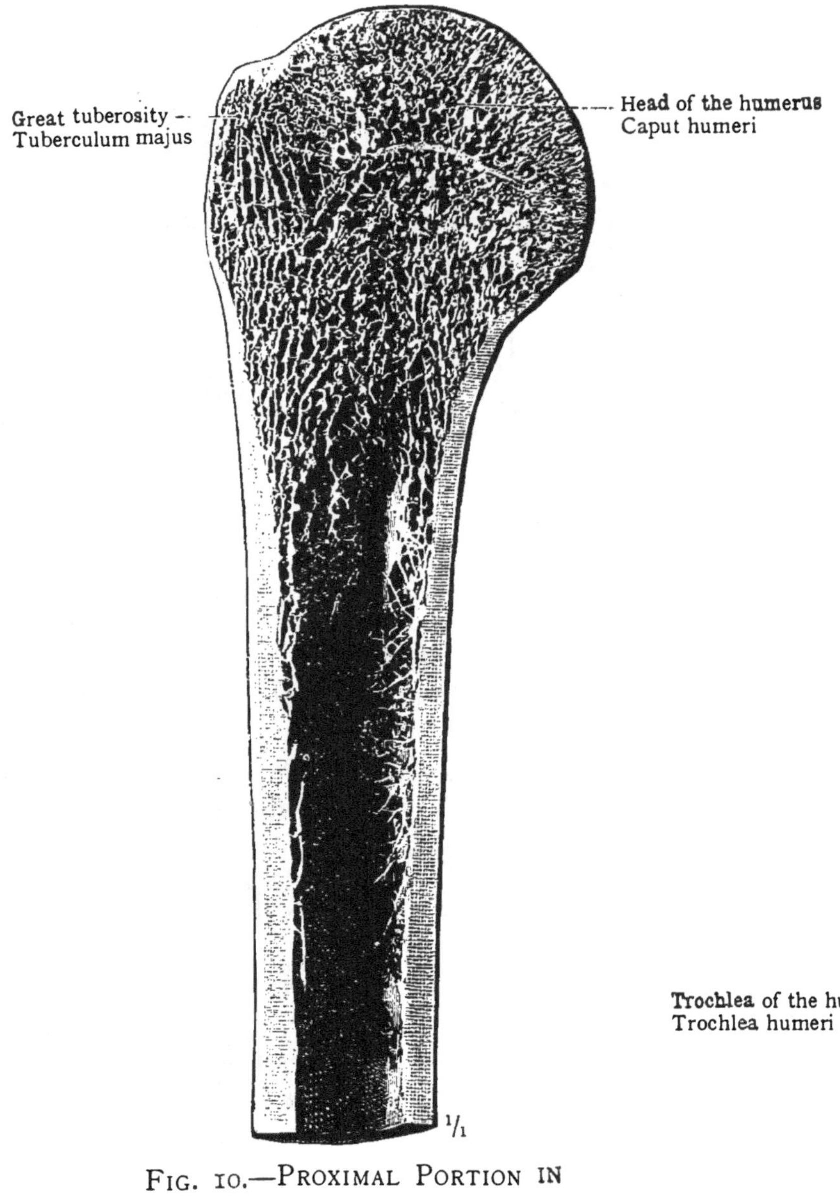

FIG. 10.—PROXIMAL PORTION IN FRONTAL SECTION.

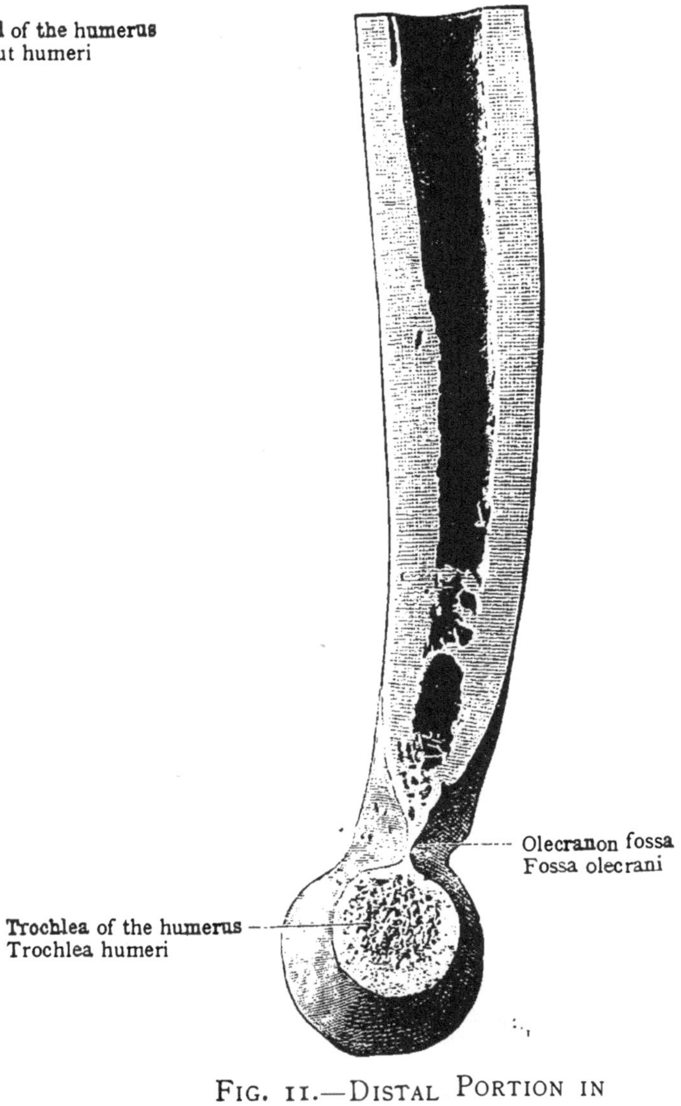

FIG. 11.—DISTAL PORTION IN SAGITTAL SECTION.

Humerus—Arm-bone: Substantia compacta et substantia spongiosa ossium—Compact and cancellous tissue of the bones.

Ossa longa—Long bones.

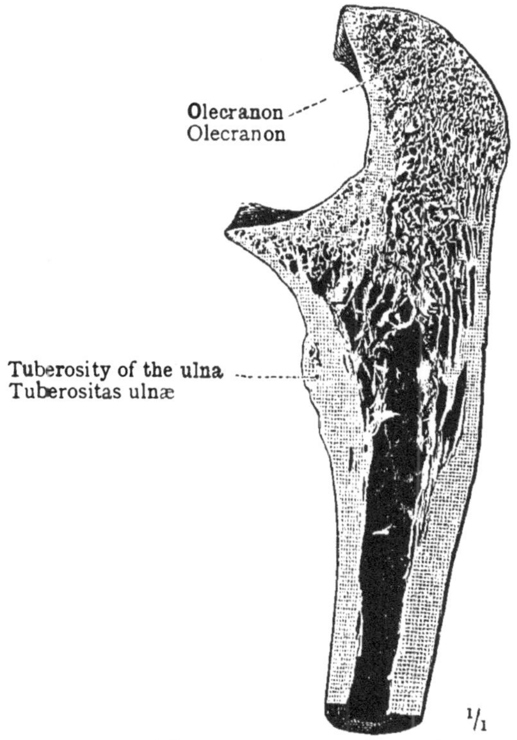

FIG. 12.—PROXIMAL PORTION IN SAGITTAL SECTION.

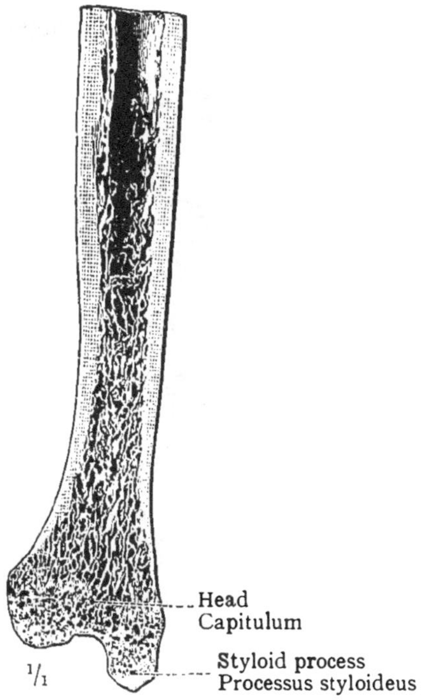

FIG. 13.—DISTAL PORTION IN FRONTAL SECTION.

Ulna.

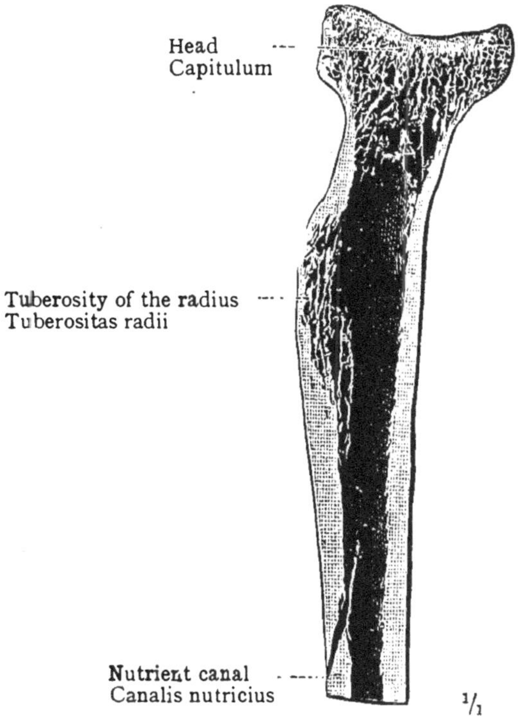

FIG. 14.—PROXIMAL PORTION.

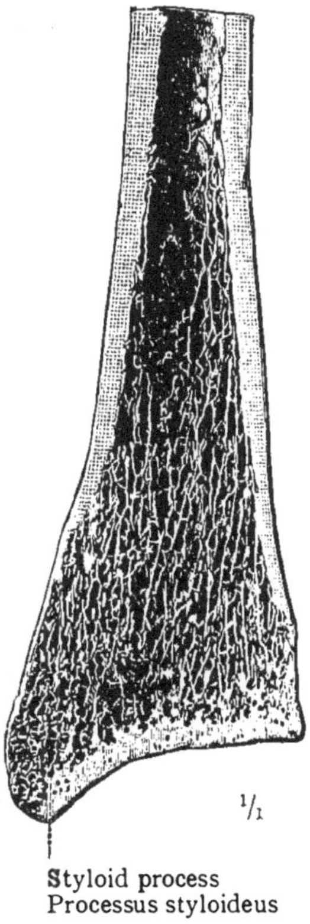

FIG. 15.—DISTAL PORTION.

Radius.

Substantia compacta et substantia spongiosa ossium—Compact and cancellous tissue of the bones.

Ossa longa—Long bones.

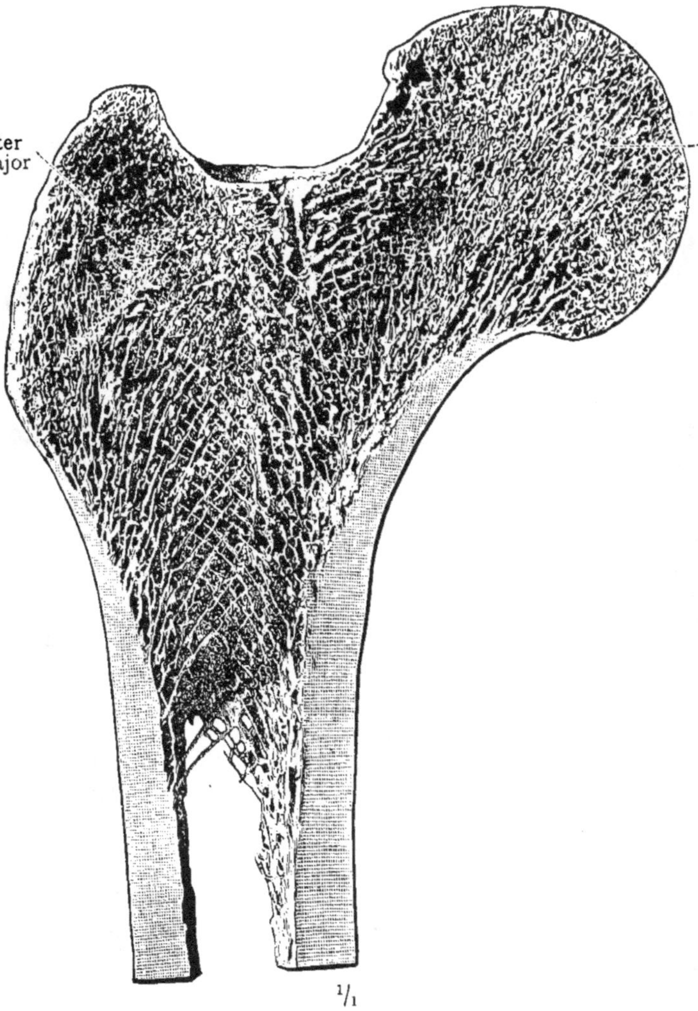

FIG. 16.—PROXIMAL PORTION IN FRONTAL SECTION.

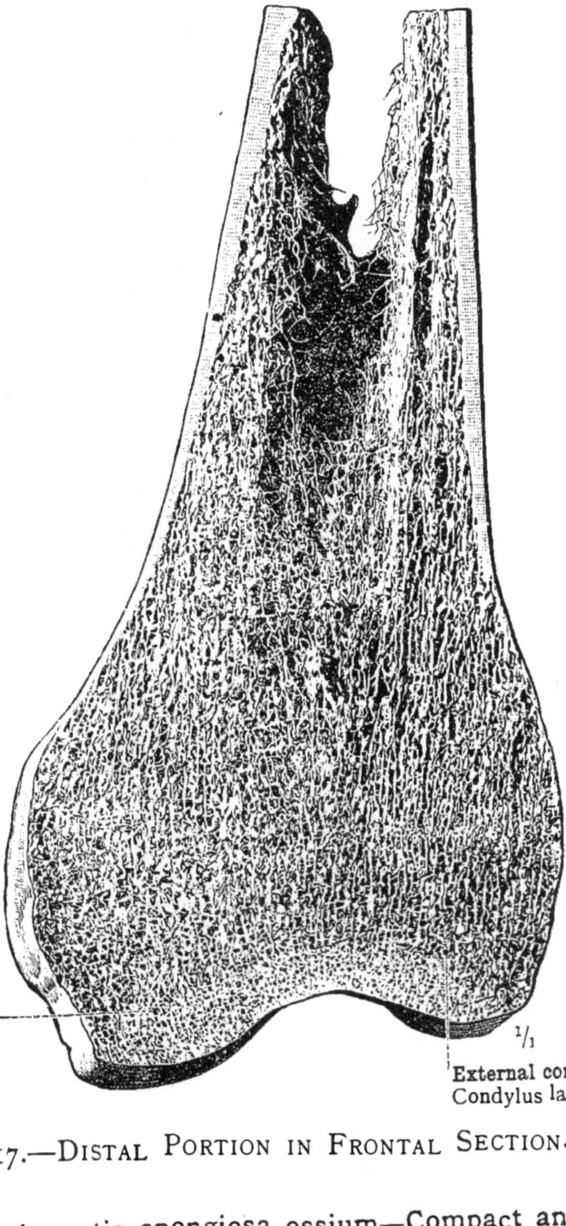

FIG. 17.—DISTAL PORTION IN FRONTAL SECTION.

Femur—Thigh-bone Substantia compacta et substantia spongiosa ossium—Compact and cancellous tissue of the bones.

Ossa longa—Long bones.

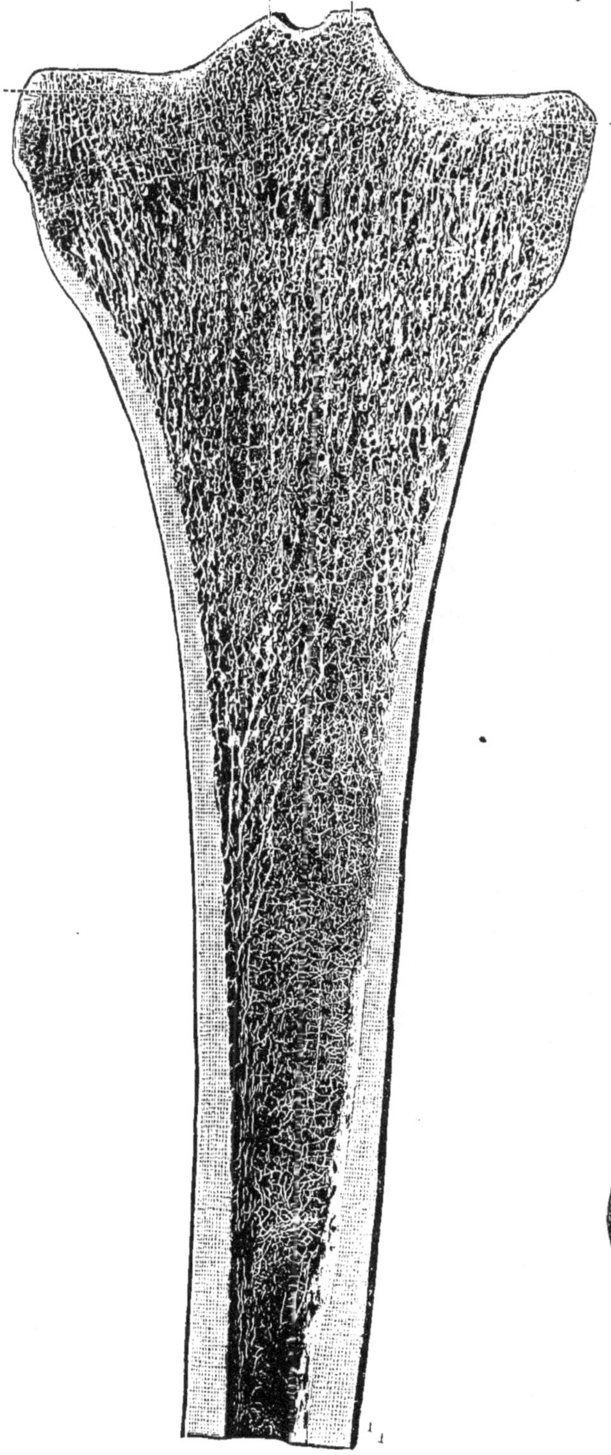

FIG. 18.—PROXIMAL PORTION IN FRONTAL SECTION.

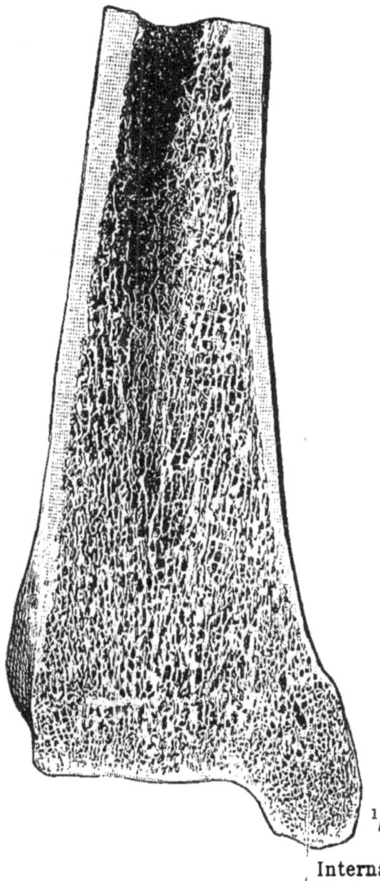

FIG. 19.—DISTAL PORTION IN FRONTAL SECTION.

Tibia—Shin-bone: Substantia compacta et substantia spongiosa ossium—Compact and cancellous tissue of the bones.

Ossa longa—Long bones.

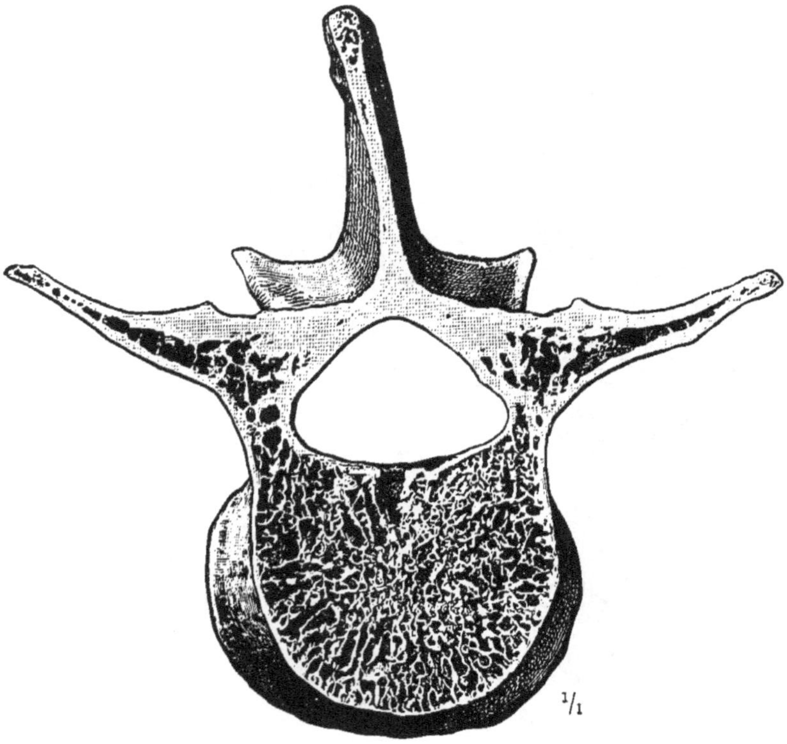

Fig. 20.—Third Lumbar Vertebra in Horizontal Section.

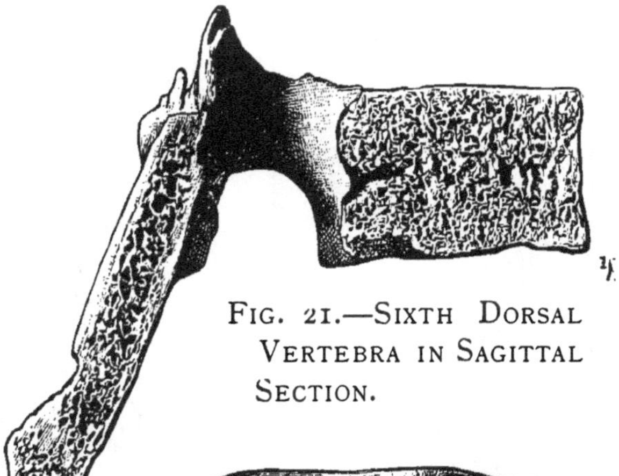

Fig. 21.—Sixth Dorsal Vertebra in Sagittal Section.

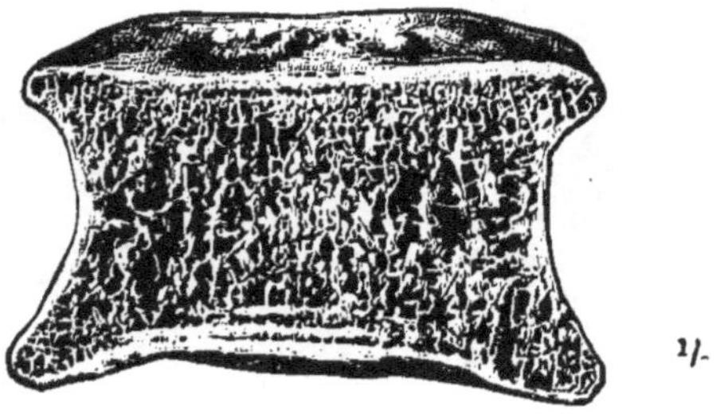

Fig. 22.—Body of the Second Lumbar Vertebra in Frontal Section.

Vertebræ **Substantia compacta et substantia spongiosa ossium—Compact and cancellous tissue of the bones.**

Ossa brevia—Short bones.

Fig. 23.—Os Cuneiforme III., the External Cuneiform Bone.

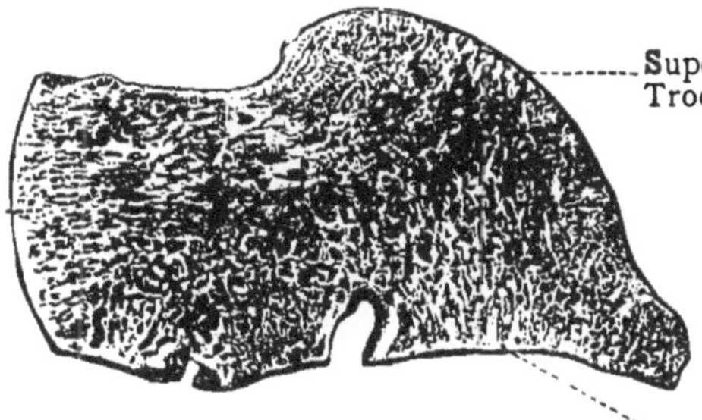

Fig. 24.—Talus, the Astragalus, in Sagittal Section.

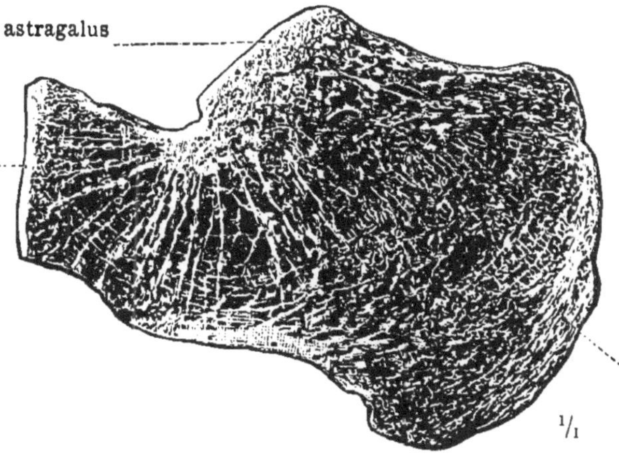

Fig. 25.—Calcaneum, the Os Calcis, in Sagittal Section.

Ossa tarsi—Tarsal bones Substantia compacta et substantia spongiosa ossium—Compact and cancellous tissue of the bones.

Ossa brevia—Short bones.

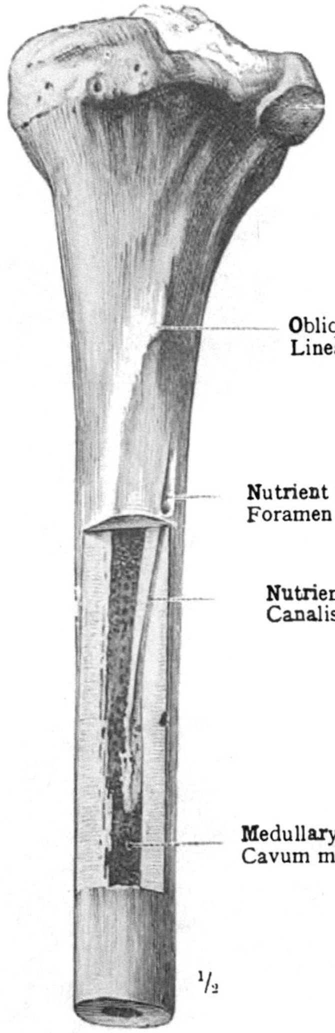

FIG. 26.—NUTRIENT FORAMEN AND NUTRIENT CANAL OF THE RIGHT TIBIA. SEEN FROM BEHIND.

By sawing away a portion of the shaft the whole length of the nutrient canal has been opened up.

Nutrient Foramen and Nutrient Canal of a Long Bone.

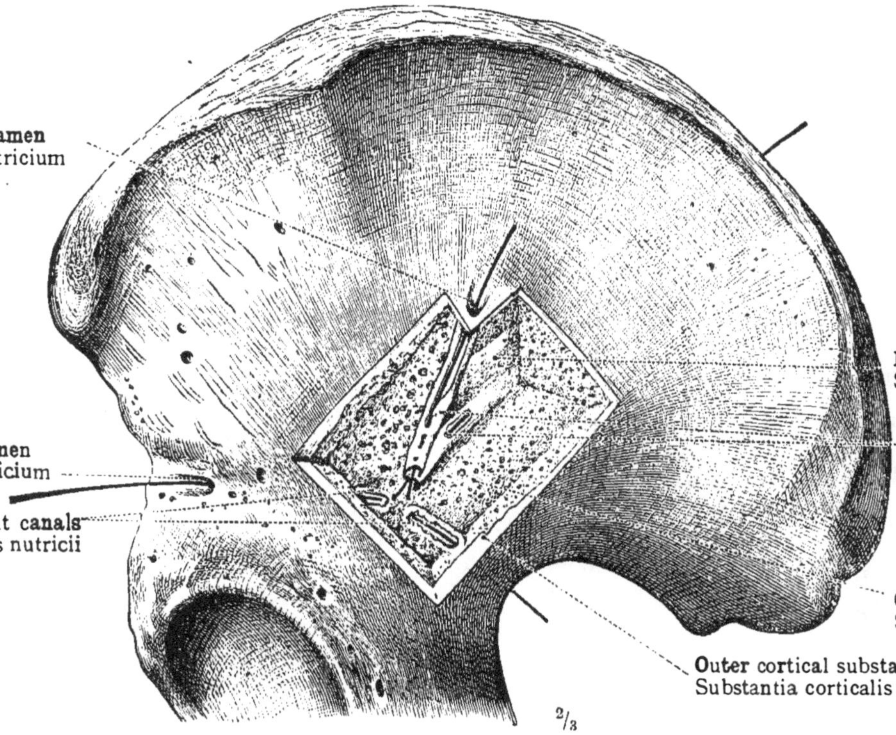

FIG. 27.—OUTER SURFACE OF LEFT ILIUM.

By the removal of the outer compact layer and the cancellous tissue of a portion of the bone, the nutrient canals have been displayed. The bristles projecting towards the right above and below show that the nutrient canals into which they have been inserted open on the inner surface of the bone—that turned away from the observer.

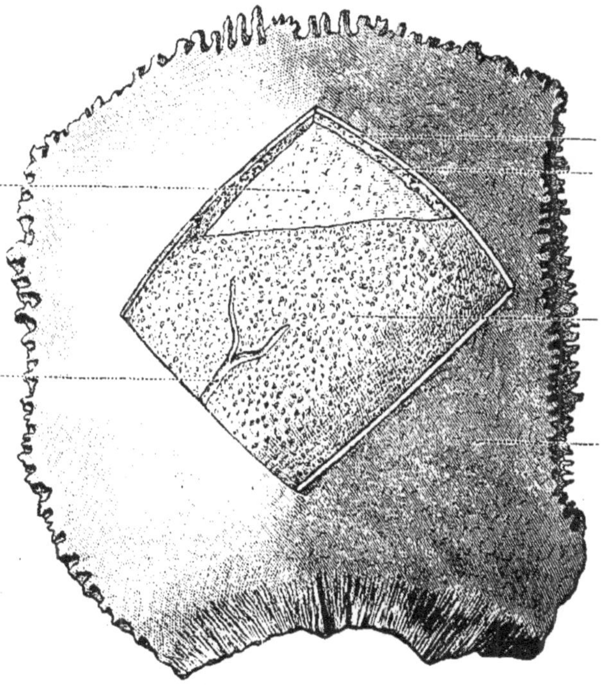

FIG. 28.—OS PARIETALE, PARIETAL BONE, PREPARED TO SHOW THE DIPLOË AND THE COMPACT INNER TABLE. SEEN FROM WITHOUT.

Substantia compacta, substantia spongiosa, et canales nutricii—Compact tissue, cancellous tissue, and nutrient canals.

Ossa plana—Flat bones.

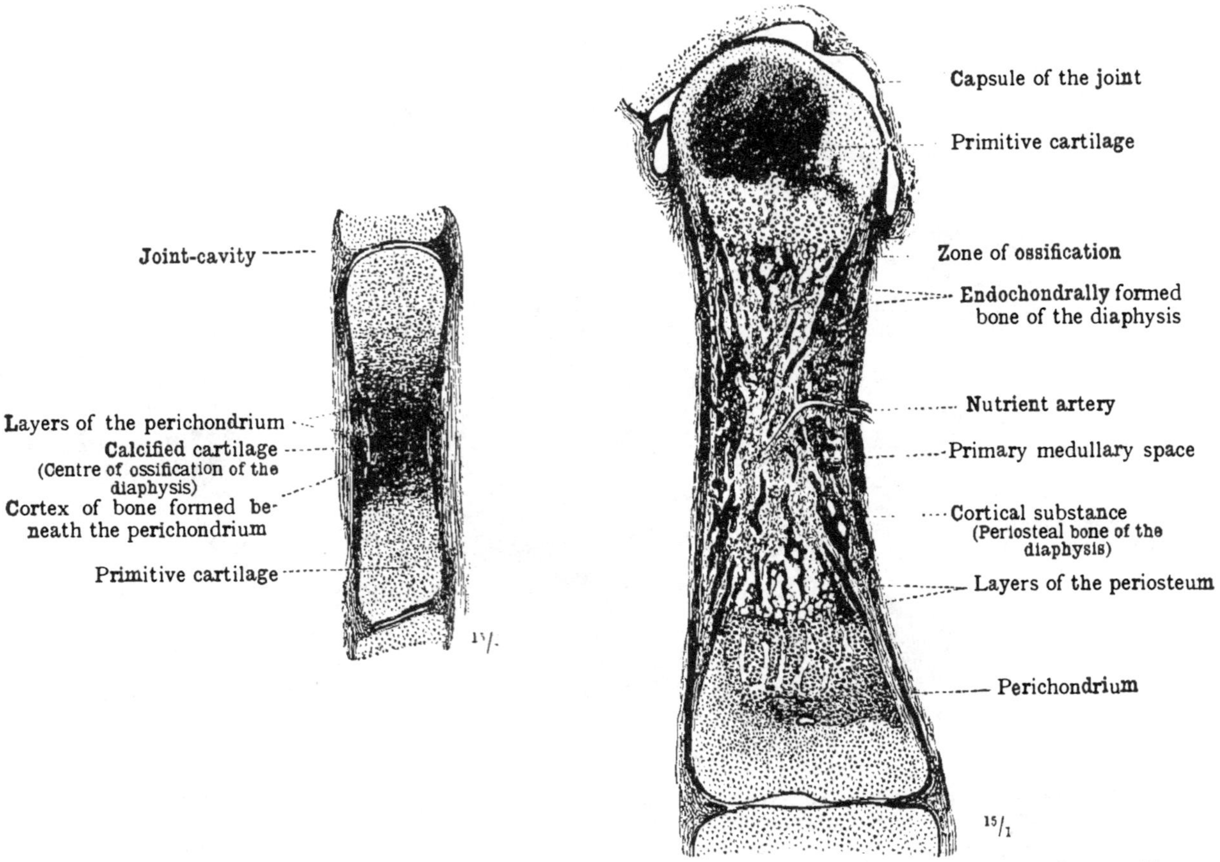

FIGS. 29 AND 30.—TWO STAGES IN THE INTRACARTILAGINOUS OSSIFICATION OF LONG BONES, AS SHOWN BY LONGITUDINAL SECTIONS OF THE PHALANGES OF A HUMAN FŒTUS.

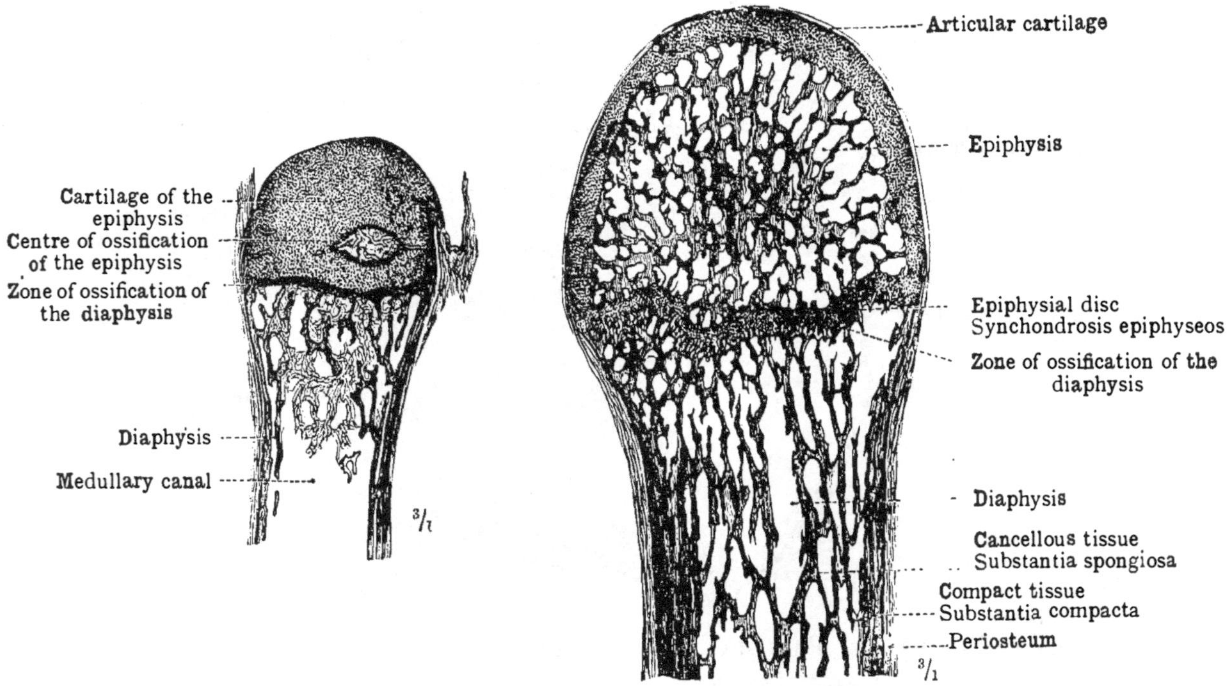

FIGS. 31 AND 32.—TWO STAGES IN THE INTRACARTILAGINOUS OSSIFICATION OF THE EPIPHYSIS OF A LONG BONE, AS SHOWN BY LONGITUDINAL SECTIONS OF THE DISTAL PORTIONS OF METACARPAL BONES.

Development of the Bones.

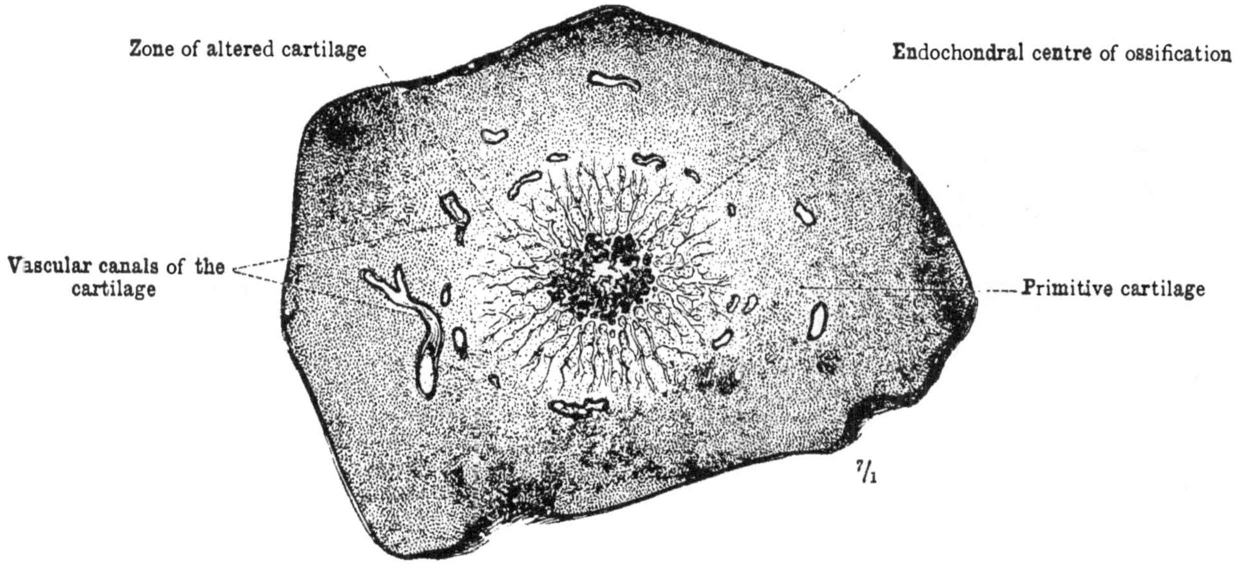

FIG. 33.—INTRACARTILAGINOUS OSSIFICATION OF A SHORT BONE.
A section of the cuboid bone of a new-born child.

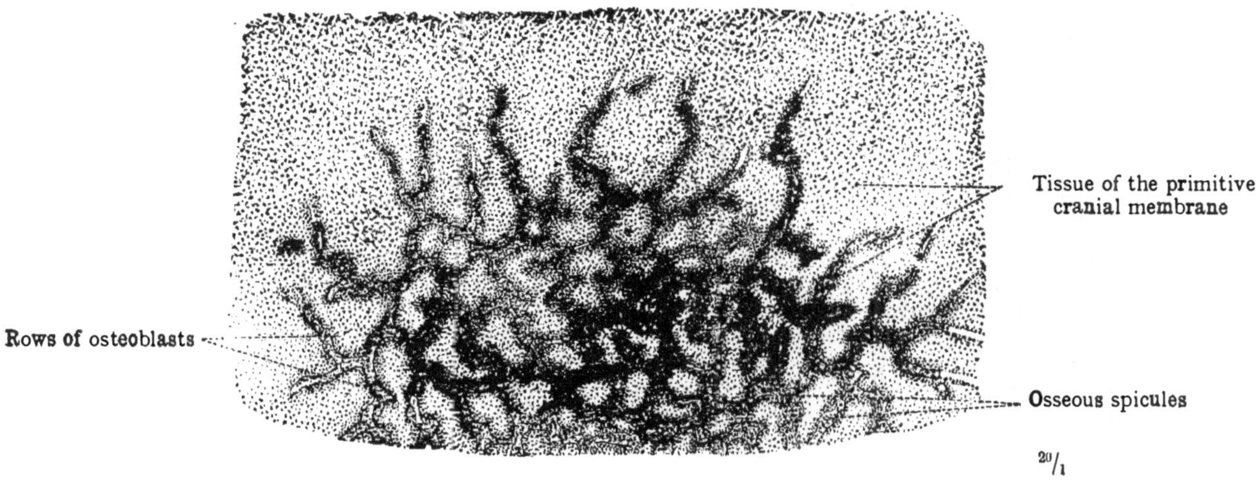

FIG. 34.—INTRAMEMBRANOUS OSSIFICATION OF THE BONES OF THE CRANIAL VAULT.
Upper half of the parietal bone of a human fœtus in the eleventh week of intra-uterine life.

Development of the Bones.

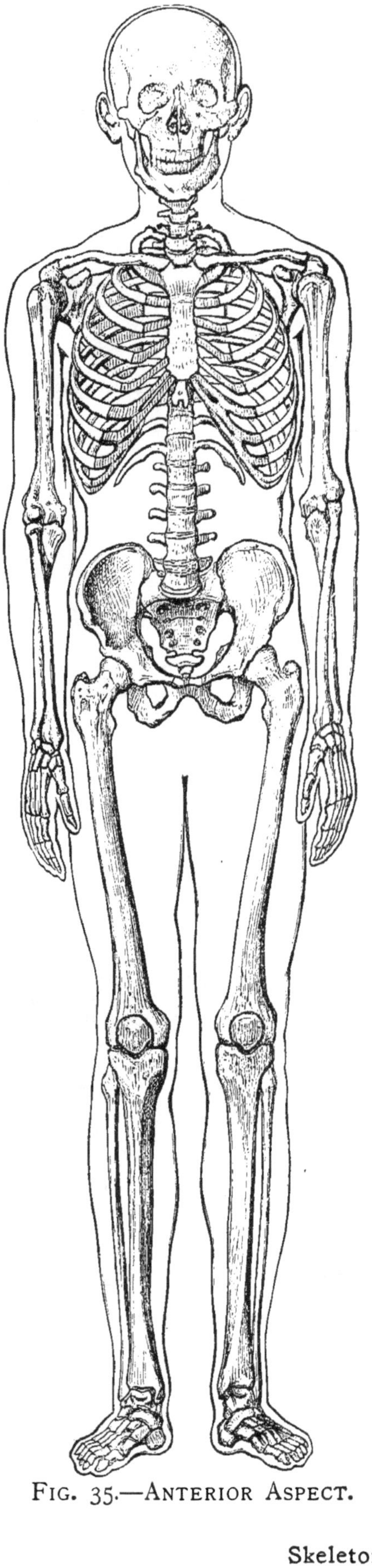

FIG. 35.—ANTERIOR ASPECT.

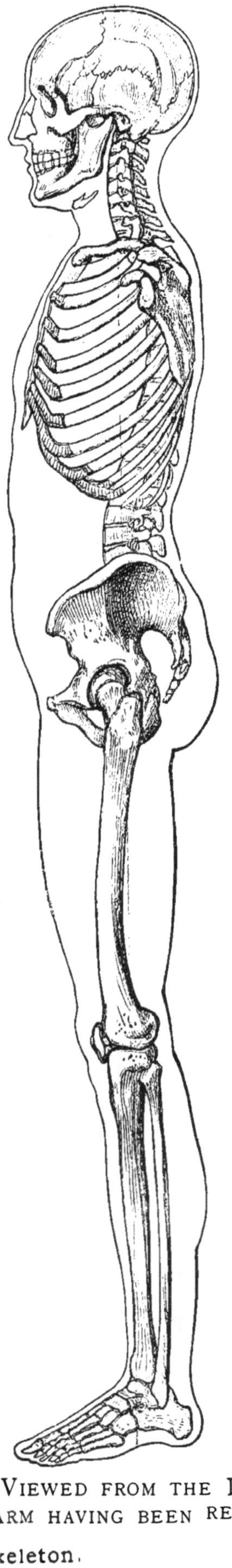

FIG. 36.—VIEWED FROM THE LEFT SIDE, THE ARM HAVING BEEN REMOVED.

Skeleton humanum—The human skeleton.

SKELETON TRUNCI

THE AXIAL SKELETON

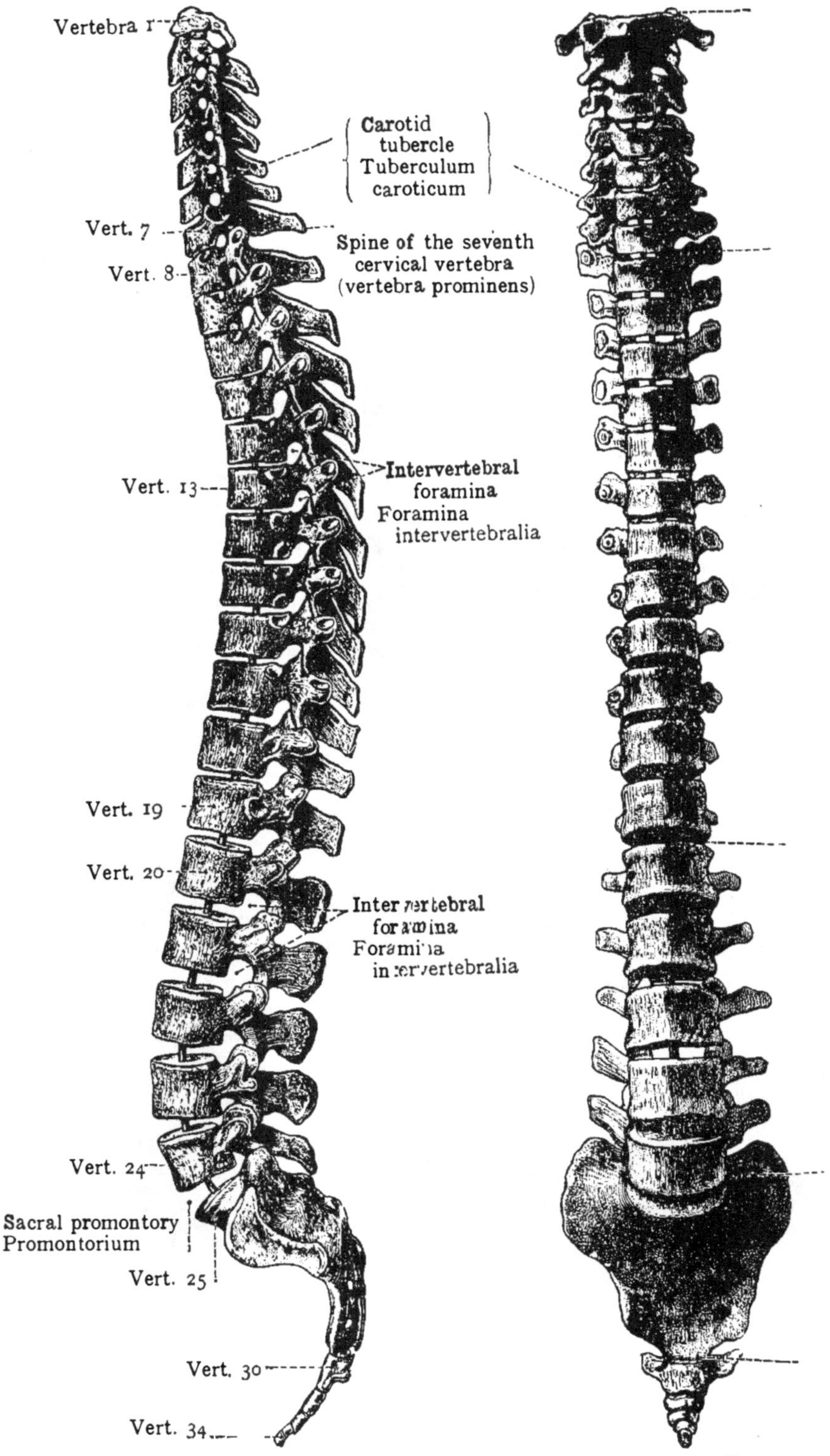

SEEN FROM THE LEFT. SEEN FROM THE FRONT.

FIG. 37.—THE VERTEBRAL COLUMN AS A WHOLE. CLASS OF THE VERTEBRÆ.

Columna vertebralis—The spinal

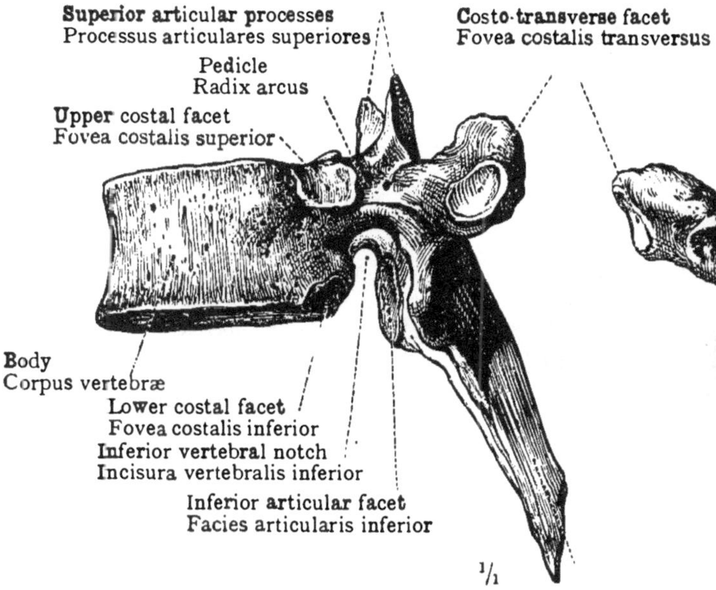

Fig. 38.—Seen from the Left Side.

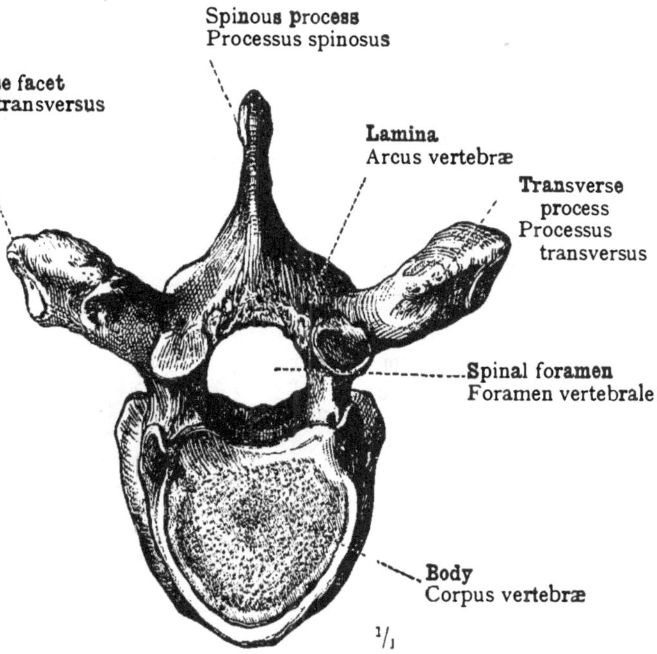

Fig. 39.—Seen from Above.

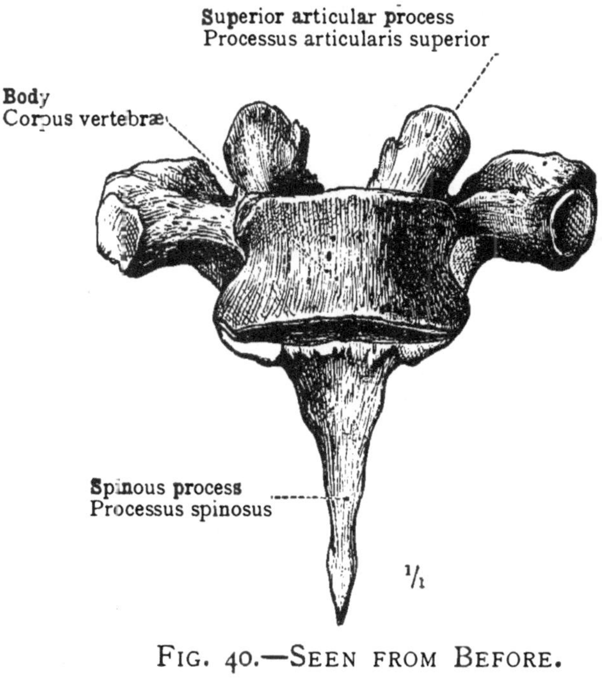

Fig. 40.—Seen from Before.

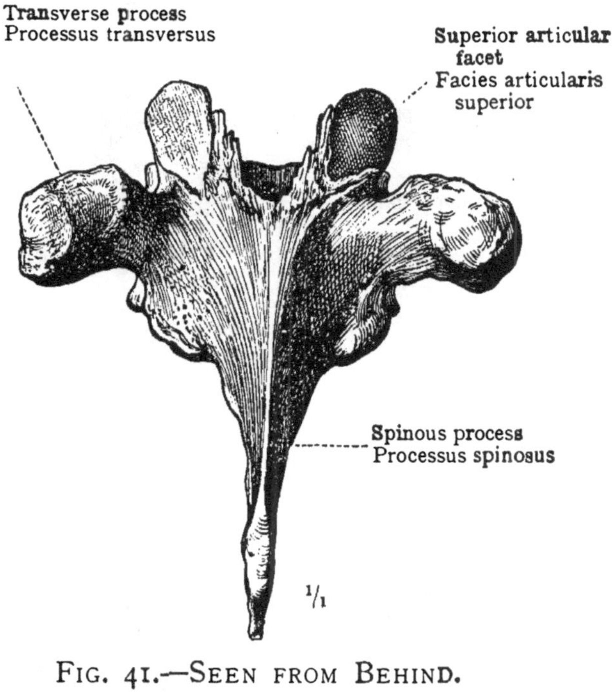

Fig. 41.—Seen from Behind.

Vertebræ: Vertebra thoracalis VI.—Sixth dorsal vertebra.

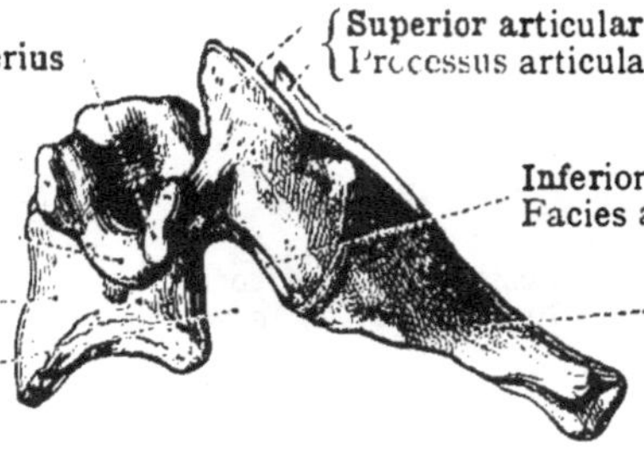

FIG. 42.—SEEN FROM THE LEFT SIDE.

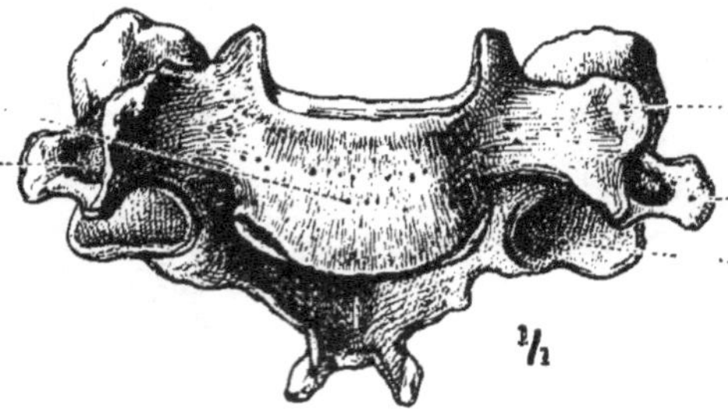

FIG. 43.—SEEN FROM BEFORE.

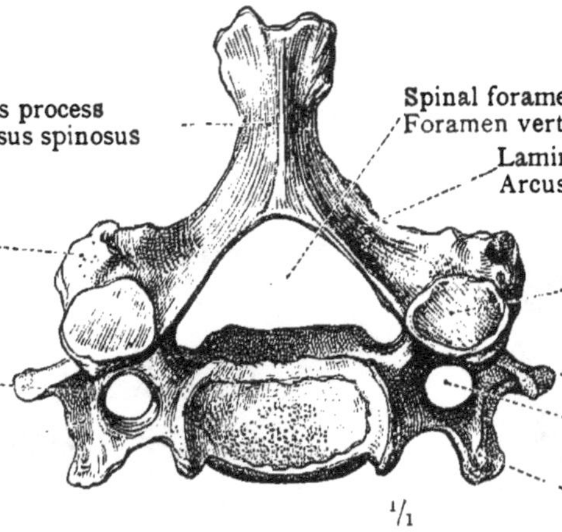

FIG. 44.—SEEN FROM ABOVE.

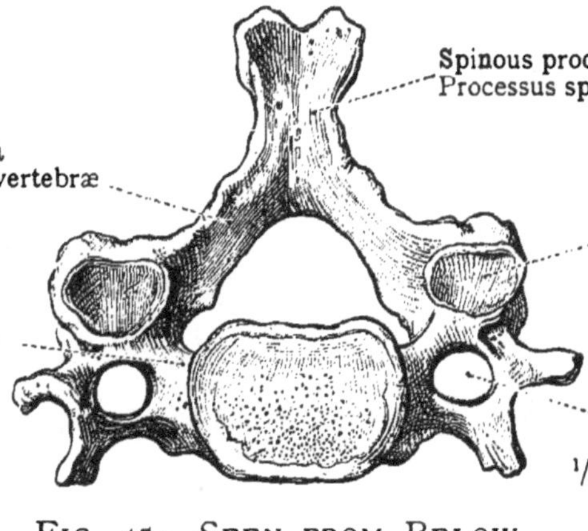

FIG. 45.—SEEN FROM BELOW.

Vertebræ: Vertebra cervicalis V.—Fifth cervical vertebra.

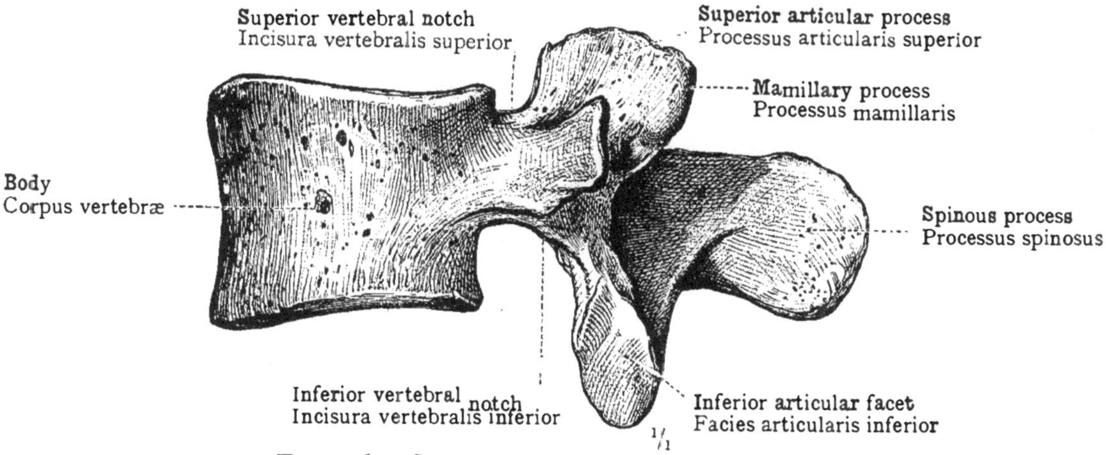

FIG. 46.—SEEN FROM THE LEFT SIDE.

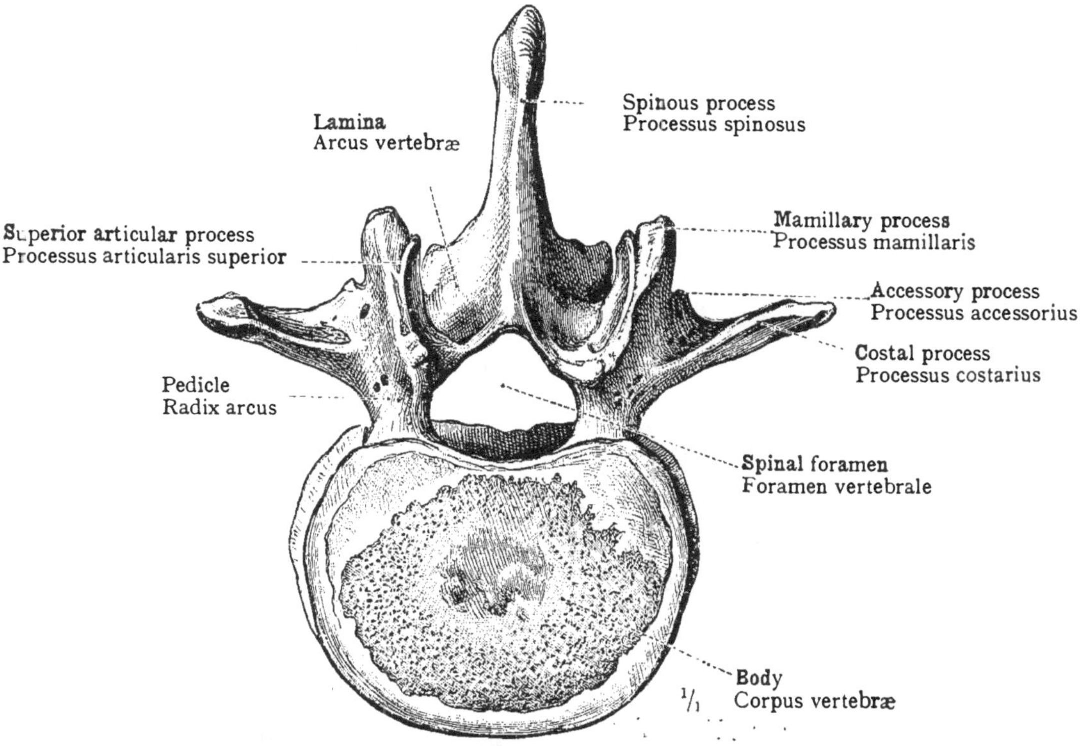

FIG. 47.—SEEN FROM ABOVE.

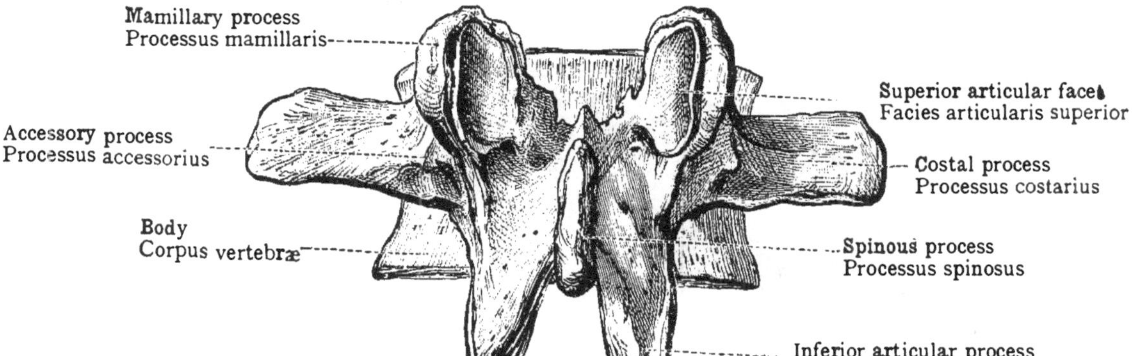

FIG. 48.—SEEN FROM BEHIND.

Vertebræ: Vertebra lumbalis II.—Second lumbar vertebra.

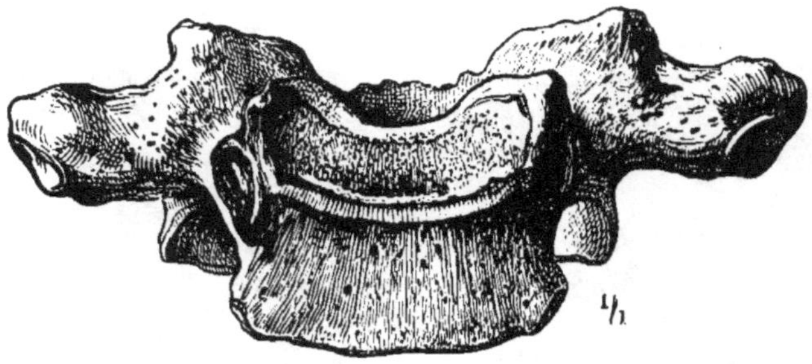

FIG. 49.—VERTEBRA THORACALIS I.—FIRST DORSAL VERTEBRA. SEEN FROM BEFORE.

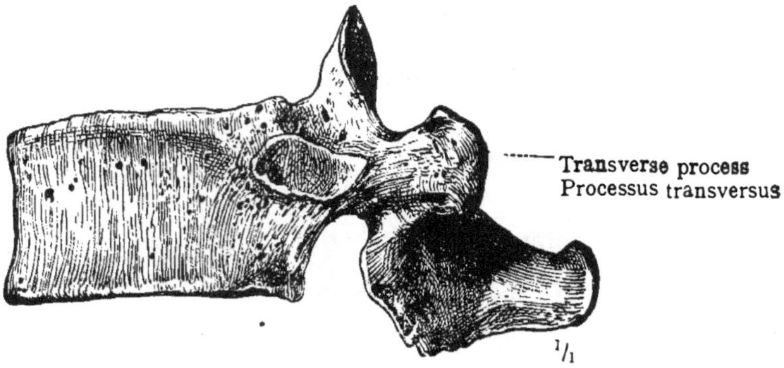

FIG. 50.—VERTEBRA THORACALIS XI.—ELEVENTH DORSAL VERTEBRA. SEEN FROM THE LEFT SIDE.

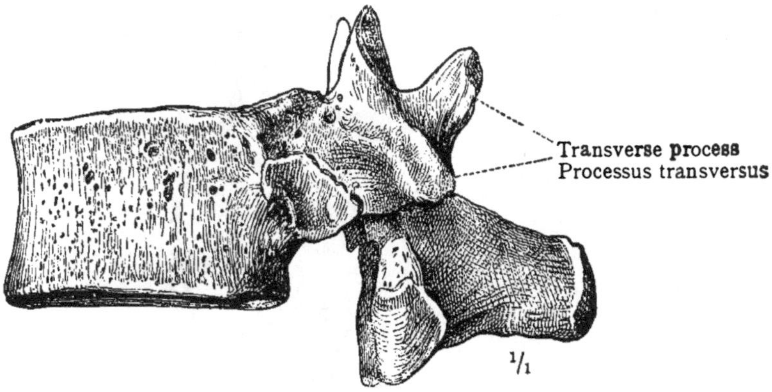

FIG. 51.—VERTEBRA THORACALIS XII.—TWELFTH DORSAL VERTEBRA. SEEN FROM THE LEFT SIDE.

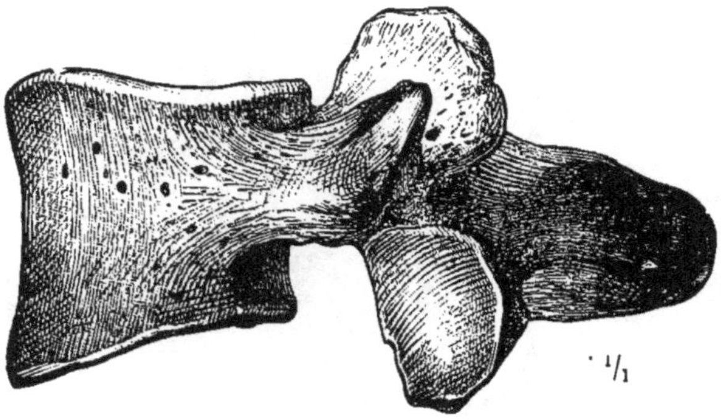

FIG. 52.—VERTEBRA LUMBALIS V.—FIFTH LUMBAR VERTEBRA. SEEN FROM THE LEFT SIDE.

Vertebræ: Transitional forms of the dorsal and lumbar vertebræ.

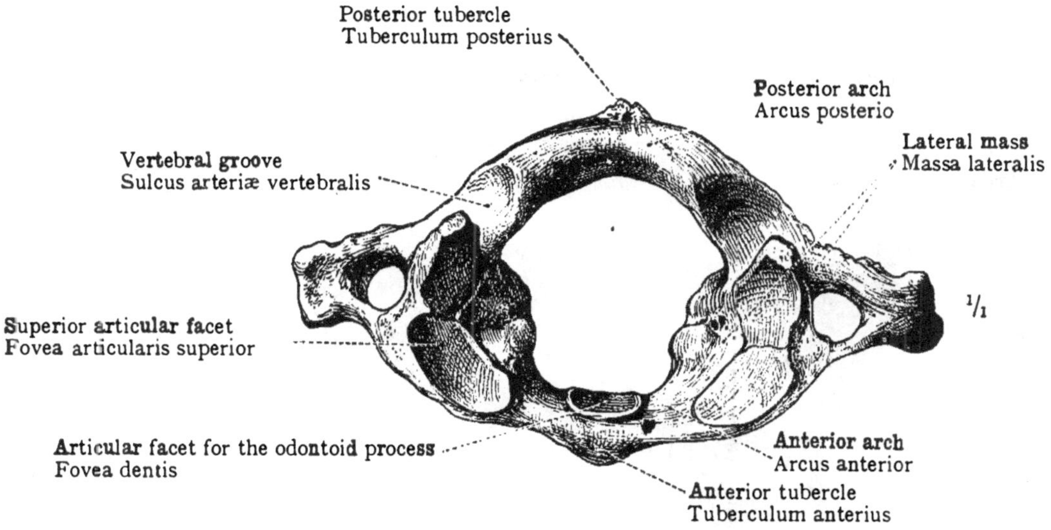

FIG. 53.—THE ATLAS, OR FIRST CERVICAL VERTEBRA. SEEN FROM ABOVE.

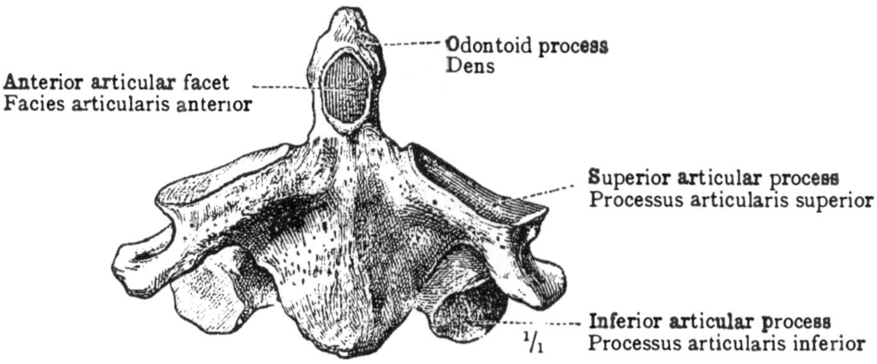

FIG. 54.—EPISTROPHEUS, THE AXIS, OR SECOND CERVICAL VERTEBRA. SEEN FROM BEFORE.

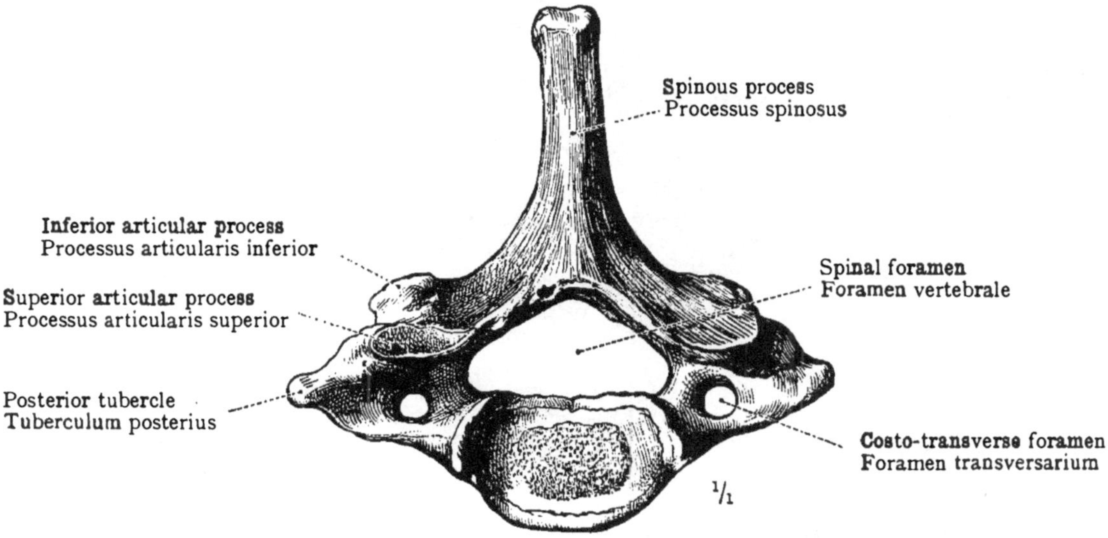

FIG. 55.—VERTEBRA CERVICALIS VII.—SEVENTH CERVICAL VERTEBRA. SEEN FROM ABOVE.

Vertebræ: The atypical cervical vertebræ.

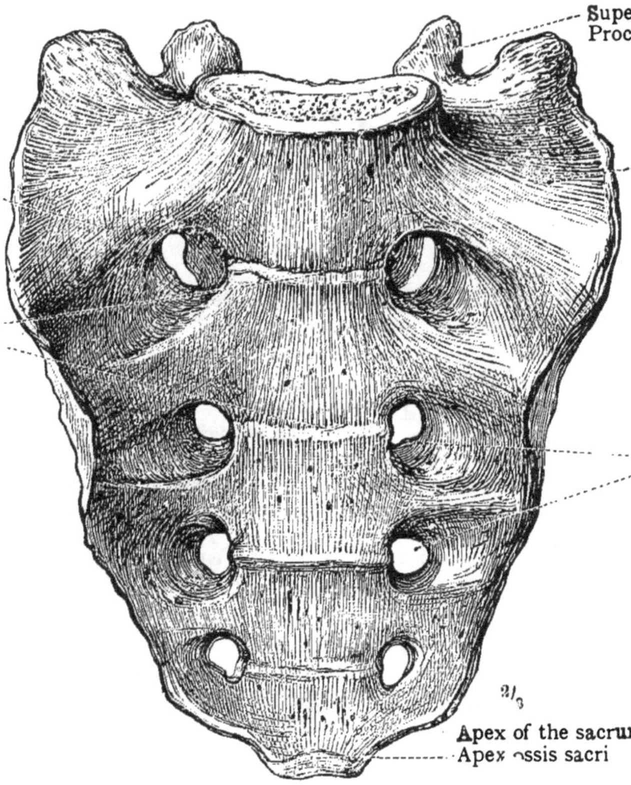

FIG. 56.—MALE SACRUM (FACIES PELVINA—PELVIC SURFACE). SEEN FROM BEFORE.

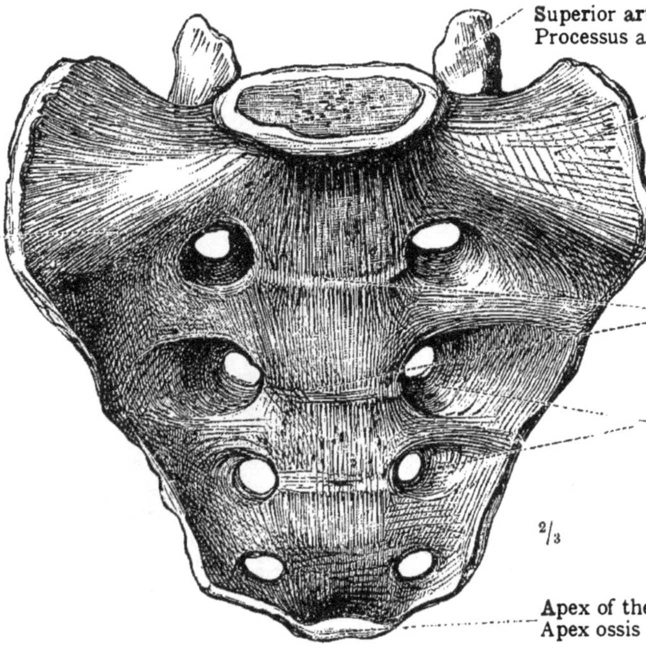

FIG. 57.—FEMALE SACRUM (FACIES PELVINA—PELVIC SURFACE). SEEN FROM BEFORE.

Os sacrum—The sacrum.

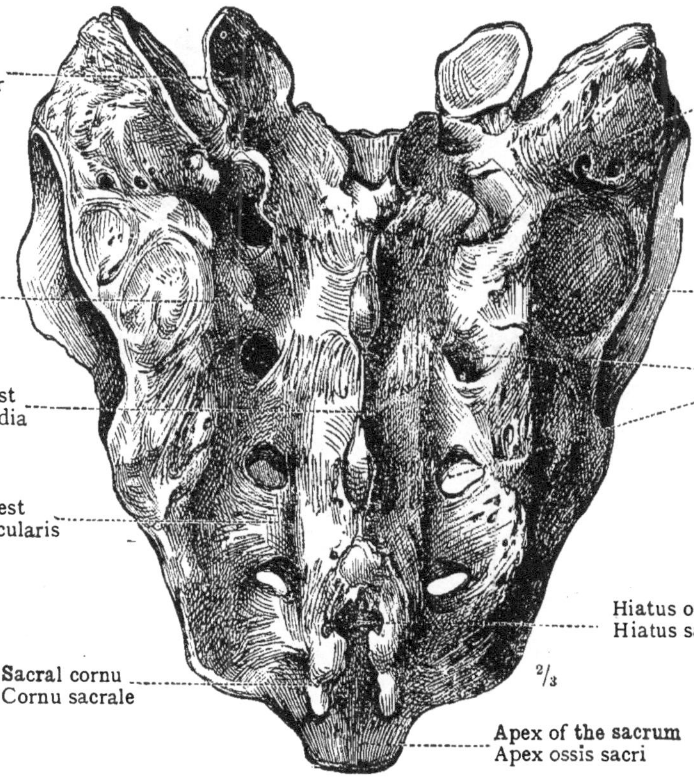

FIG. 58.—MALE SACRUM (FACIES DORSALIS—DORSAL SURFACE). SEEN FROM BEHIND.

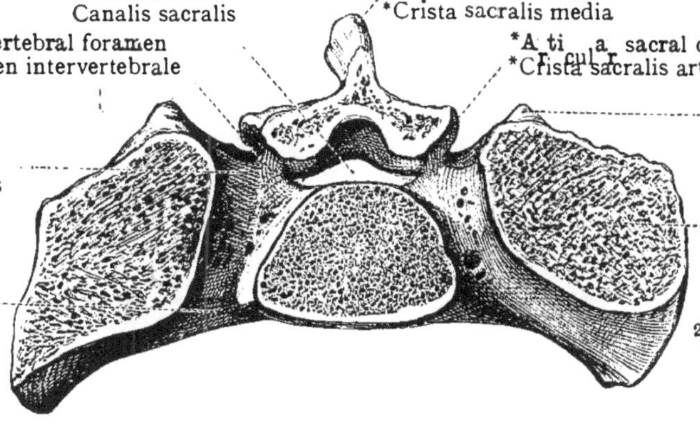

FIG. 59.—TRANSVERSE SECTION THROUGH THE SACRUM AT THE LEVEL OF THE FIRST SET OF SACRAL FORAMINA.

Os sacrum—The sacrum.

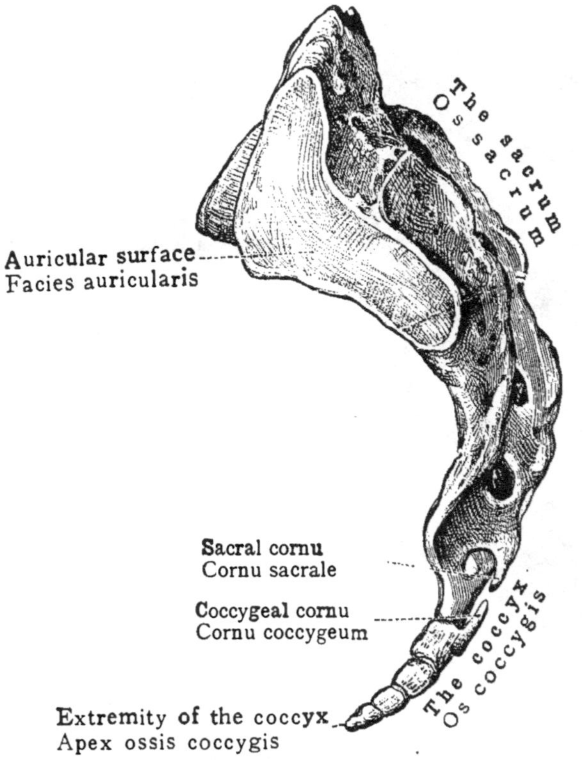

FIG. 60.—SACRUM AND COCCYX. SEEN FROM THE LEFT SIDE.

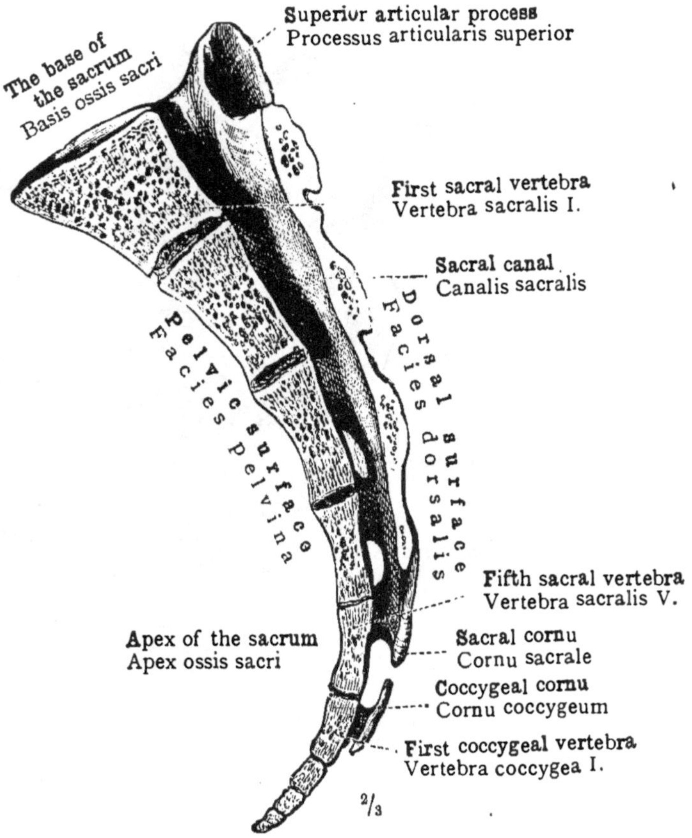

FIG. 61.—SACRUM AND COCCYX IN SAGITTAL SECTION THROUGH THE MEDIAN LINE.

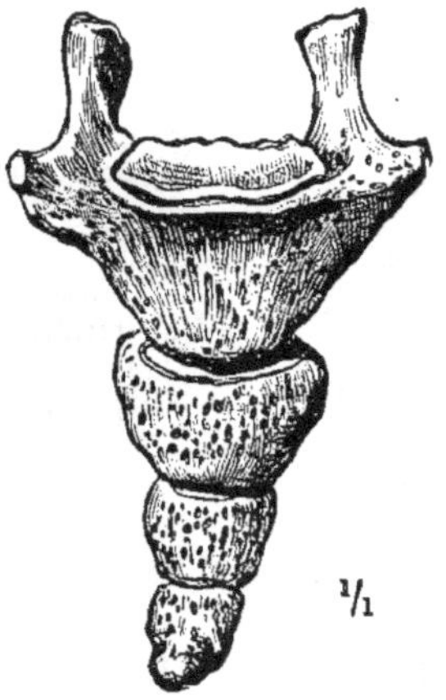

FIG. 62.—COCCYX SEEN FROM BEFORE.

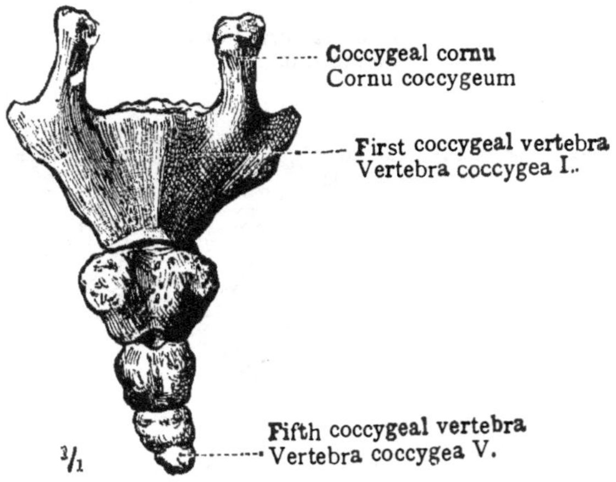

FIG. 63.—COCCYX SEEN FROM BEHIND.

Os sacrum et os coccygis—Sacrum and coccyx.

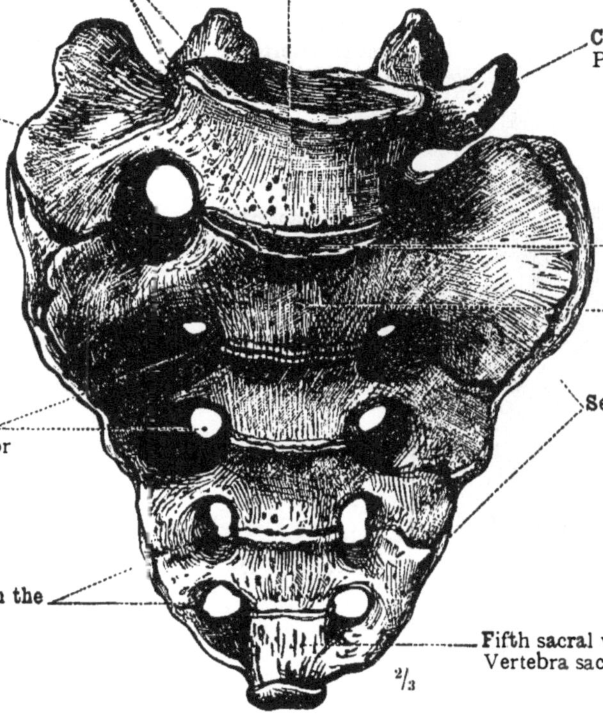

FIG. 64.—UNILATERAL ASSIMILATION AND COMMENCING ANKYLOSIS OF THE FIFTH LUMBAR VERTEBRA WITH THE SACRUM. SEEN FROM BEFORE.

From a boy seventeen years of age. Epiphyses on the bodies of the sacral vertebra, and along the lateral margins of the sacrum.

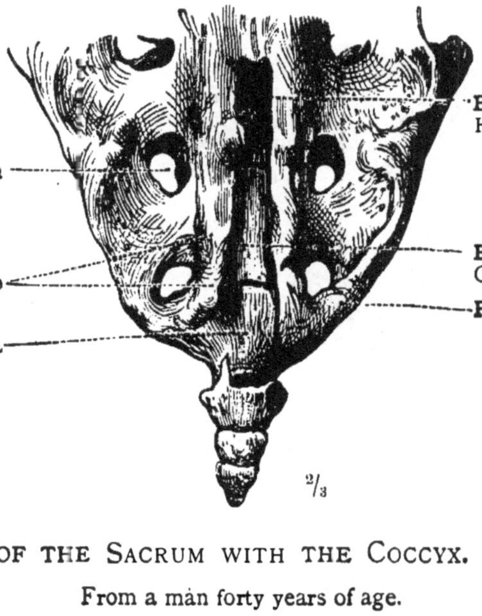

FIG. 65.—ANKYLOSIS OF THE SACRUM WITH THE COCCYX. SEEN FROM BEHIND.

From a man forty years of age.

Anomalous Ankyloses of the Sacrum.

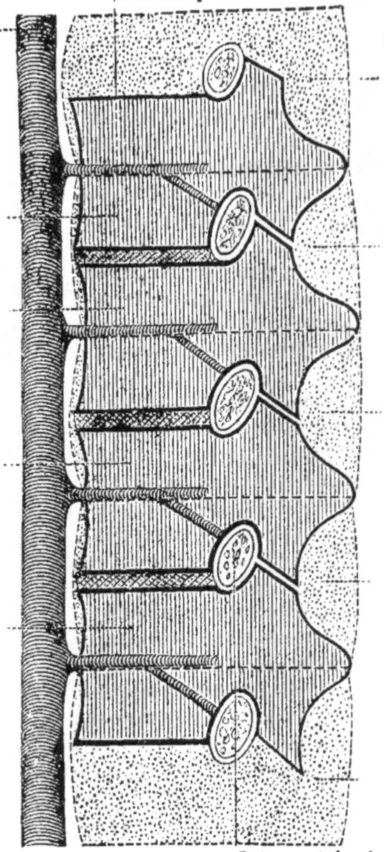

FIG. 66.—DIAGRAM SHOWING THE RELATIONS OF THE PROTOVERTEBRÆ TO THE VERTEBRÆ. (FROM VON EBNER.)

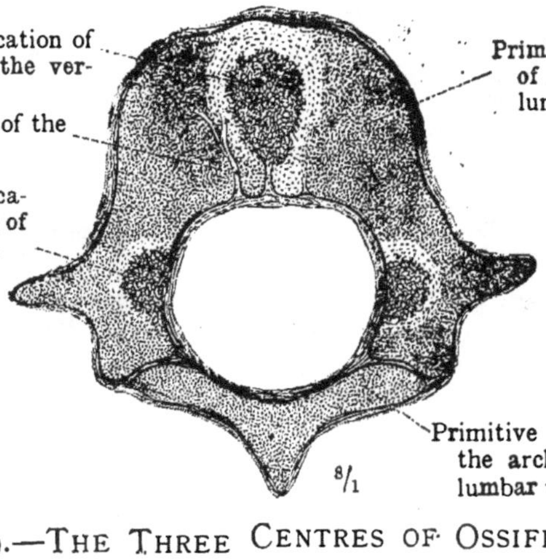

FIG. 69.—THE THREE CENTRES OF OSSIFICATION OF A VERTEBRA.

Horizontal section through the second and a portion of the first lumbar vertebræ of a human fœtus in the beginning of the fifth month (months of four weeks each). (Length of fœtus, $5\frac{1}{2}$ inches.)

Development of the Ver

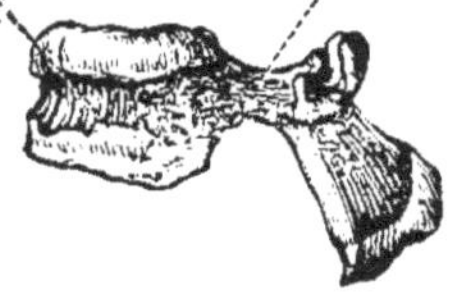

FIG. 70.—FIRST LUMBAR VERTEBRA OF A NEW-BORN CHILD.

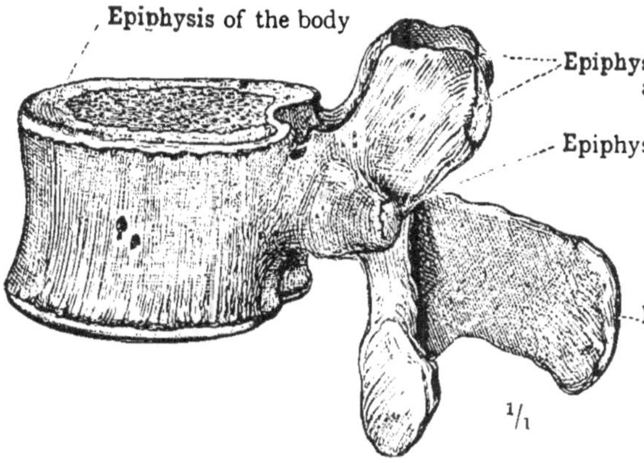

FIG. 71.—FIRST LUMBAR VERTEBRA IN THE EIGHTEENTH YEAR.

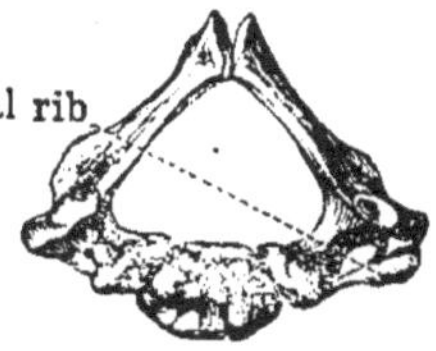

FIG. 72.—THE SEVENTH CERVICAL VERTEBRA OF A NEW-BORN CHILD.

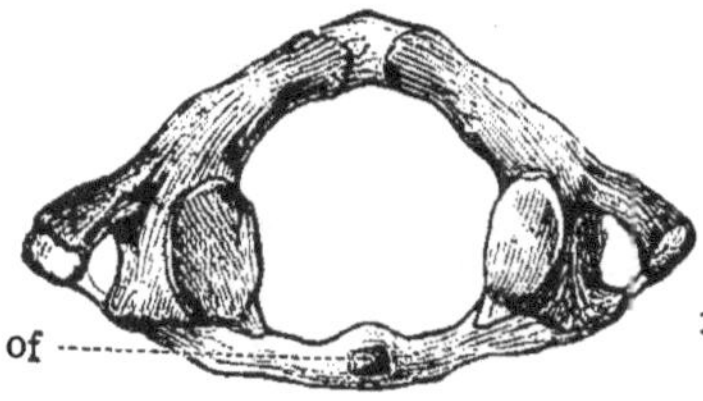

FIG. 73.—THE ATLAS AT THE END OF THE FIRST YEAR.

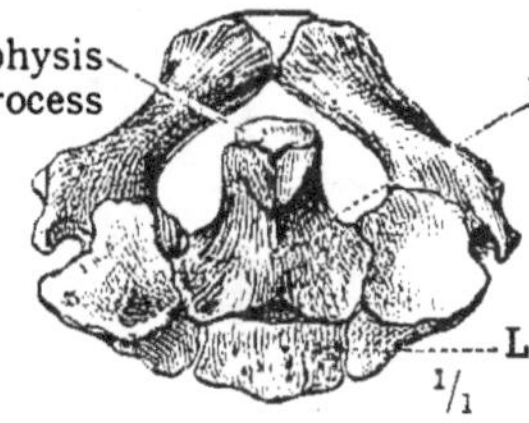

FIG. 74.—THE AXIS AT THE END OF THE FIRST YEAR.

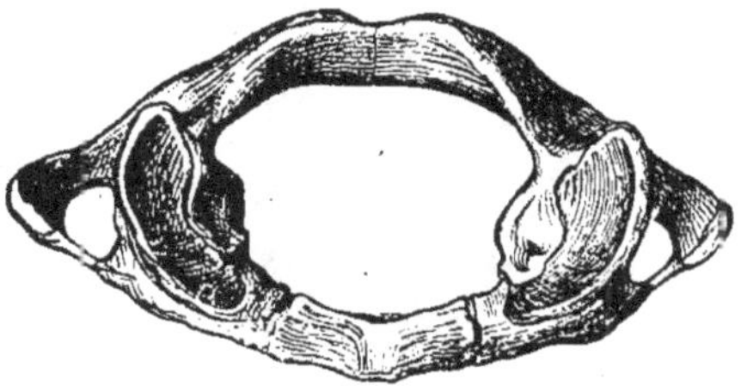

FIG. 75.—THE ATLAS IN THE FOURTH YEAR.

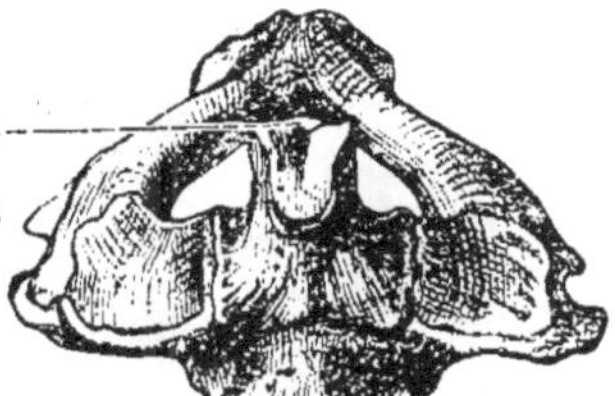

FIG. 76.—THE AXIS IN THE FOURTH YEAR.

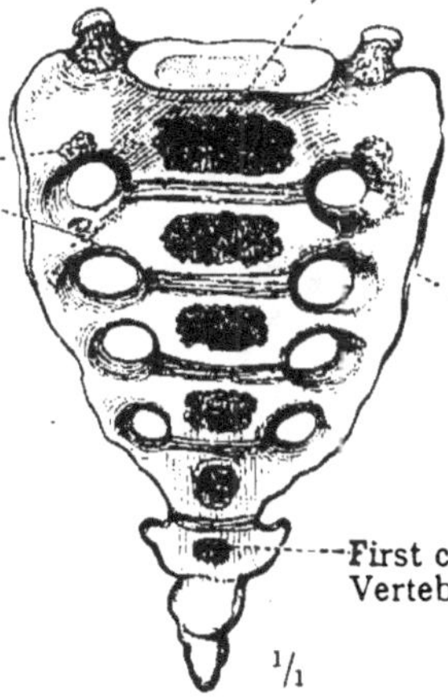

FIG. 77.—SEEN FROM BEFORE.

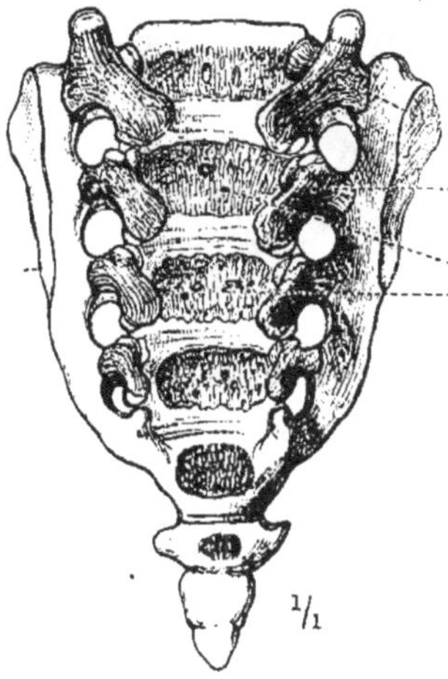

FIG. 78.—SEEN FROM BEHIND.

Development of the Vertebræ: The centres of ossification in the sacrum and coccyx of a child at the age of two months.

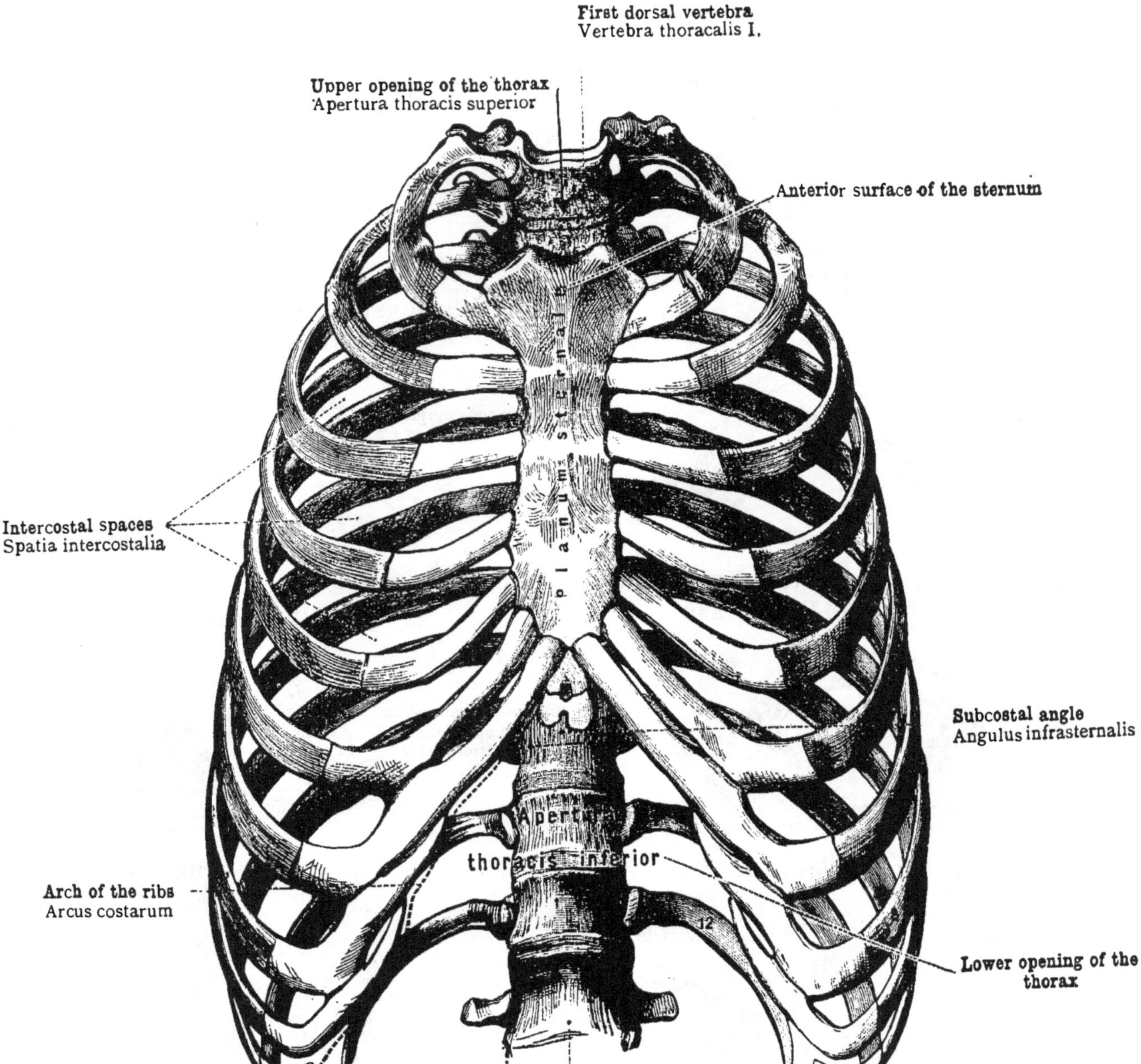

(1—7, Costæ veræ, sternal or true ribs; 8—12, Costæ spuriæ, asternal or false ribs; 11 and 12, Costæ fluctuantes, floating ribs.)

FIG. 79.—THE THORAX SEEN FROM BEFORE.

The Thorax.

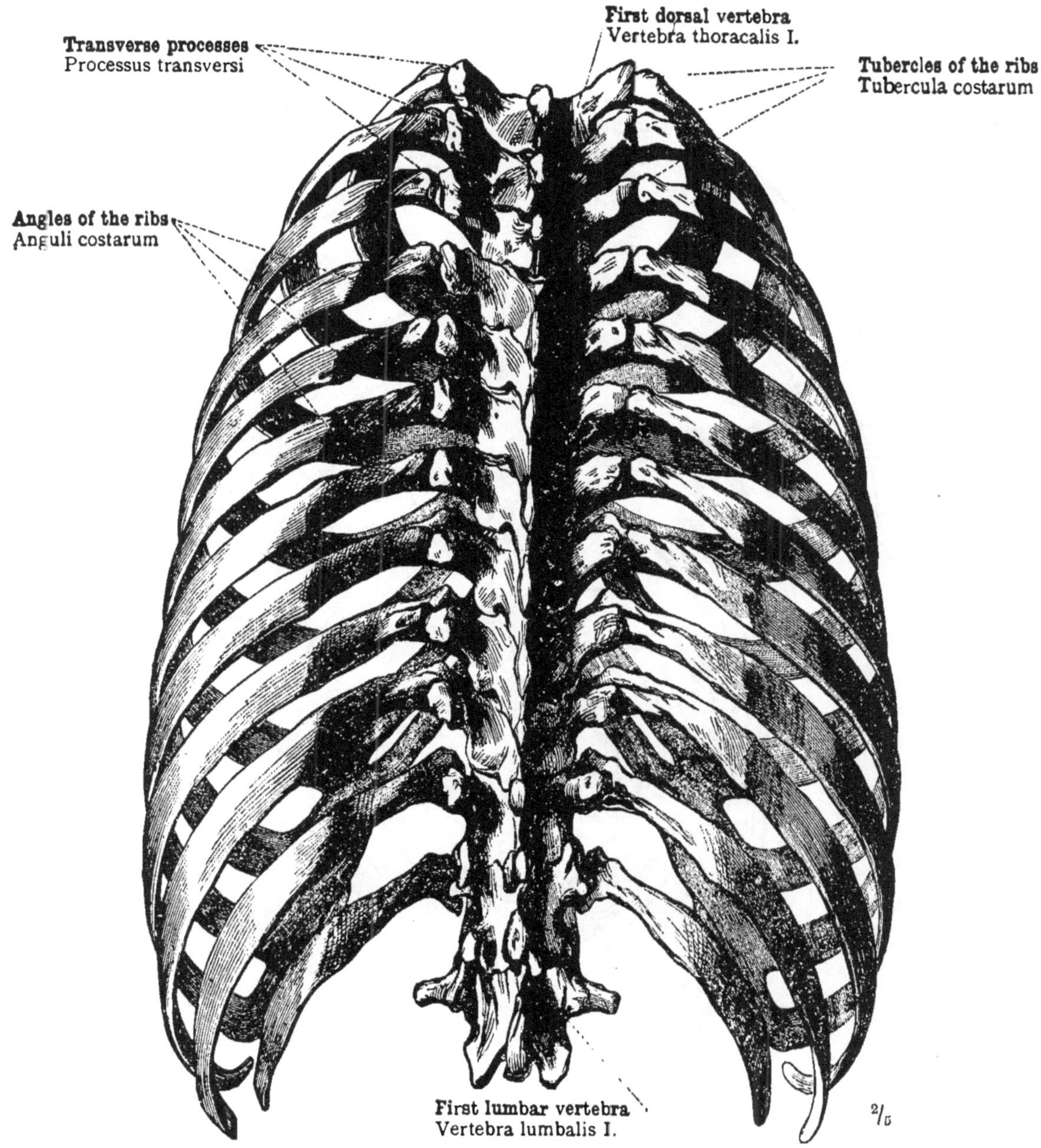

FIG. 80.—THE THORAX SEEN FROM BEHIND.

The Thorax.

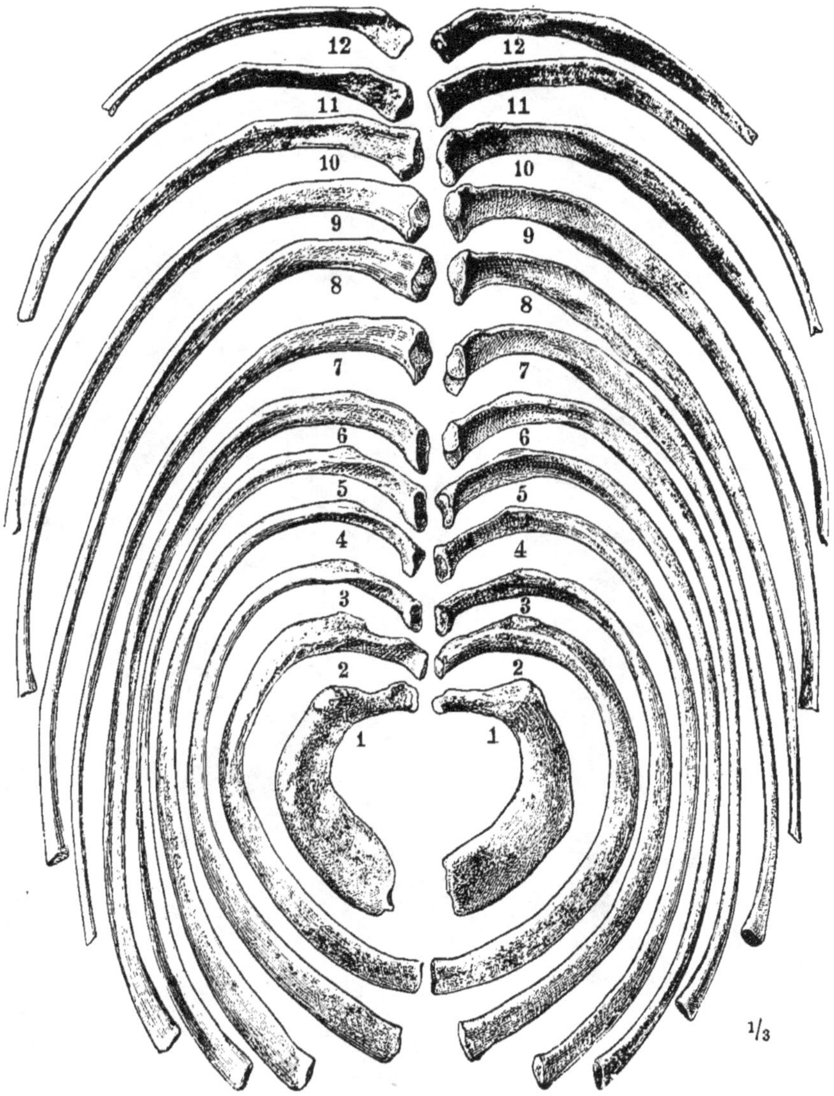

FIG. 81.—THE TWELVE PAIRS OF RIBS.

Ossa costalia—The ribs.

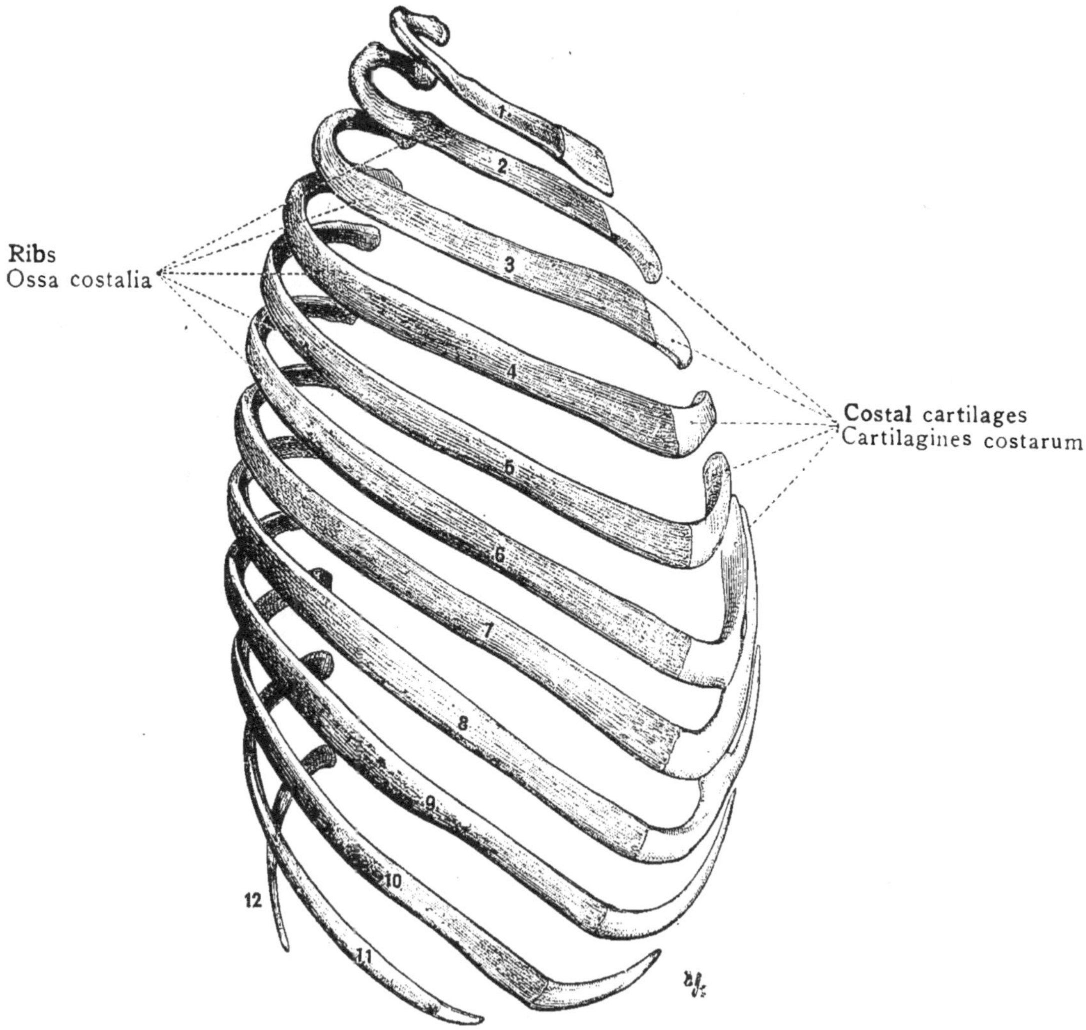

FIG. 82.—THE TWELVE RIBS OF THE RIGHT SIDE IN THEIR NATURAL POSITION. SEEN FROM THE RIGHT.

Costæ—The ribs.

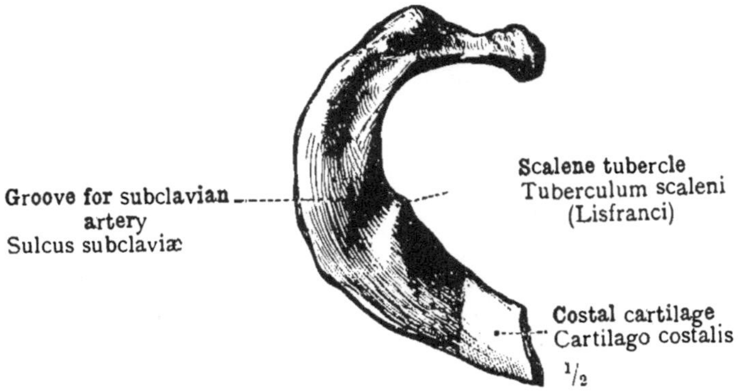

FIG. 83.—FIRST (RIGHT) RIB. SEEN FROM ABOVE.

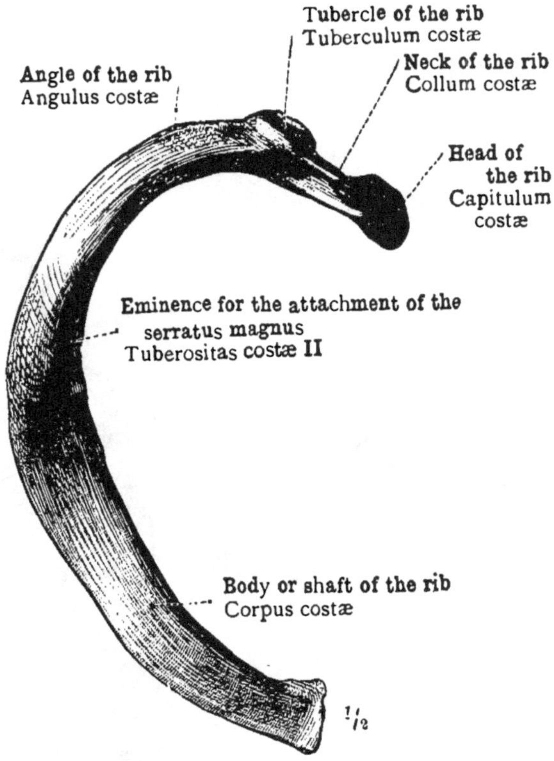

FIG. 84.—SECOND (RIGHT) RIB. SEEN FROM ABOVE.

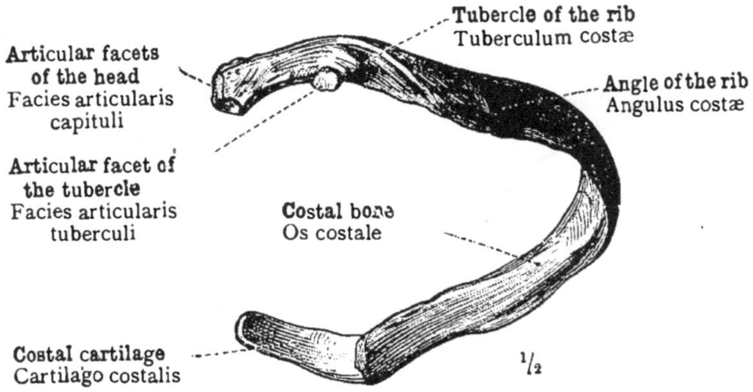

FIG. 85.—FOURTH (RIGHT) RIB. SEEN FROM BEHIND

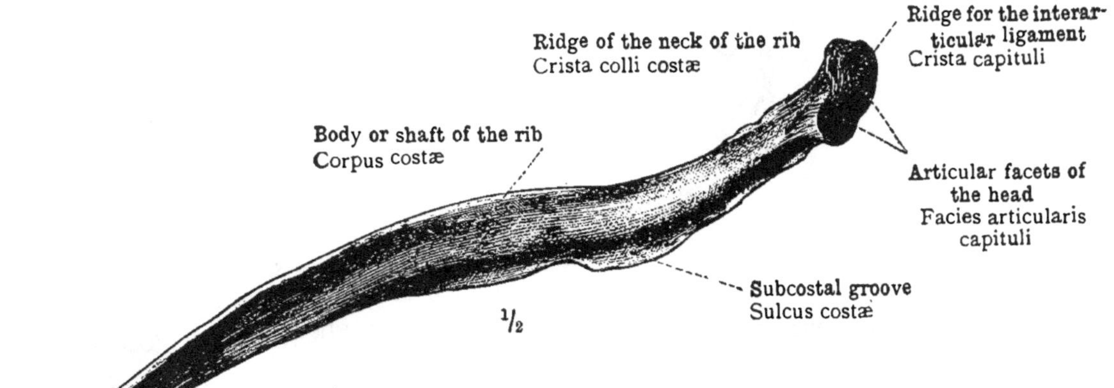

FIG. 86.—SEVENTH (RIGHT) RIB. SEEN FROM WITHIN.

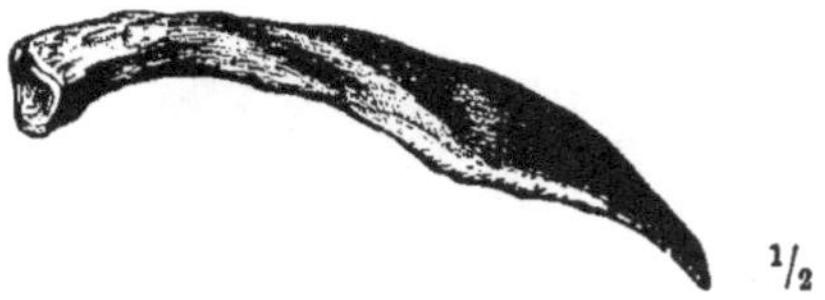

FIG. 87.—TWELFTH (RIGHT) RIB. SEEN FROM WITHIN.

Costæ—The ribs.

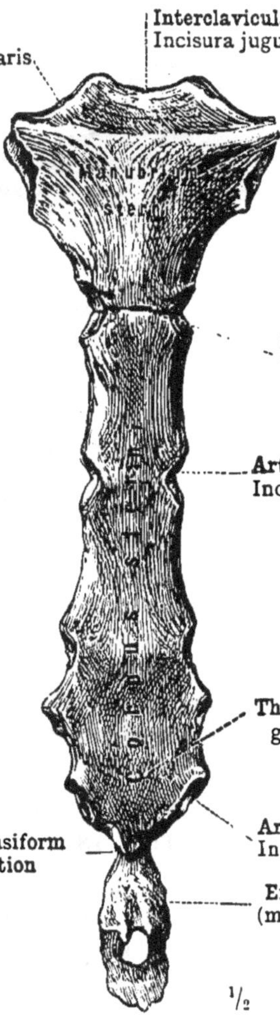

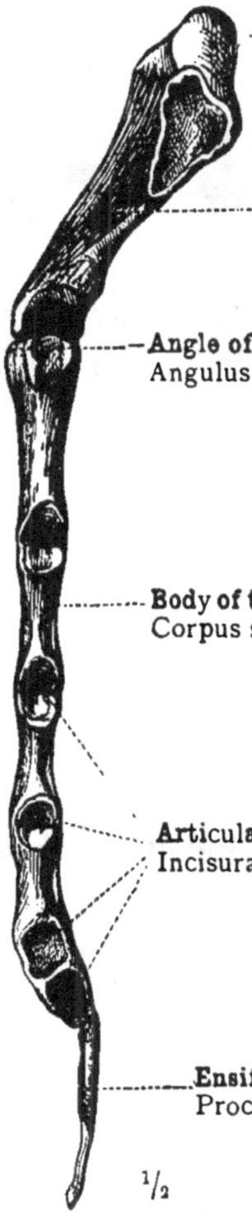

[1] In certain pathological conditions the angle between the manubrium and the body of the sternum becomes less obtuse, and therefore more prominent. It is then known as *angulus Ludovici*, or Ludwig's angle.—Tr.

Fig. 88.—The Sternum seen from Before.

Fig. 89.—The Sternum seen from the Left Side.

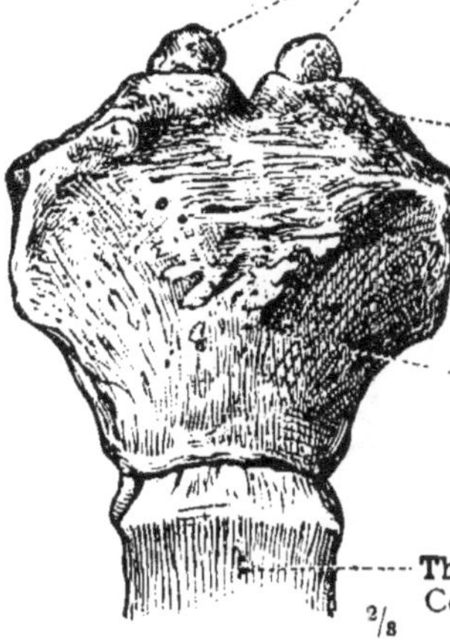

Fig. 90.—The Upper Portion of the Sternum with the Suprasternal Bones (a Rare Variety). Seen from Before.

Sternum—The breast-bone.

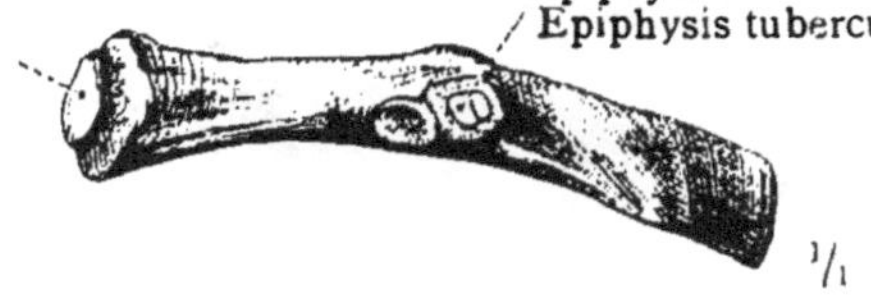

FIG. 91.—POSTERIOR PORTION OF THE SIXTH RIB, IN THE FIFTEENTH YEAR.

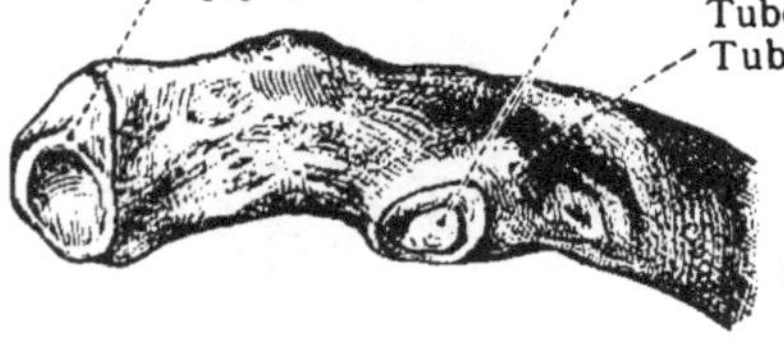

FIG. 92.—POSTERIOR PORTION OF THE SIXTH RIB, IN THE EIGHTEENTH YEAR.

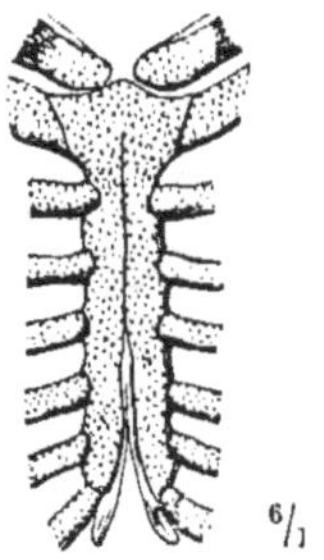

FIG. 93.—DIVIDED PRIMITIVE CARTILAGE OF THE STERNUM.

From a human fœtus of two months (mouths of four weeks each).

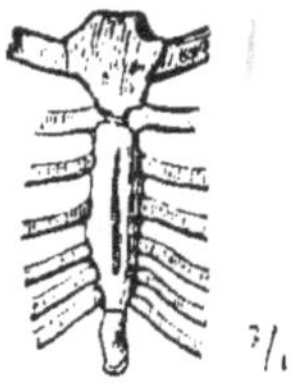

FIG. 94.—PRIMITIVE CARTILAGE OF THE STERNUM.

From a human fœtus of four months (months of four weeks each).

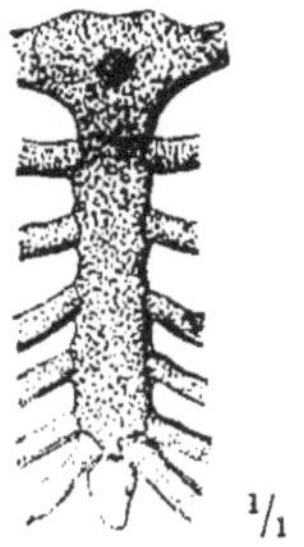

FIG. 95.—PRIMITIVE CARTILAGE OF THE STERNUM WITH THE FIRST CENTRE OF OSSIFICATION IN THE MANUBRIUM.

From a human fœtus in the second half of the sixth month (months of four weeks each).

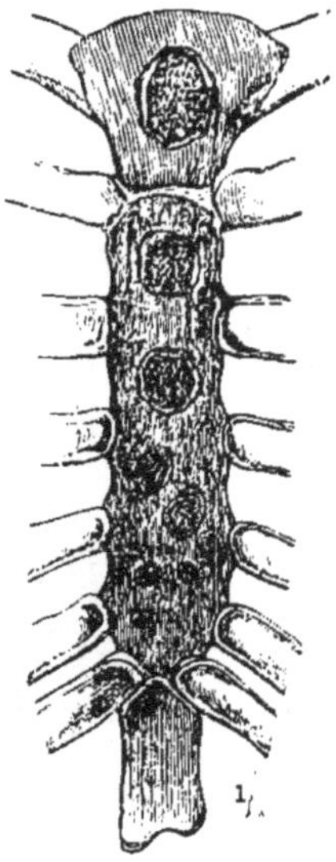

FIG. 96.—CENTRES OF OSSIFICATION IN THE STERNUM OF A NEW-BORN CHILD.

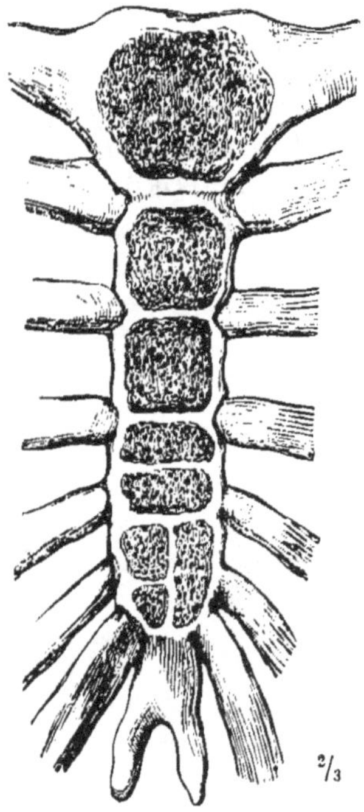

FIG. 97.—STERNUM OF A BOY AT THE AGE OF ELEVEN YEARS.

Development of the Ribs and the Sternum.

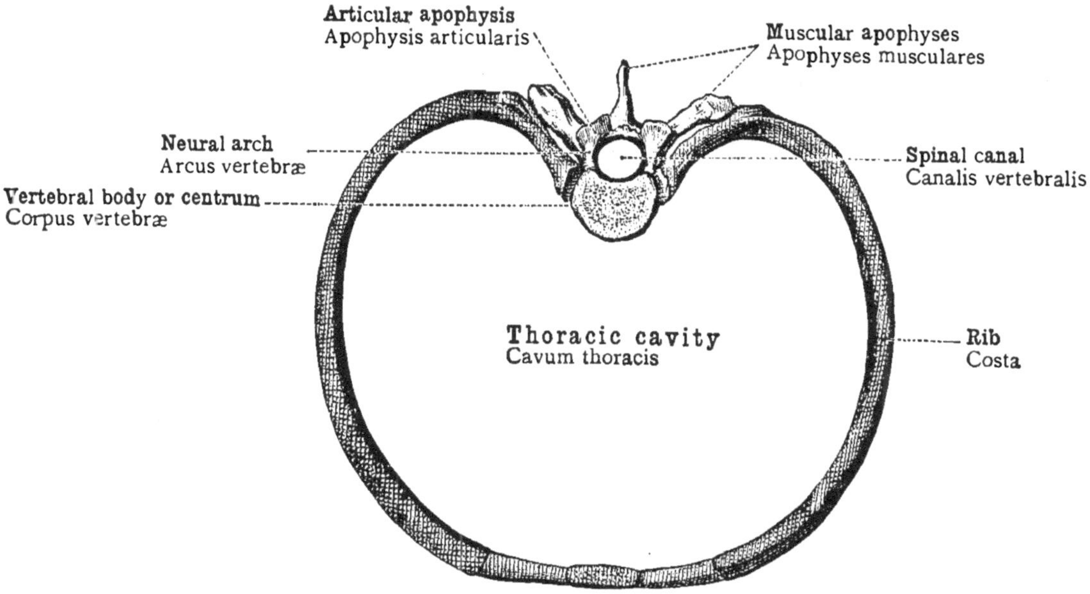

Fig. 98.—Skeleton of a Thoracic Segment.

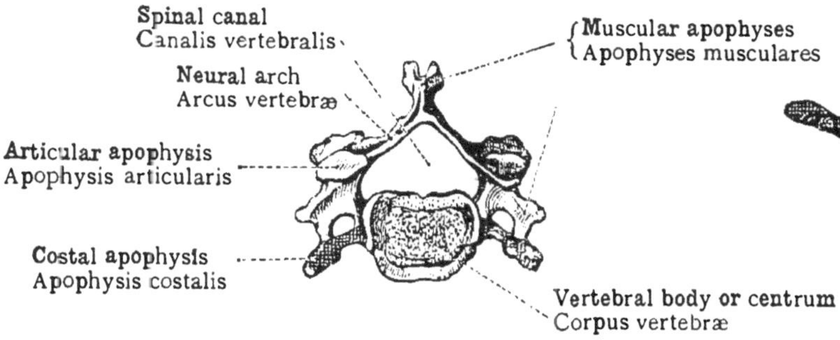

Fig. 99.—Skeleton of a Cervical Segment.

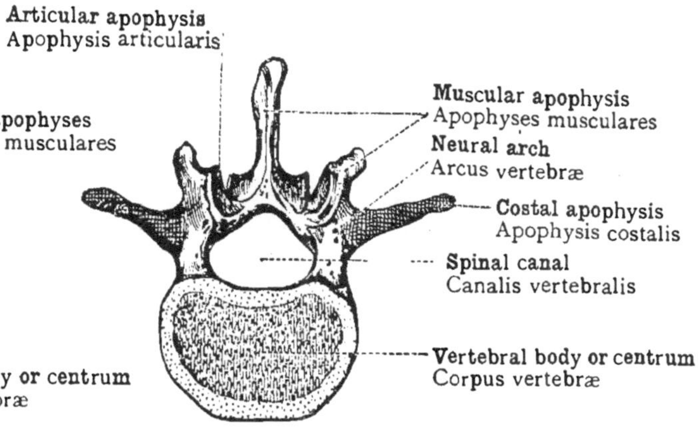

Fig. 100.—Skeleton of a Lumbar Segment.

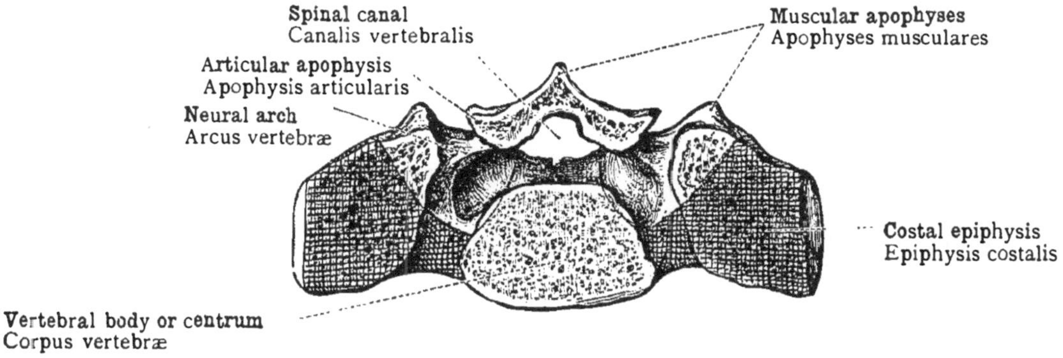

Fig. 101.—Skeleton of a Sacral Segment.

The Homologous Skeletal Parts of the Segments of the Body.

CRANIUM ET OSSA CRANII

THE SKULL
AND THE BONES OF THE SKULL

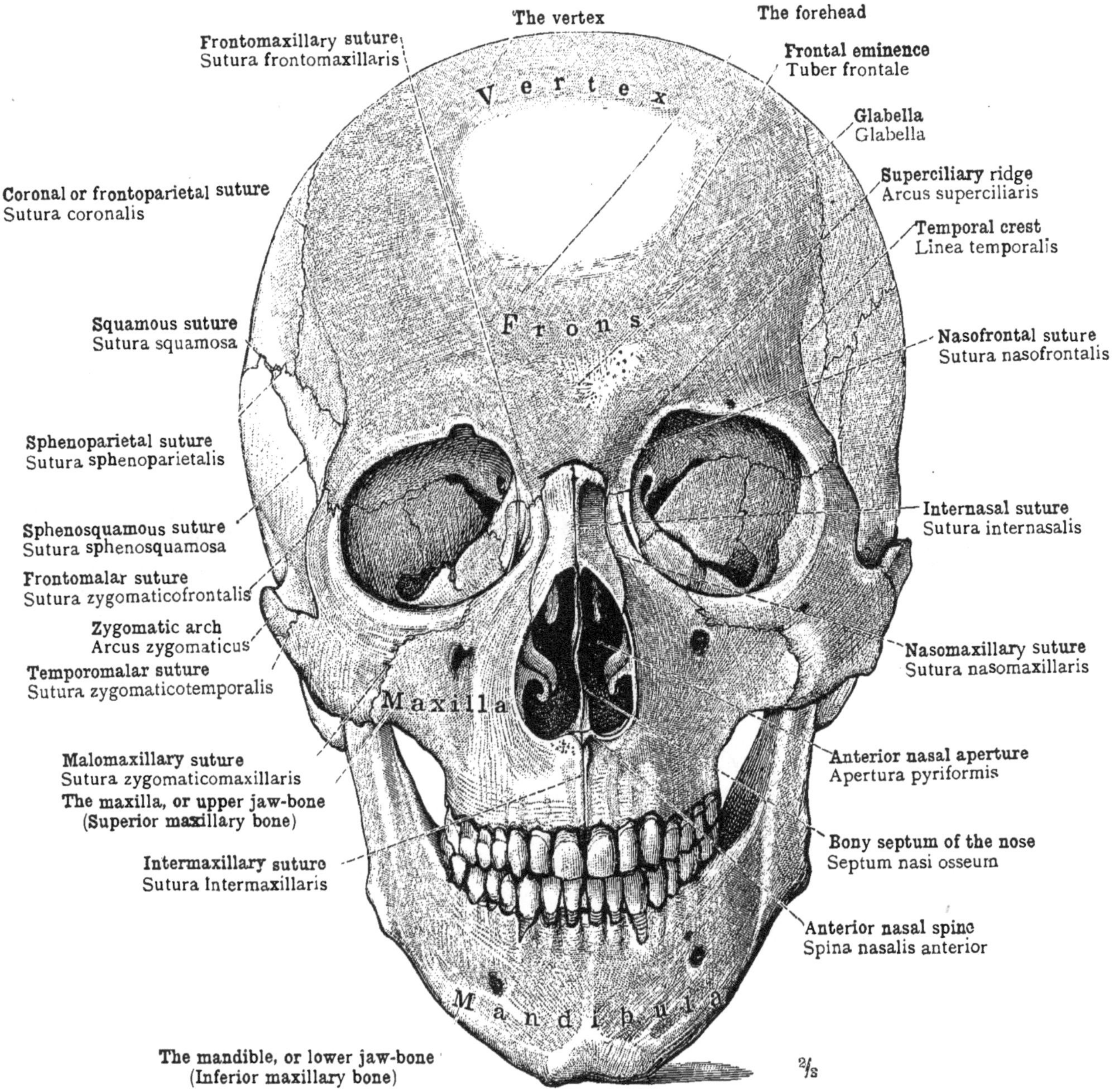

FIG. 102.—THE SKULL SEEN FROM BEFORE: NORMA FRONTALIS.

Cranium—The skull.

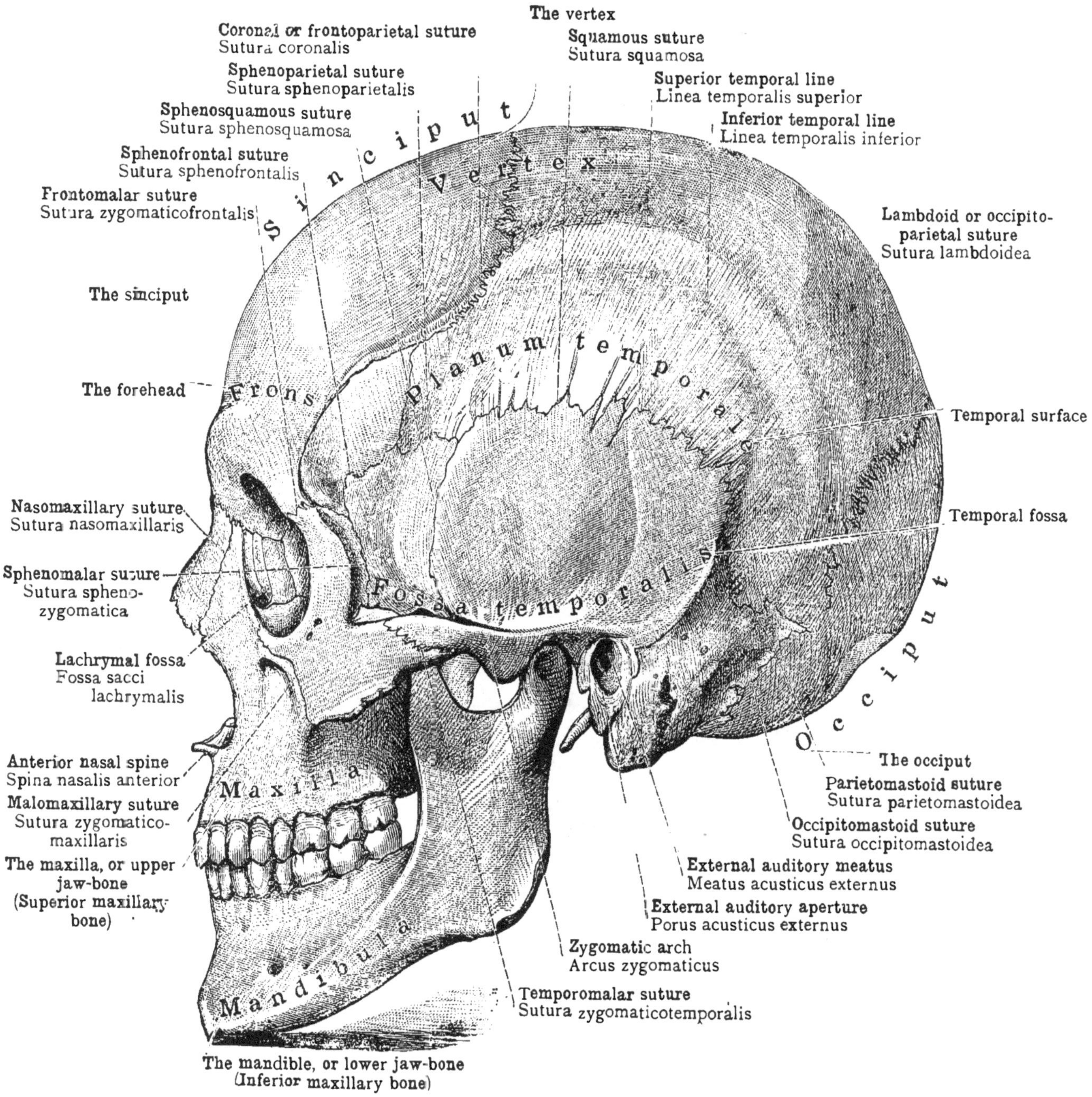

FIG. 103.—THE SKULL SEEN FROM THE LEFT SIDE: NORMA LATERALIS.

Cranium—The skull.

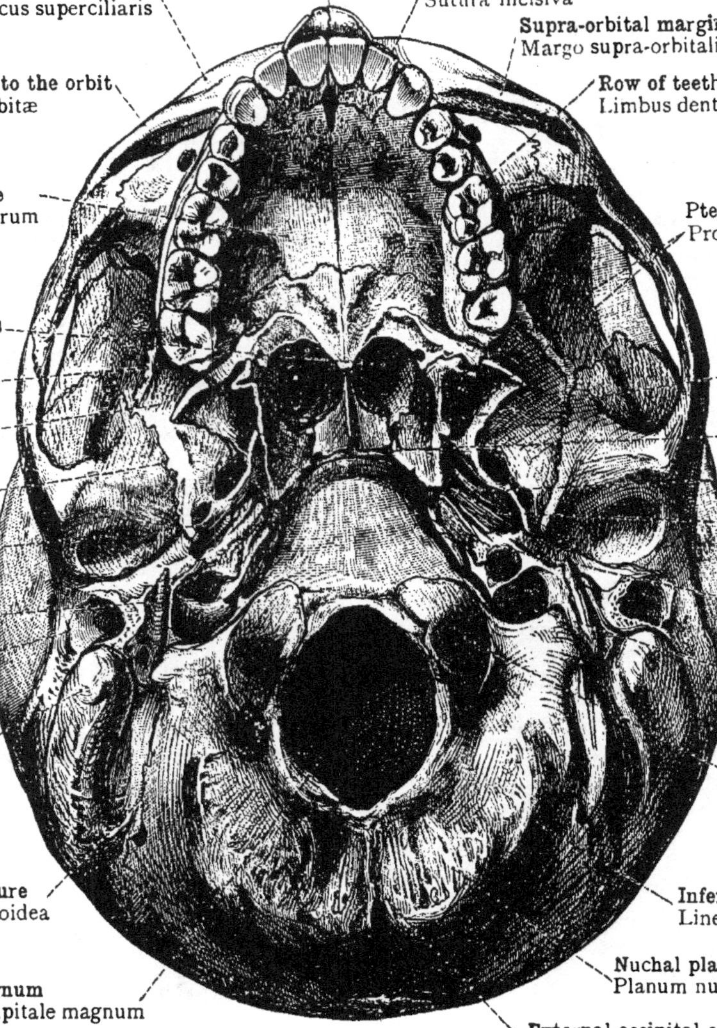

[1] **Canalis basipharyngeus,** basipharyngeal canal: This term is not often used by English anatomists, nor even is the canal itself mentioned by Quain. Macalister, however, in his description of the vomer, writes (p. 233): "In the region of its sphenoidal articulation there are three canals transmitting small vessels in the young skull, which usually become obliterated with advancing age; these are—one median vomerine canal between the vomer and the root of the rostrum, and a lateral on each side between the extremity of the ala vomeris and the vaginal process. These run parallel to, and may communicate with, the pterygopharyngeal [pterygopalatine] canal in the vaginal process." The two lateral canals here mentioned are those called by Toldt **canales basipharyngei.*—Tr.

FIG. 104.—EXTERNAL ASPECT OF THE BASE OF THE SKULL: BASIS CRANII EXTERNA.

Cranium—The skull.

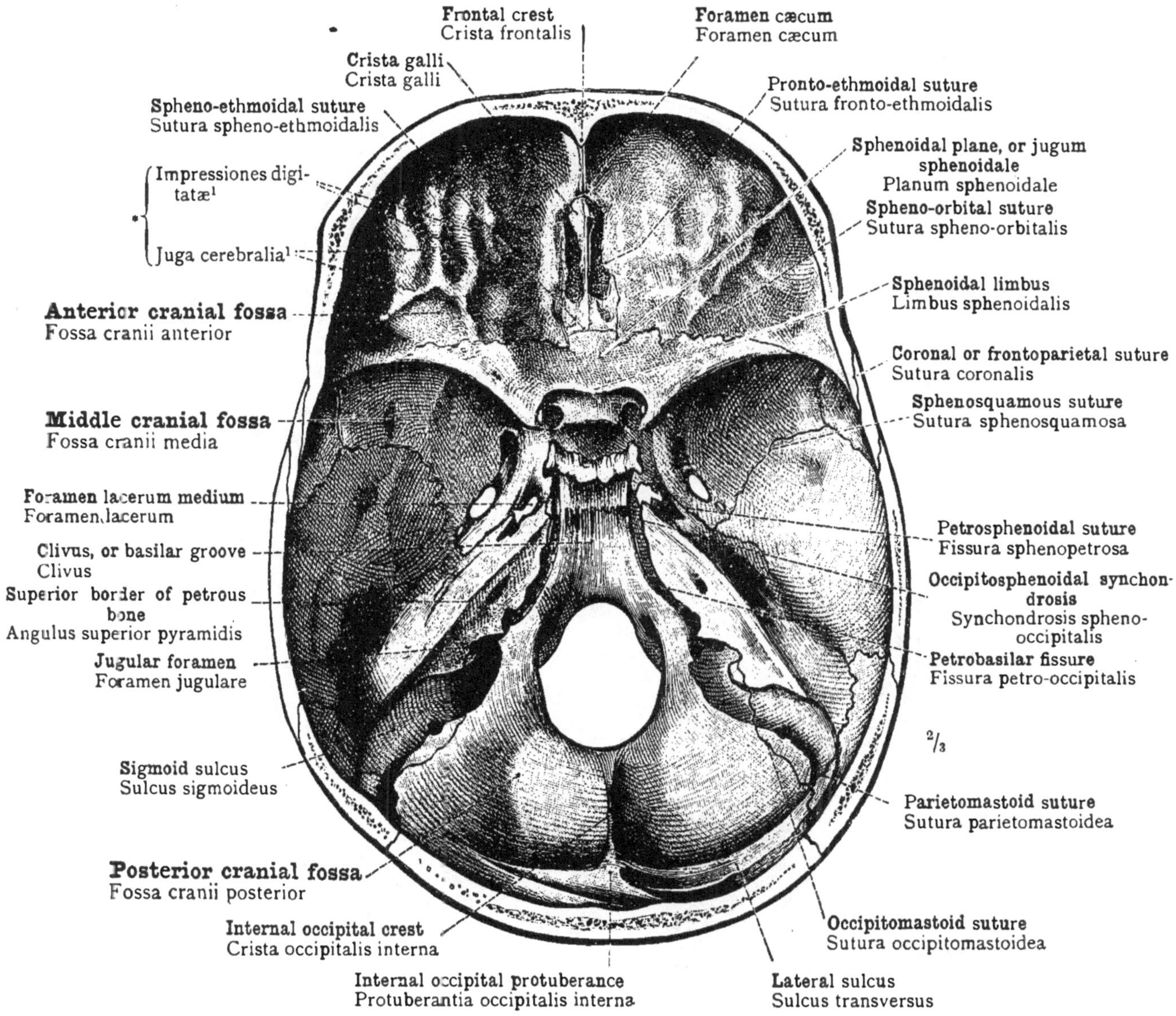

[1] Mouldings of the bone corresponding with the sulci and convolutions of the inferior surface of the frontal lobe of the cerebrum.

FIG. 105.—INTERNAL ASPECT OF THE BASE OF THE SKULL—BASIS CRANII INTERNA: FOSSÆ CRANII ANTERIOR, MEDIA, ET POSTERIOR—THE ANTERIOR, MIDDLE, AND POSTERIOR CRANIAL FOSSÆ. SEEN FROM ABOVE.

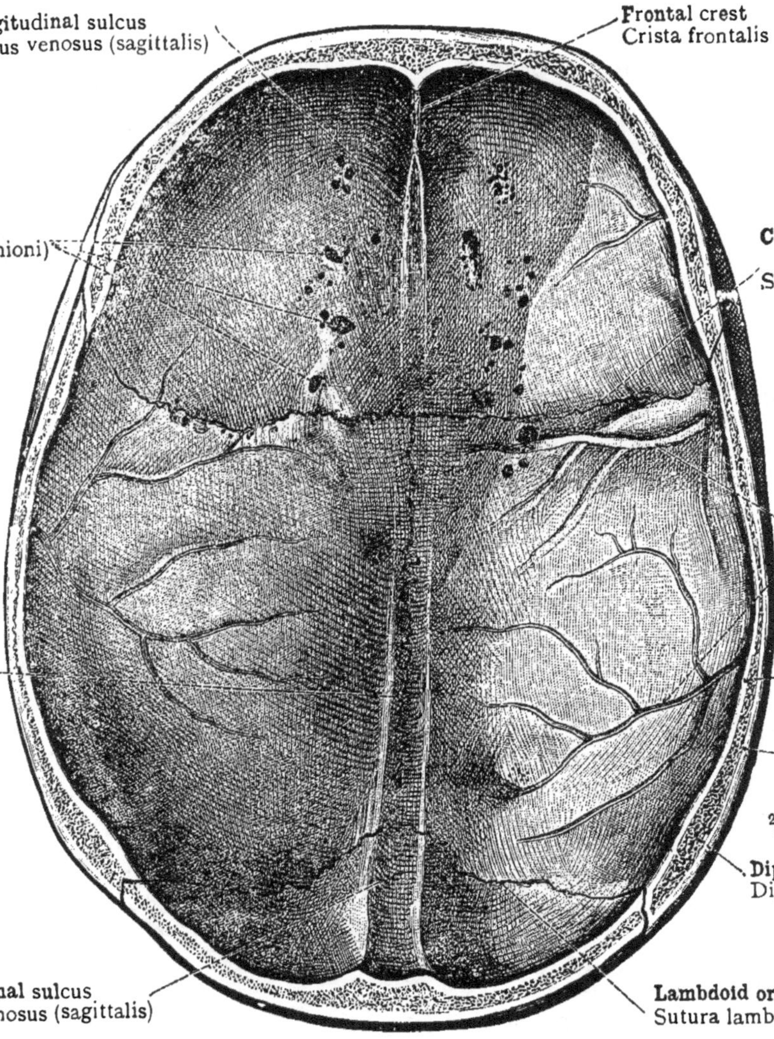

FIG. 106.—CALVARIA—THE SKULLCAP, OR ROOF OF THE SKULL. INNER ASPECT.

Cranium—The skull.

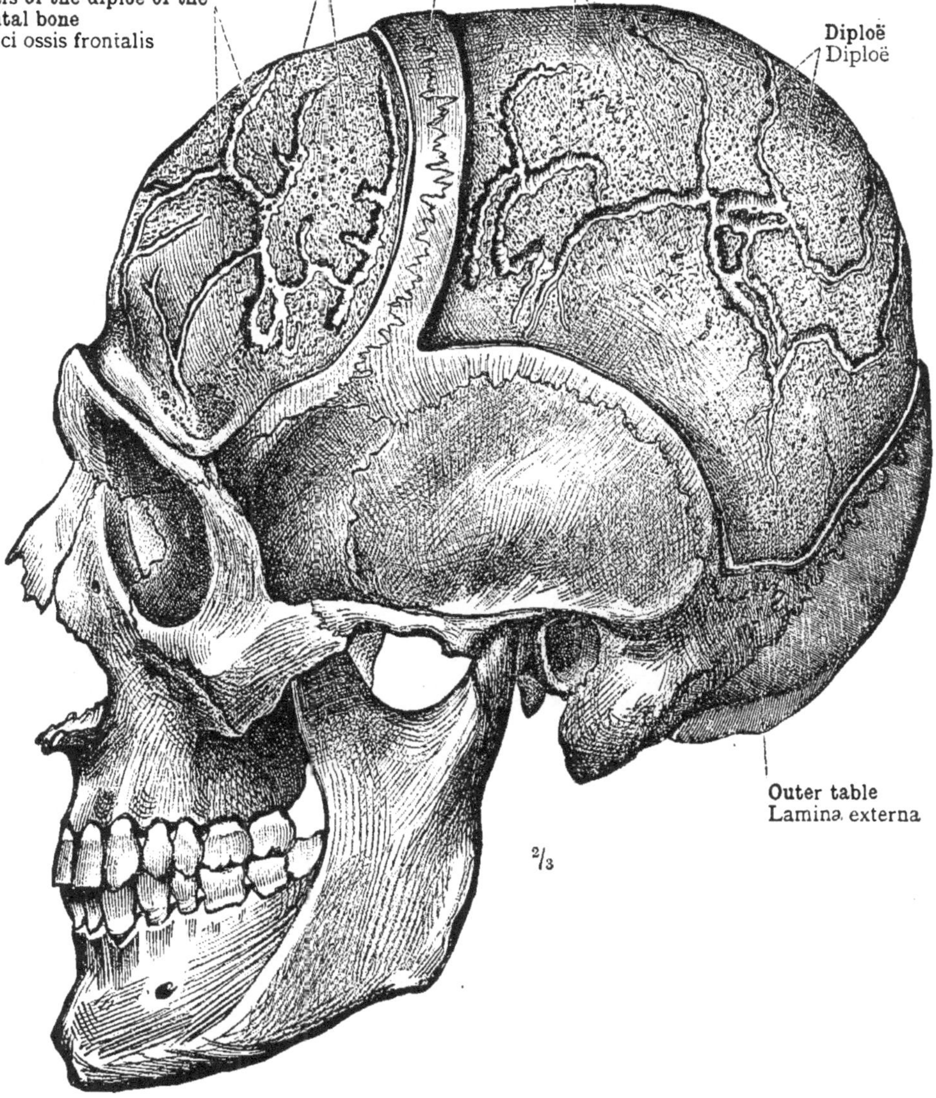

FIG. 107.—VASCULAR CANALS OF THE DIPLOË OF THE ROOF OF THE SKULL, SHOWN BY REMOVAL OF THE OUTER TABLE OF COMPACT BONE FROM THE FRONTAL BONE AND THE PARIETAL BONE: CANALES DIPLOICI (BRESCHETI). SEEN FROM THE LEFT SIDE.

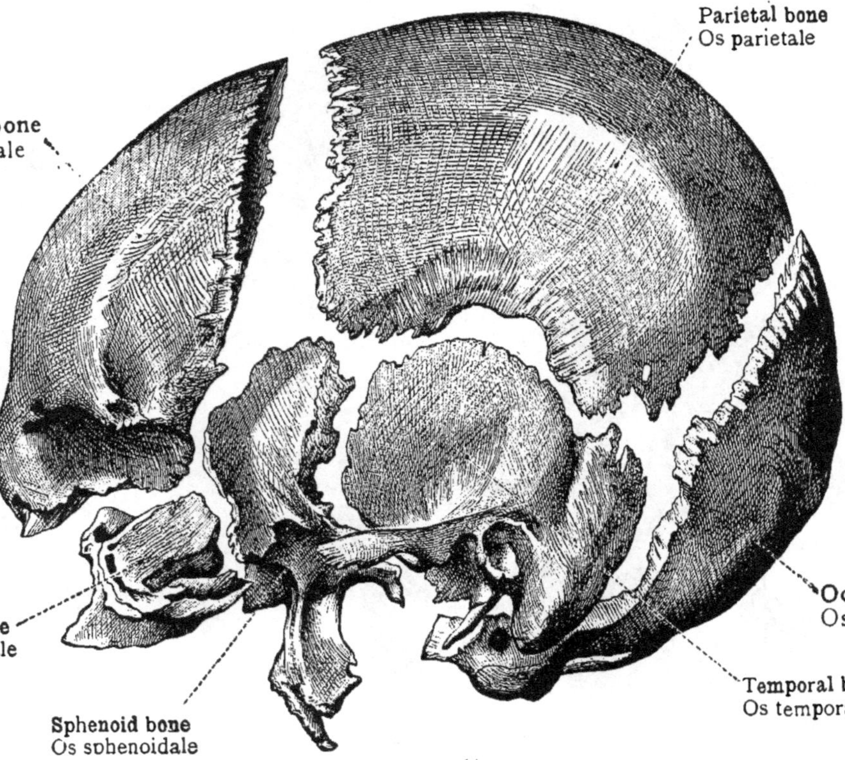

1/2

FIG. 108.—THE SEPARATE BONES OF WHICH THE CRANIUM CEREBRALE OR CRANIUM PROPER CONSISTS.

Ossa cranii cerebralis—Bones of the cranium proper.

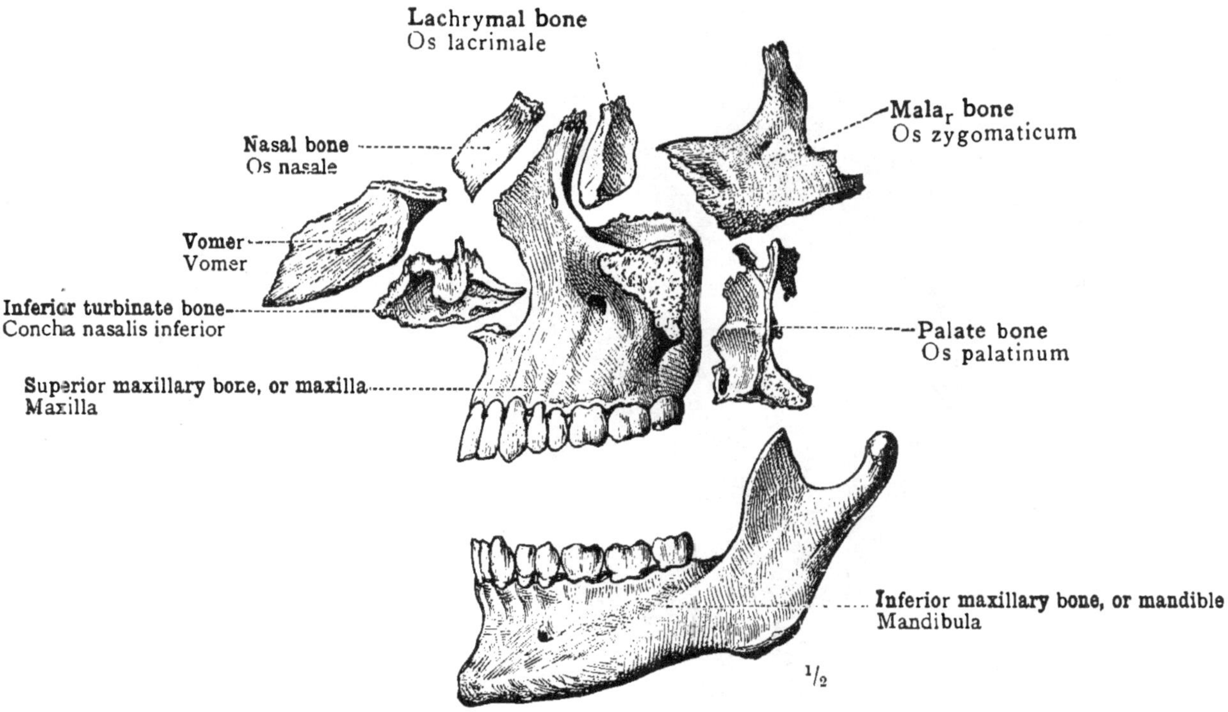

FIG. 109.—THE SEPARATE BONES OF WHICH THE CRANIUM VISCERALE (FACIES OSSEA), OR FACIAL PORTION OF THE SKULL, CONSISTS.

Ossa faciei—Bones of the face.

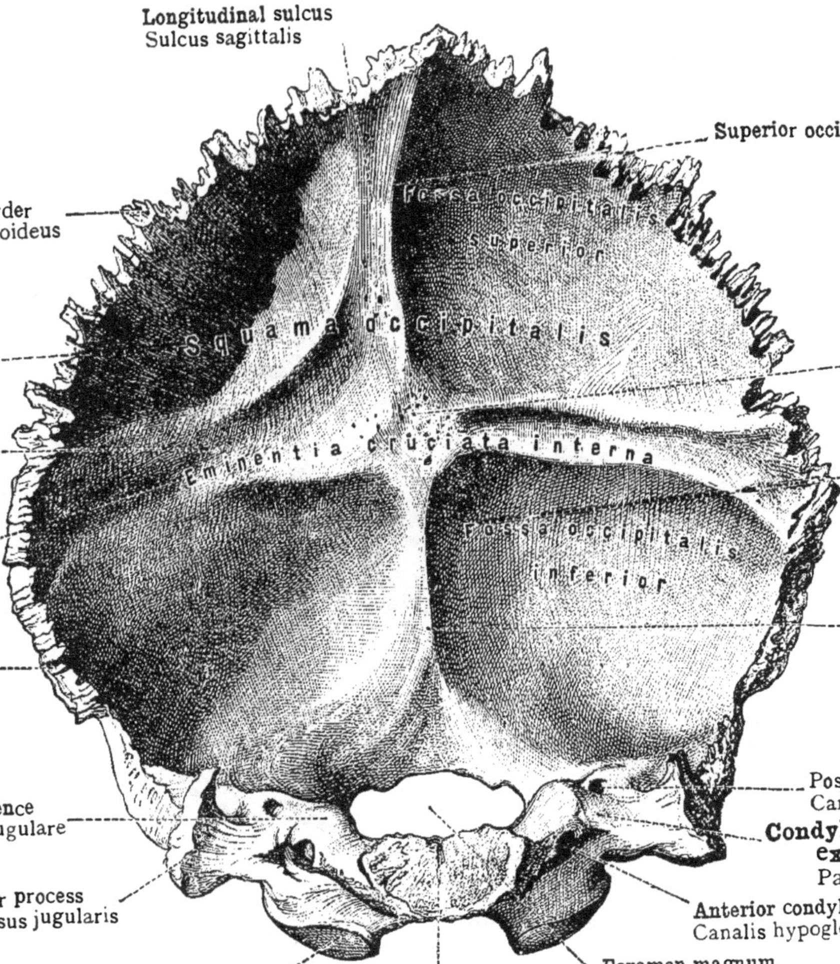

FIG. 110.—ANTERIOR (INTERNAL) ASPECT OF THE OCCIPITAL BONE.

Os occipitale—The occipital bone.

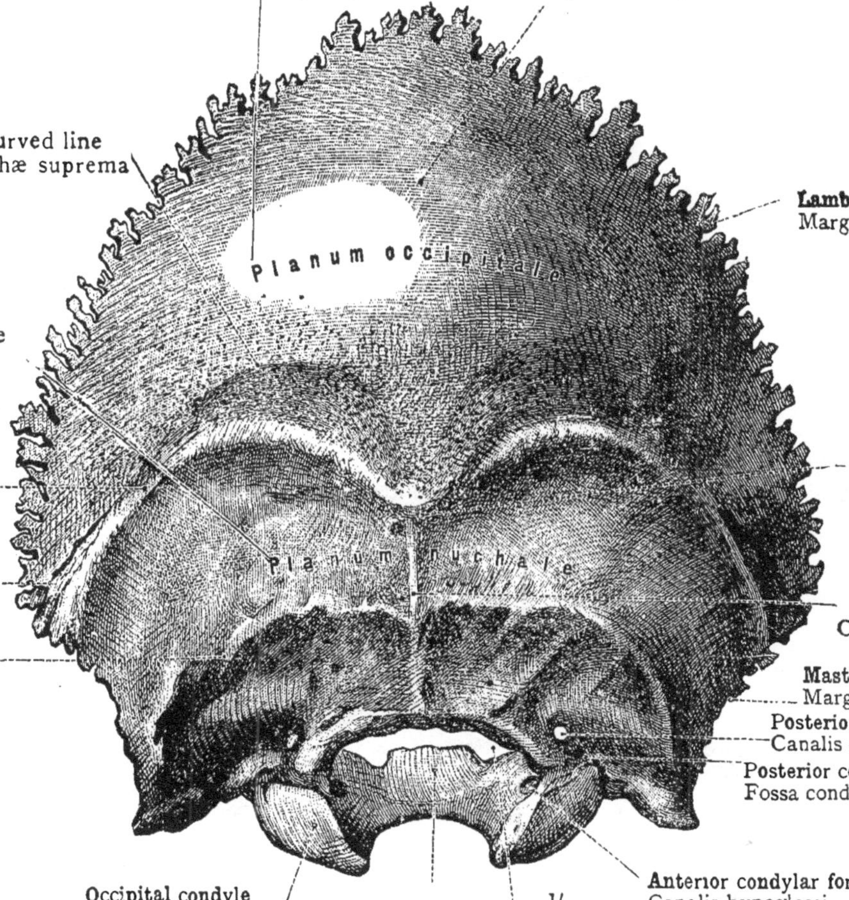

[1] See foot-note to p. 57.

FIG. 111.—POSTERIOR (EXTERNAL) ASPECT OF THE OCCIPITAL BONE.

Os occipitale—The occipital bone.

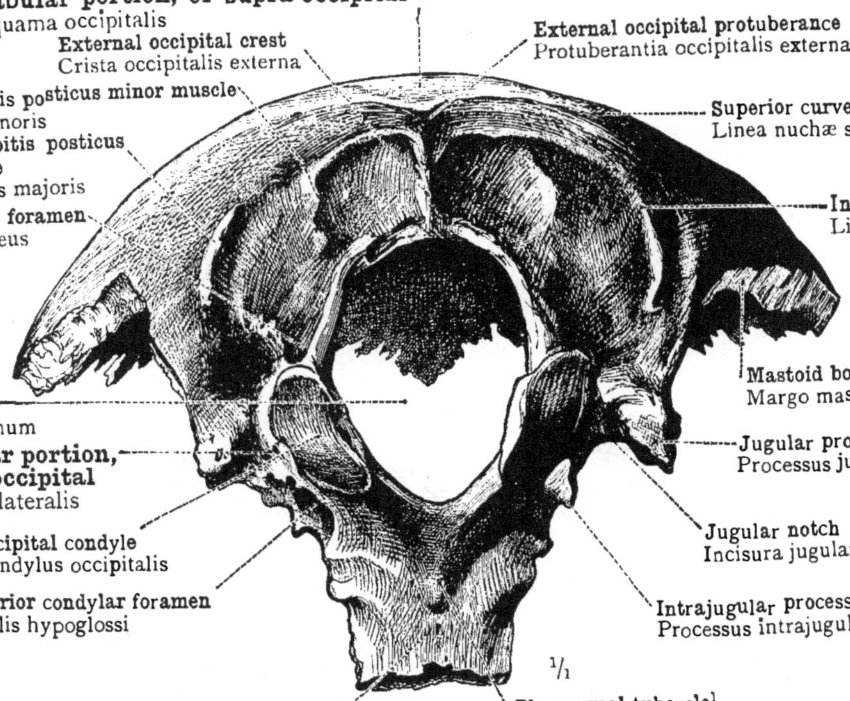

[1] Pharyngeal spine.—U.S.

FIG. 112.—THE OCCIPITAL BONE SEEN FROM BELOW (EXTERNAL BASAL SURFACE).

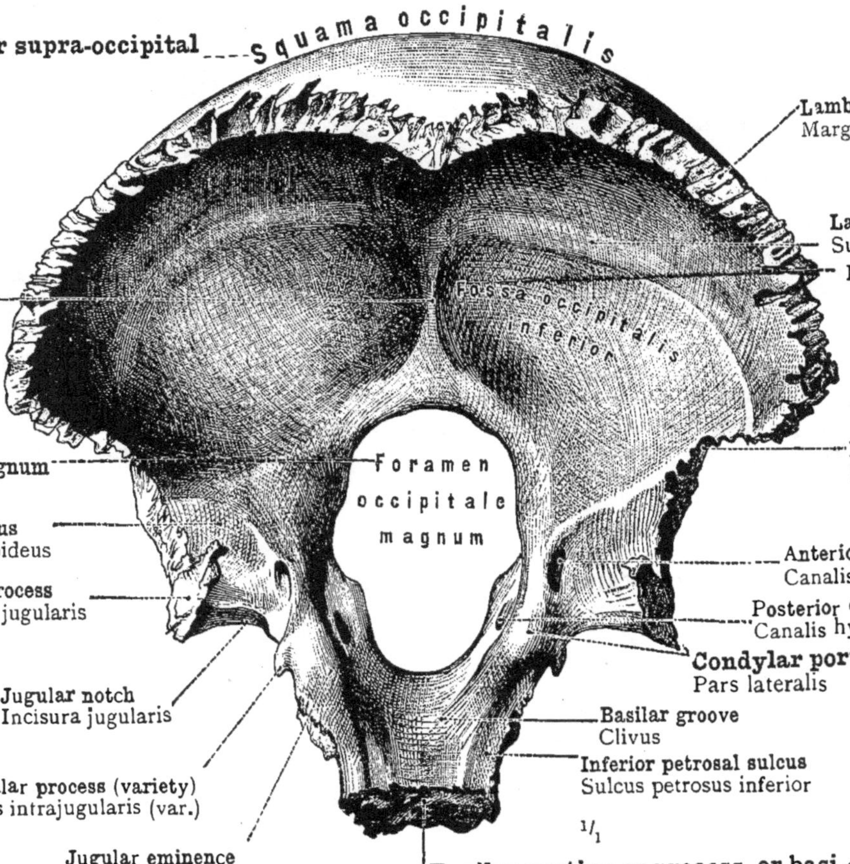

FIG. 113.—THE OCCIPITAL BONE SEEN FROM ABOVE (INTERNAL BASAL SURFACE).

Os occipitale—The occipital bone.

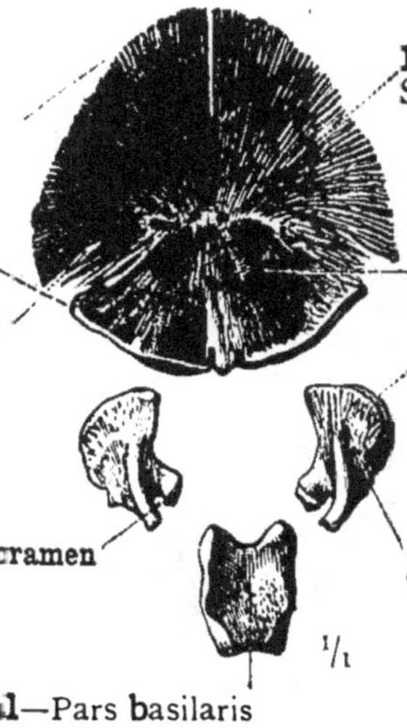

FIG. 114.—THE PORTIONS OF THE OCCIPITAL BONE FROM A HUMAN FŒTUS AT THE END OF THE SIXTH MONTH (MONTHS OF FOUR WEEKS EACH). SEEN FROM WITHIN.

Body-length, 12 inches.

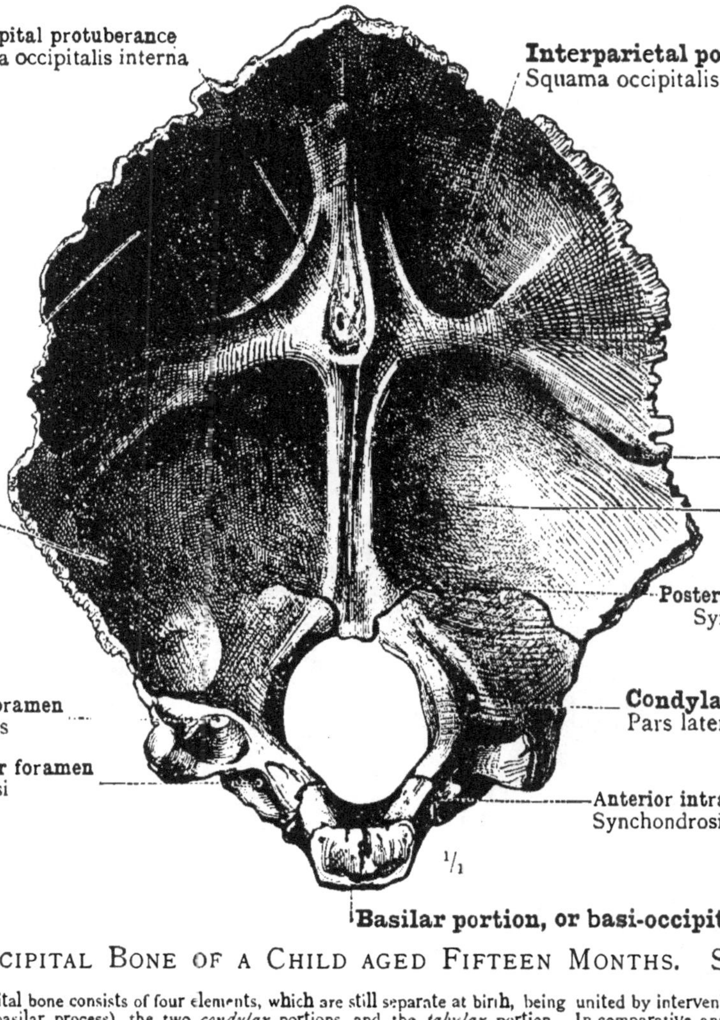

FIG. 115.—THE OCCIPITAL BONE OF A CHILD AGED FIFTEEN MONTHS. SEEN FROM WITHIN.

[1] The human occipital bone consists of four elements, which are still separate at birth, being united by intervening cartilage; these are, the *basilar* portion (basilar process), the two *condylar* portions, and the *tabular* portion. In comparative anatomy these are known respectively as *basi-occipital, exoccipitals*, and *supra-occipital*. The basi-occipital and the exoccipitals ossify each from a single nucleus; the supra-occipital ossifies from four nuclei, an upper pair and a lower. These soon unite, but leave for some time fissures running in along the superior curved line. Not uncommonly this fissure persists on one or both sides through life, and in rare cases there is a persistent suture running right across and dividing the tabular portion of the occipital bone into two parts (*Sutura mendosa; see Figs. 111 and 114). Of these two parts, the lower, which belongs to the base of the skull and ossifies in cartilage, is the proper *supra-occipital* element, homologous with the *supra-occipital bone* of other vertebrata; whilst the upper, which belongs to the vertex of the skull and ossifies in membrane, represents the *interparietal bone* of many animals. This part alone is entitled to the name *squama occipitalis*, a term, however, little used by English anatomists. The occasional persistence of the suture between the interparietal and supra-occipital elements of the occipital bone is of surgical importance, since, in cases of injury to the back of the head, it is, if present, liable to be mistaken for fracture.—TR.

Development of the Occipital Bone.

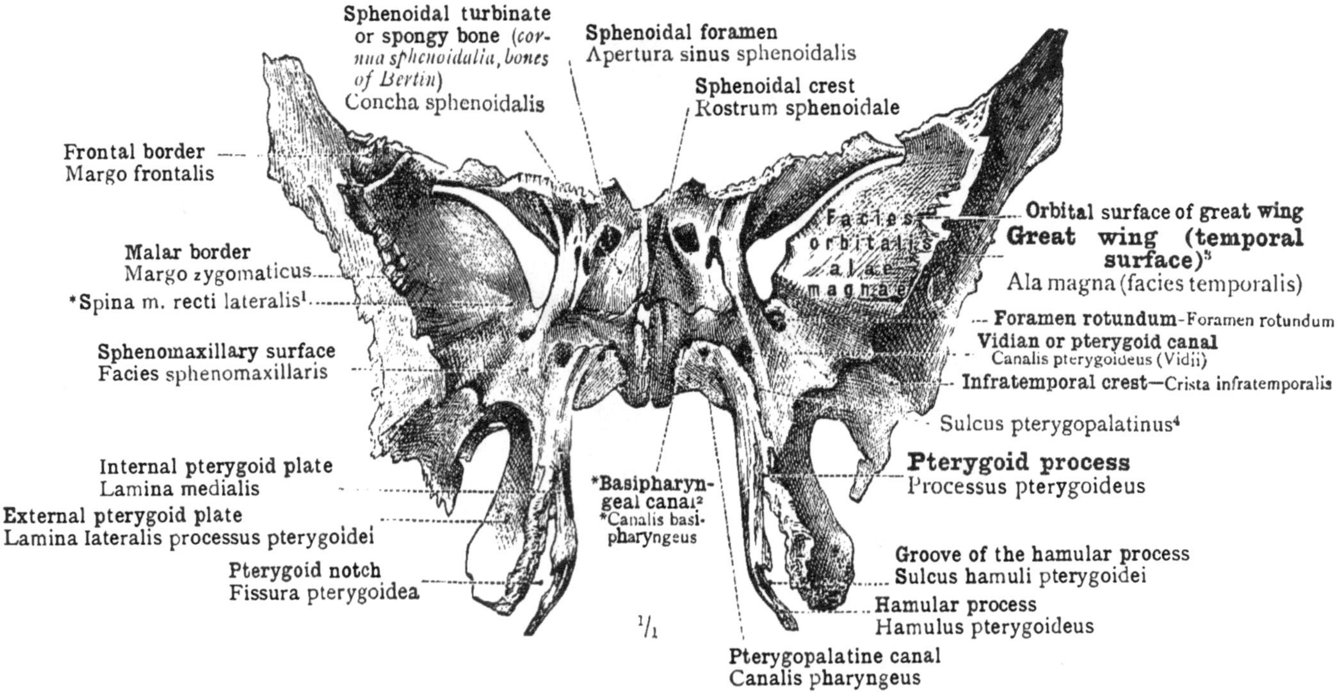

[1] Spine for the attachment of the lower head of the external rectus muscle of the eyeball.
[2] See note to p. 48. [3] See note to p. 59.
[4] As mentioned in the Preface, the canal called by English anatomists *palatomaxillary* or *posterior palatine canal* is by Toldt called *pterygopalatine canal*. The inner grooved portion of the sphenomaxillary surface, which he here calls the *pterygopalatine groove*, leads down into that canal, but does not form a part of it, since it lies between the palate bone and the superior maxillary bone.—Tr.

FIG. 116.—THE SPHENOID BONE SEEN FROM BEFORE

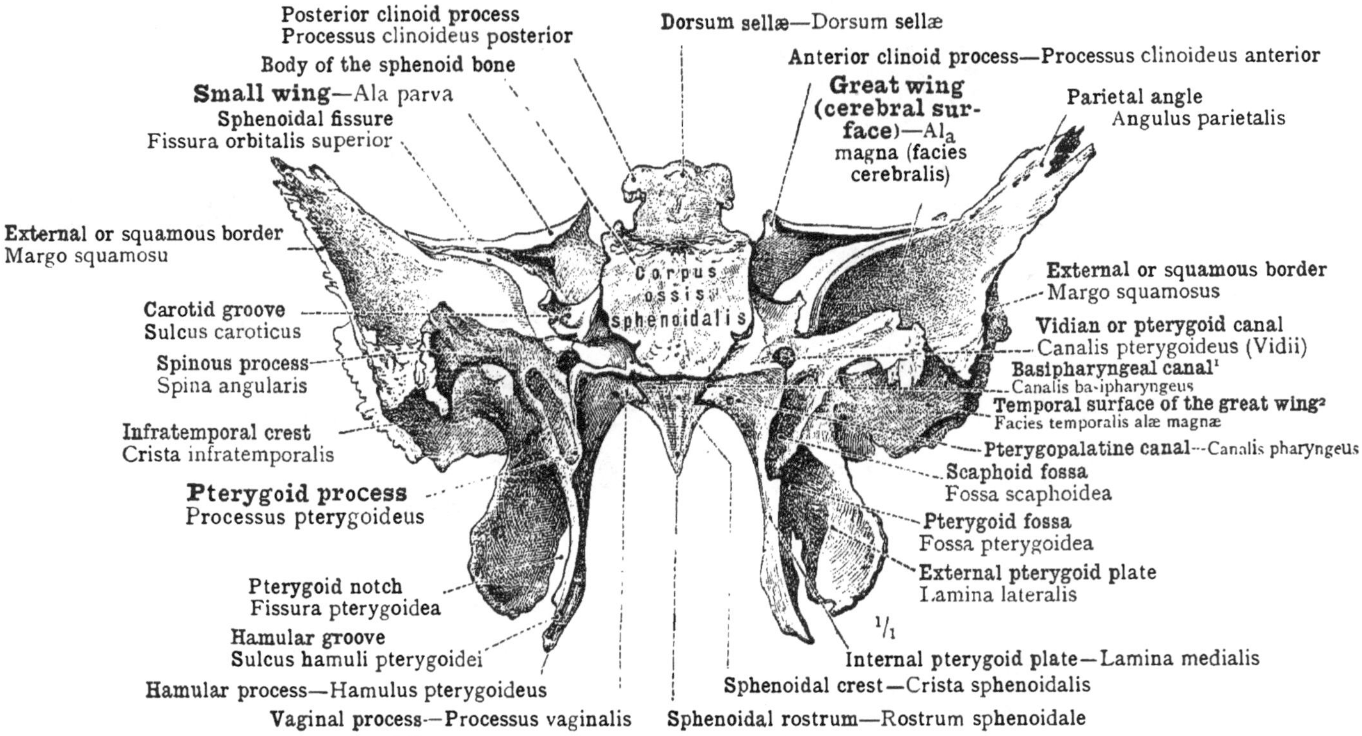

[1] See note to p. 48. [2] See note to p. 59.

FIG. 117.—THE SPHENOID BONE SEEN FROM BEHIND.

Os sphenoidale—The sphenoid bone.

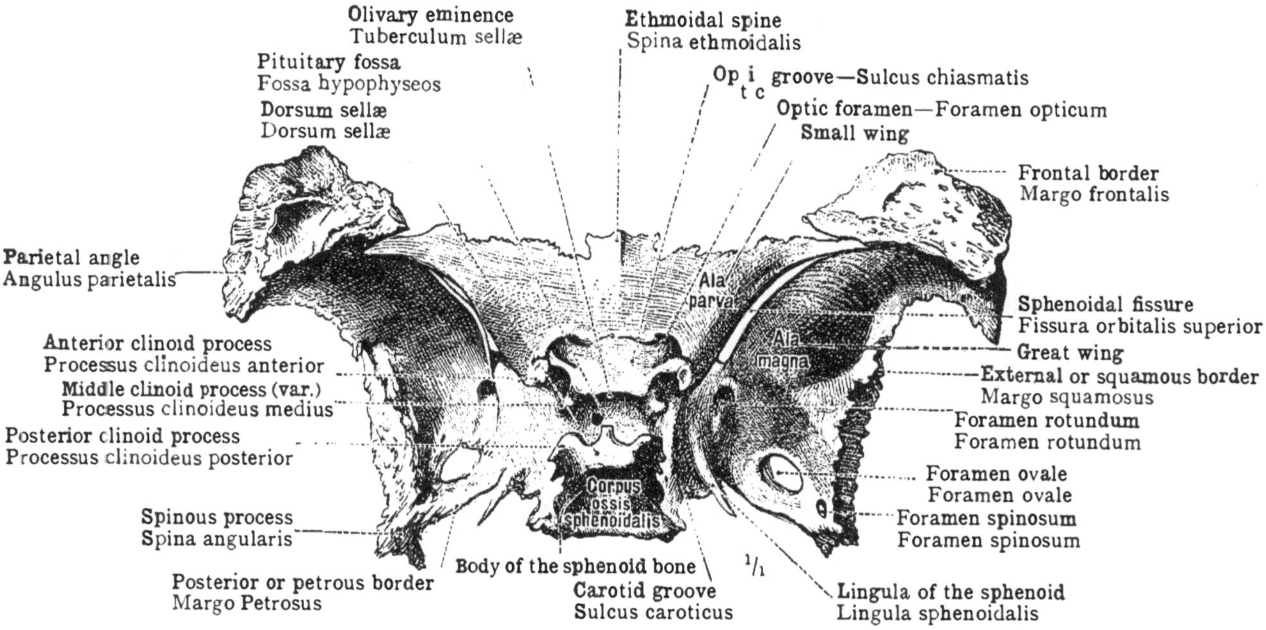

FIG. 118.—THE SPHENOID BONE SEEN FROM ABOVE (CEREBRAL ASPECT).

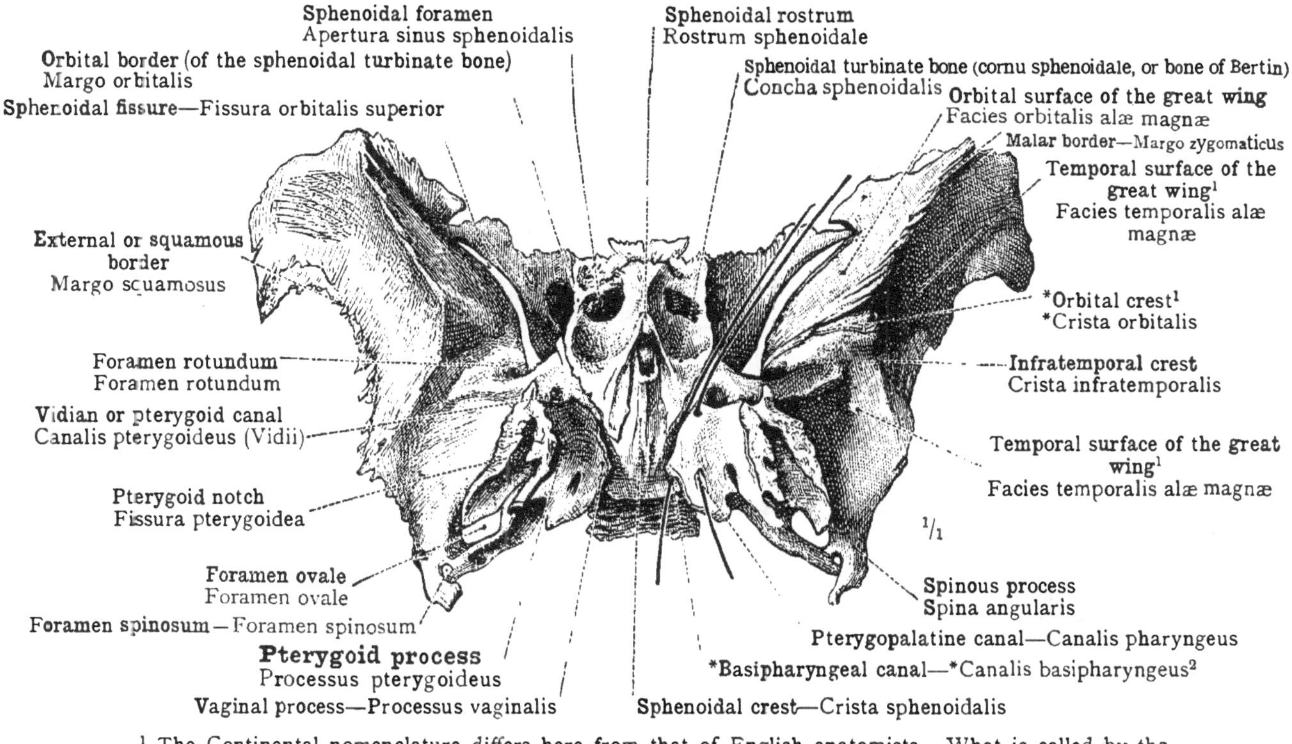

[1] The Continental nomenclature differs here from that of English anatomists. What is called by the author *facies temporalis alæ magnæ*, the temporal surface of the great wing, is in England known as the *temporozygomatic surface*, being divided by the *infratemporal crest* into an upper *temporal surface* and a lower *sphenomaxillary surface*. As regards the term *crista orbitalis*, the crest, this is not used by Quain at all, while Macalister applies it to the *lower margin of the sphenoidal fissure*, the free border separating the orbital from the cerebral surface of the great wing. Toldt, on the other hand, as an examination of Fig. 119 shows, means by *crista orbitalis* the *posterior margin of the sphenomaxillary fissure*, free border separating the orbital from the zygomatic surface of the great wing.—TR.

[2] See note to p. 48.

FIG. 119.—THE SPHENOID BONE SEEN FROM BELOW (EXTERNAL ASPECT).

Os sphenoidale—The sphenoid bone.

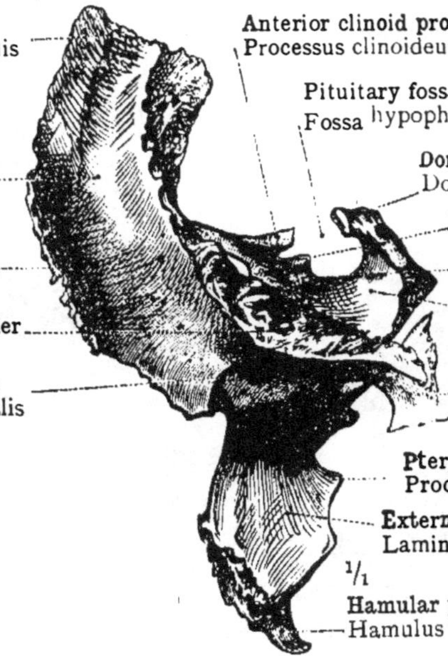

[1] See note to p. 59.

[2] English anatomists use the terms *pituitary fossa* and *sella turcica* as synonyms; Toldt, more accurately, distinguishes between them, meaning by *pituitary fossa* (Fossa hypophyseos) the deep pit on the upper surface of the body of the sphenoid bone which lodges the pituitary body or hypophysis cerebri, and by *sella turcica* the saddle-shaped surface which forms the floor of that fossa.—TR.

FIG. 120.—THE SPHENOID BONE SEEN FROM THE LEFT SIDE (TEMPOROZYGOMATIC SURFACE).[1]

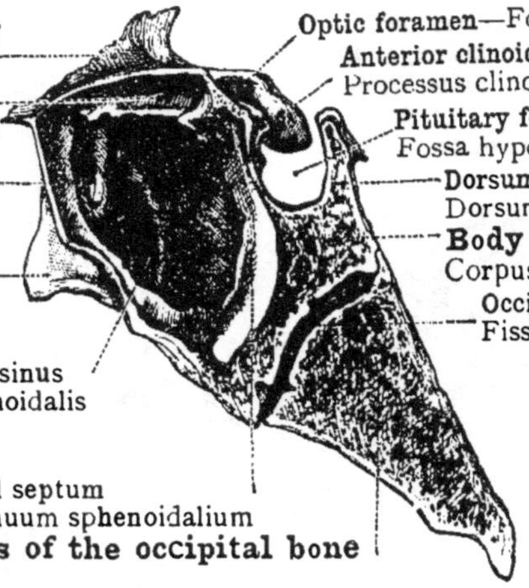

FIG. 121.—THE SPHENOIDAL SINUSES IN MEDIAN SAGITTAL SECTION, THE GREATER PART OF THE SPHENOIDAL SEPTUM HAVING BEEN REMOVED. SEEN FROM THE LEFT SIDE.

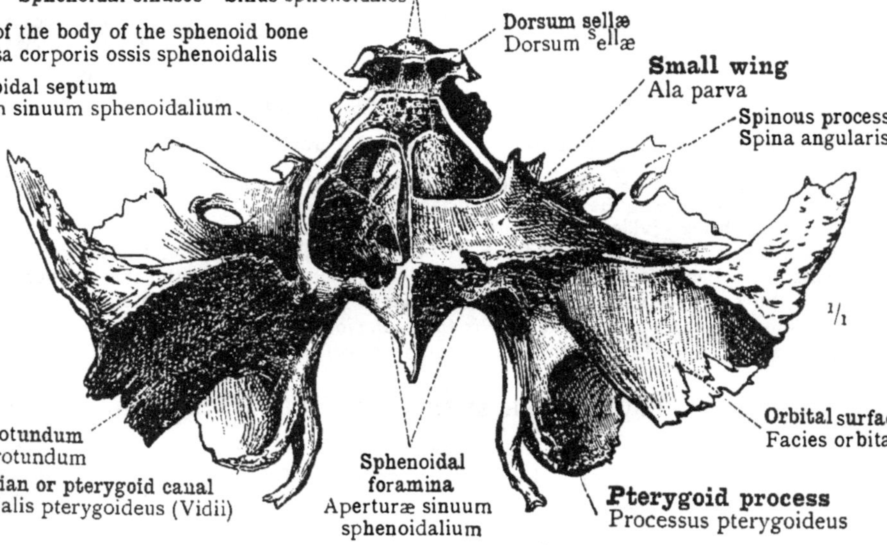

FIG. 122.—THE SPHENOIDAL SINUSES, EXPOSED FROM ABOVE BY THE REMOVAL OF THE INNER LAMELLA OF COMPACT BONE.

The right sinus is opened from above; the left is unopened.

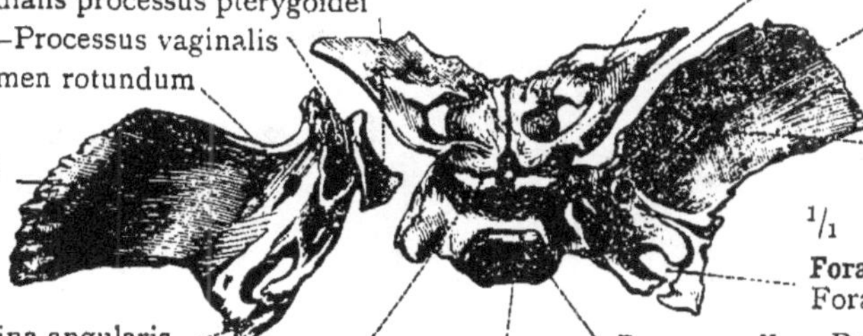

FIG. 123.—THE SPHENOID BONE OF A BOY BORN AT FULL TERM, SEEN FROM ABOVE.
Body-length, 19 inches.

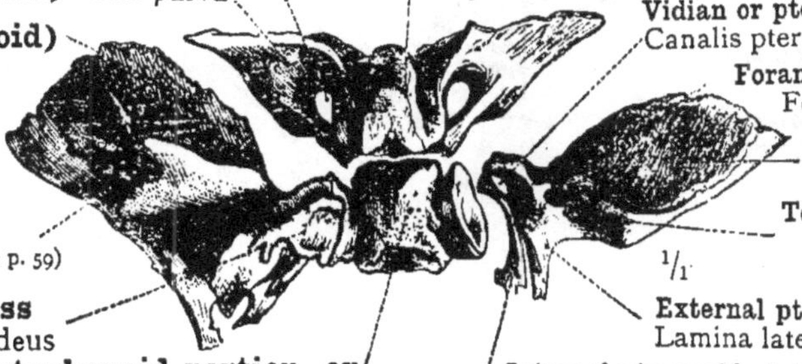

FIG. 124.—THE SPHENOID BONE OF A BOY BORN AT FULL TERM, SEEN FROM BELOW.
Body-length, 19 inches.

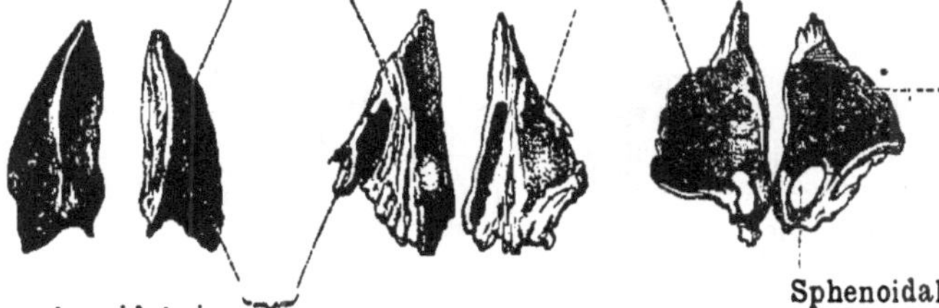

FIG. 125.—CONCHÆ SPHENOIDALES—THE SPHENOIDAL TURBINATE BONES. SEEN FROM ABOVE.

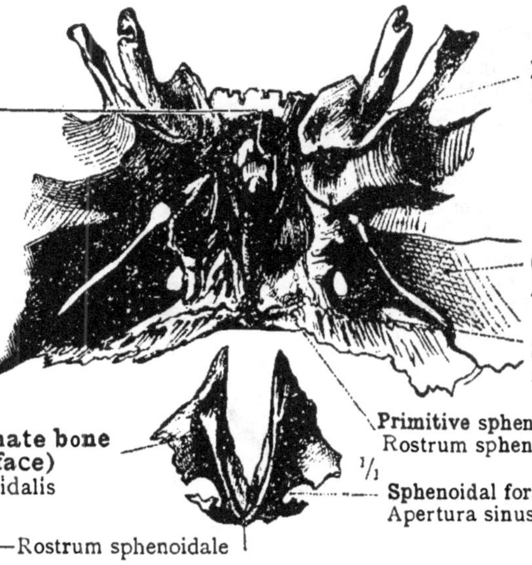

FIG. 126.—THE RELATION OF THE SPHENOIDAL TURBINATE BONES TO THE INFERIOR SURFACE OF THE SPHENOID BONE IN THE SIXTH YEAR OF LIFE.

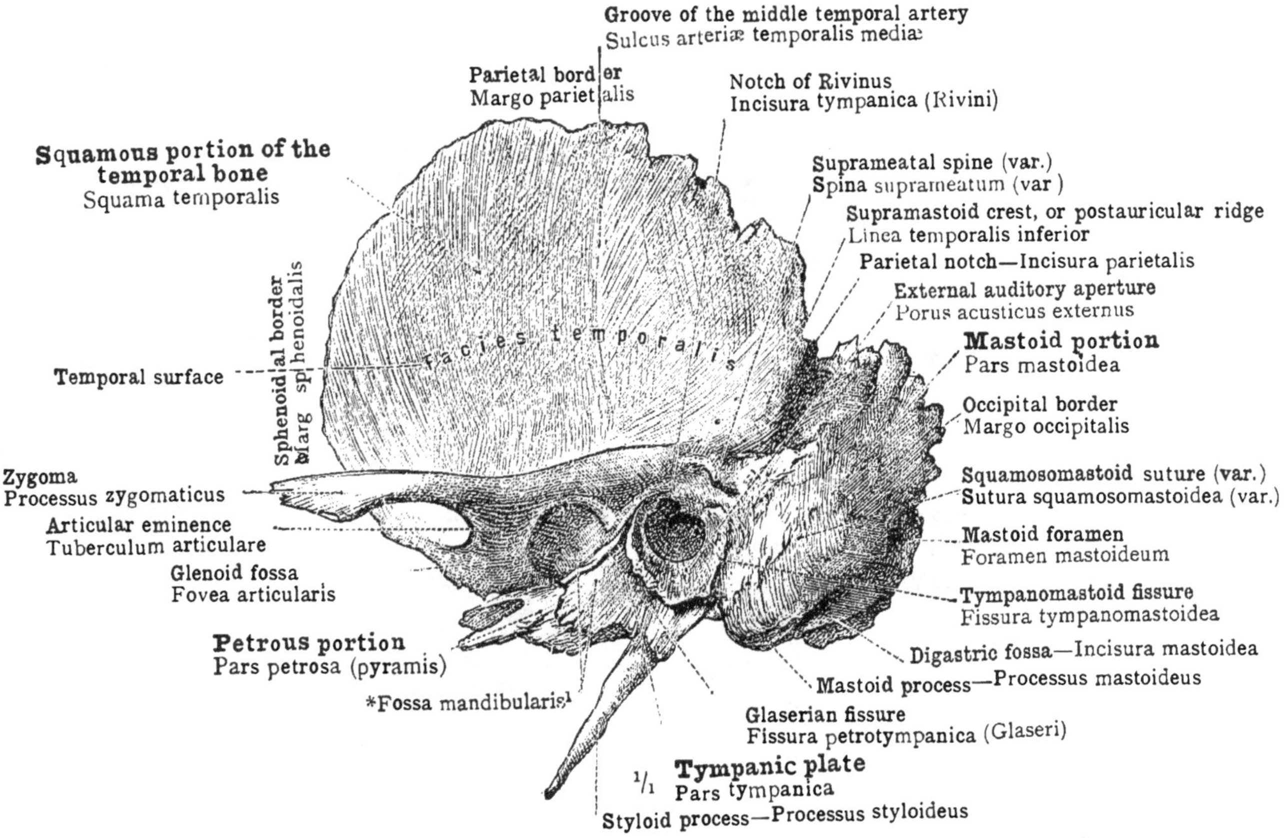

1 What is called the mandibular fossa by Toldt is the posterior non-articular portion of the glenoid fossa (separated from the articular portion by the Glaserian fissure). Its floor is formed by the tympanic plate, and it lodges a portion of the parotid gland.—Tr.

FIG. 127.—THE LEFT TEMPORAL BONE SEEN FROM THE OUTER SIDE (TEMPORAL SURFACE).

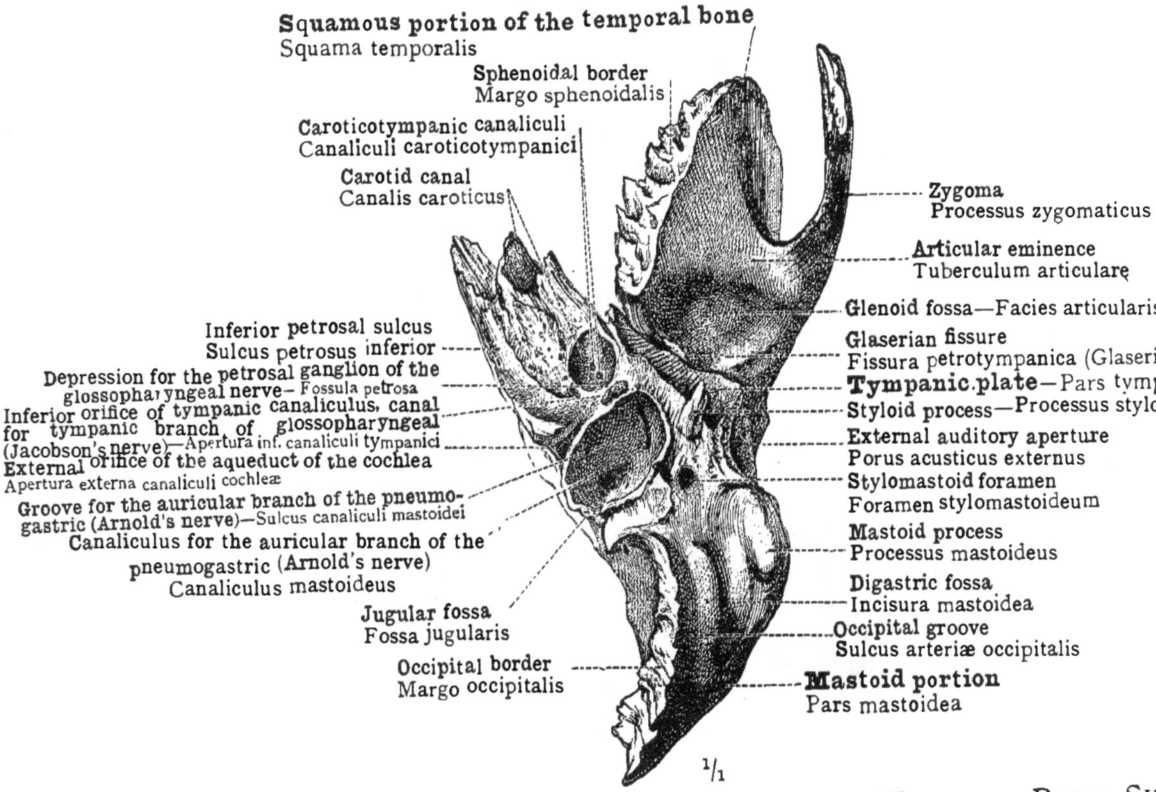

FIG. 128.—THE LEFT TEMPORAL BONE SEEN FROM BELOW (EXTERNAL BASAL SURFACE).

Os temporale—The temporal bone.

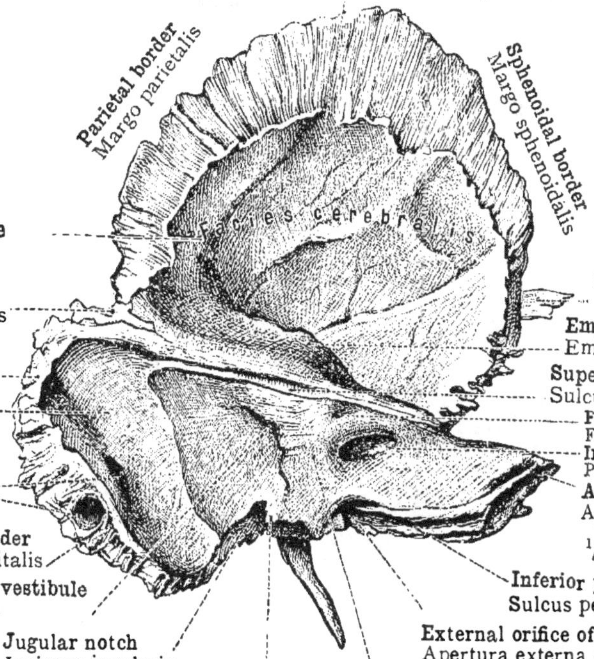

FIG. 129.—THE LEFT TEMPORAL BONE SEEN FROM WITHIN (CEREBRAL SURFACE).

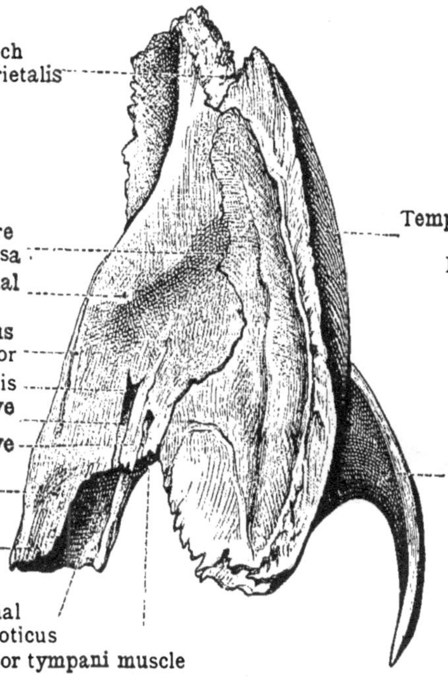

FIG. 130.—THE LEFT TEMPORAL BONE SEEN FROM ABOVE (INTERNAL BASAL SURFACE).

Os temporale—The temporal bone.

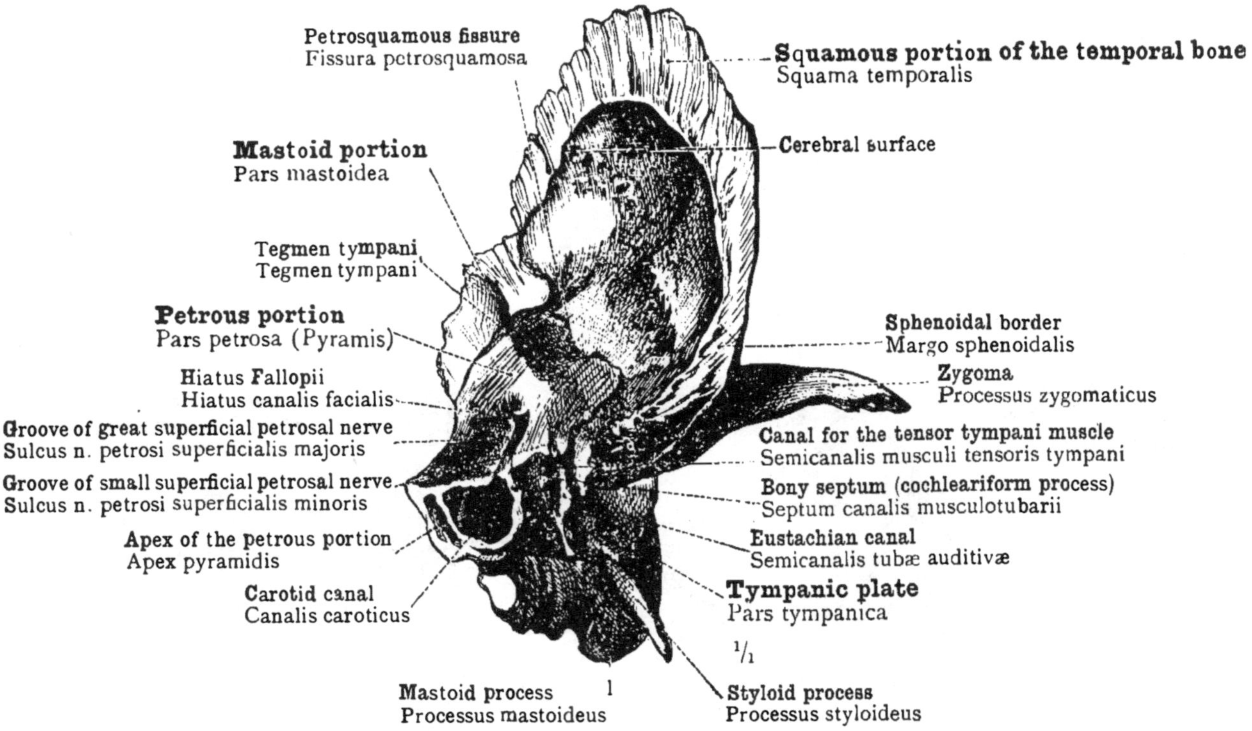

FIG. 131.—THE LEFT TEMPORAL BONE SEEN FROM BEFORE.

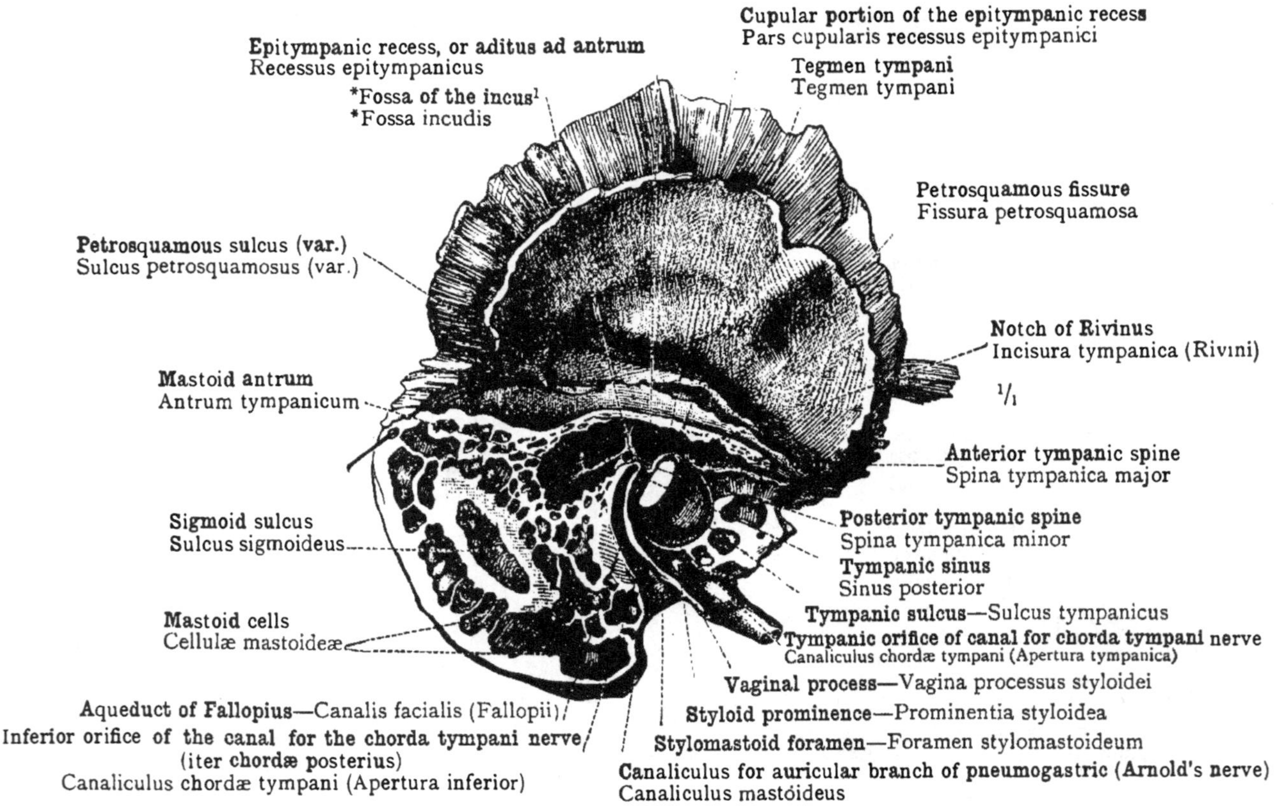

[1] *Fossa of the incus.—'The *shorter process* (*crus breve*) of the incus projects backwards. Its extremity is tipped with cartilage and is . . . articulated by ligamentous fibres (ligament of the incus) with the posterior and partly with the outer wall of the tympanum near the entrance to the mastoid cells. The place where the ligamentous fibres are attached to the wall of the tympanum is somewhat depressed, and has a covering of cartilage.'—Quain's 'Anatomy,' tenth edition, vol. iii., part iii., p. 90. *Fossa of the incus* is a most suitable name for this depressed cartilage-covered area, and may well be adopted by English anatomists.—TR.

FIG. 132.—THE EXTERNAL WALL OF THE TYMPANUM AND THE MASTOID CELLS DISPLAYED BY A SECTION THROUGH THE LEFT TEMPORAL BONE IN A PLANE PARALLEL WITH THE SQUAMOUS PORTION OF THAT BONE.

The petrosquamous sulcus (along which a sound has been passed) is in this specimen partly bridged over by bone ; anteriorly it communicates with the outer surface of the bone by means of a spurious jugular foramen—foramen jugulare spurium (Variety).

Os temporale—The temporal bone.

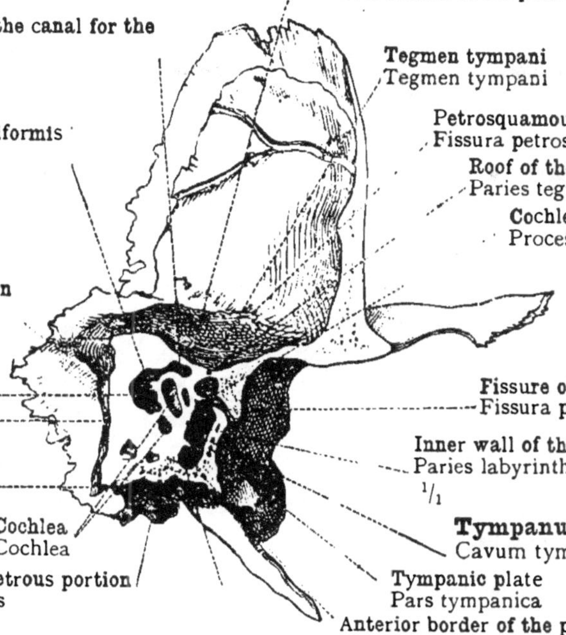

FIG. 133.—VERTICAL SECTION THROUGH THE PETROUS PORTION OF THE LEFT TEMPORAL BONE AND THROUGH THE ANTERIOR PART OF THE SQUAMOUS PORTION. (NOMENCLATURE OF THE SURFACE AND BORDERS OF THE PETROUS PORTION.)

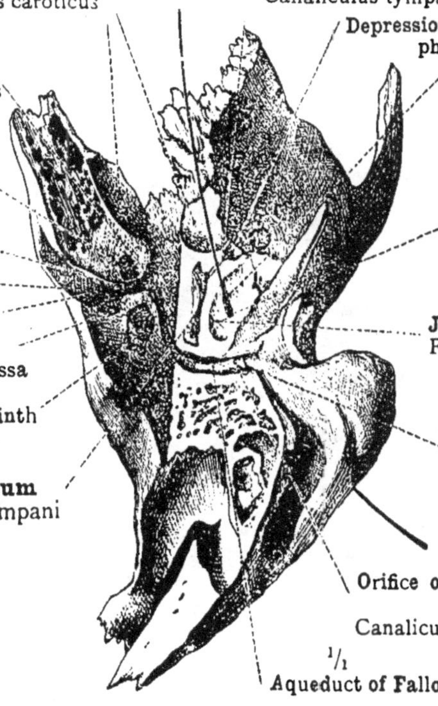

FIG. 134.—AQUEDUCTUS FALLOPII, OR CANAL FOR THE FACIAL NERVE, SHOWN FROM BENEATH BY THE REMOVAL OF A WEDGE-SHAPED PIECE FROM THE PETROUS PORTION OF THE LEFT TEMPORAL BONE.

The canaliculus tympanicus, for the tympanic branch of the glossopharyngeal nerve (Jacobson's nerve), is also opened up throughout its whole length. A sound has been passed through the canaliculus for the auricular branch of the pneumogastric nerve (nerve of Arnold). In the Continental nomenclature this canaliculus is known as the *canaliculus mastoideus*.

Os temporale—Temporal bone.

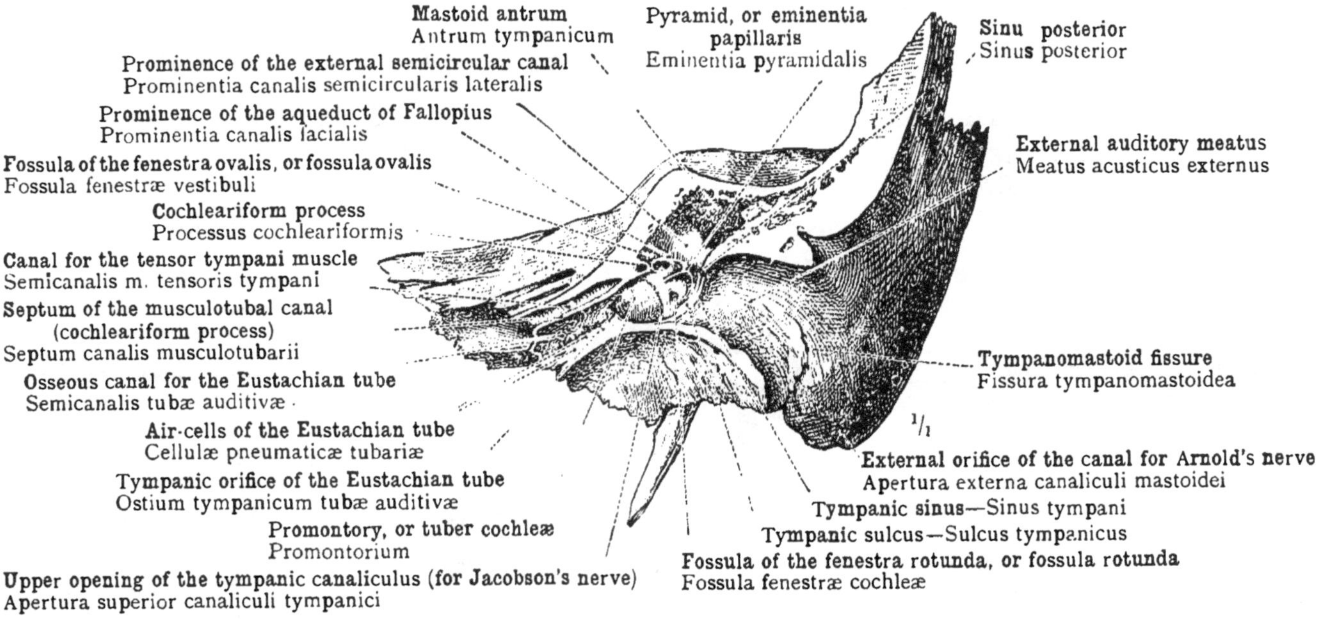

FIG. 135.—VERTICAL SECTION THROUGH THE LEFT TEMPORAL BONE IN A PLANE PARALLEL WITH THE SUPERIOR BORDER OF THE PETROUS PORTION, AND PASSING THROUGH THE MIDDLE OF THE EXTERNAL AUDITORY MEATUS, TO DEMONSTRATE THE TYMPANIC CAVITY, CAVUM TYMPANI, AND THE ADJOINING PARTS.

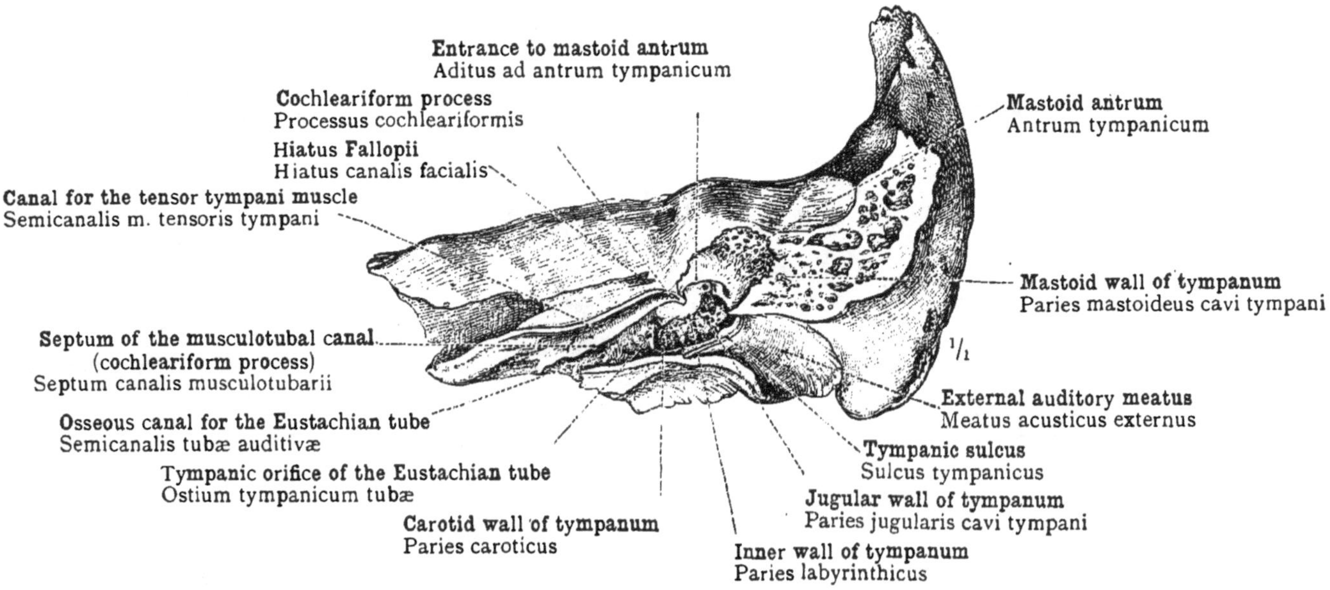

FIG. 136. VERTICAL SECTION THROUGH THE LEFT TEMPORAL BONE IN A PLANE PARALLEL WITH THE SUPERIOR BORDER OF THE PETROUS PORTION, THE SECTION PASSING ALONG THE POSTERIOR WALL OF THE EXTERNAL AUDITORY MEATUS, TO DEMONSTRATE THE TYMPANIC CAVITY, CAVUM TYMPANI, AND THE ADJOINING PARTS.

Os temporale—Temporal bone.

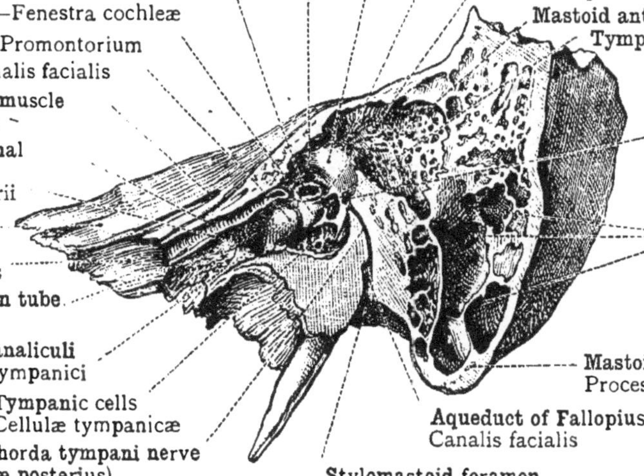

FIG. 137.—VERTICAL SECTION THROUGH THE LEFT TEMPORAL BONE, CROSSING OBLIQUELY THE SUPERIOR BORDER OF THE PETROUS PORTION, AND PASSING THROUGH THE ANTERIOR PORTION OF THE MASTOID PROCESS, TO DEMONSTRATE THE TYMPANIC CAVITY, CAVUM TYMPANI, AND THE ADJOINING PARTS (ESPECIALLY THE MASTOID ANTRUM AND THE MASTOID CELLS).

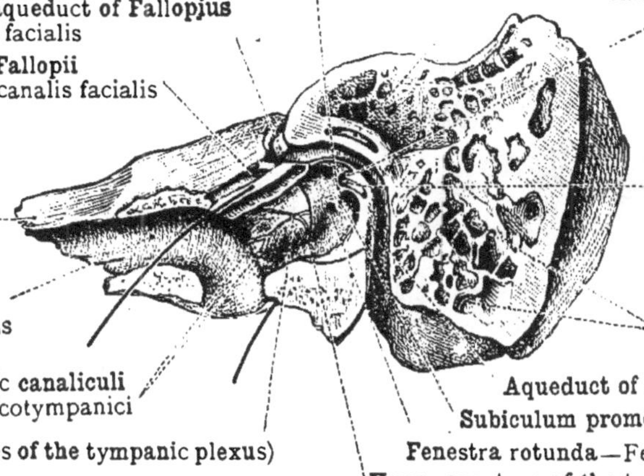

FIG. 138.—VERTICAL SECTION THROUGH THE LEFT TEMPORAL BONE, CROSSING OBLIQUELY THE SUPERIOR BORDER OF THE PETROUS PORTION, AND PASSING THROUGH THE POSTERIOR PORTION OF THE MASTOID PROCESS, TO DEMONSTRATE THE TYMPANIC CAVITY, CAVUM TYMPANI, AND THE ADJOINING PARTS.

A bristle has been passed through the canaliculus tympanicus (the canal for Jacobson's nerve—the tympanic branch of the glossopharyngeal nerve) into the tympanum, and, after traversing this cavity, leaves it by the canaliculus that opens into the groove for the small superficial petrosal nerve.

Os temporale—Temporal bone.

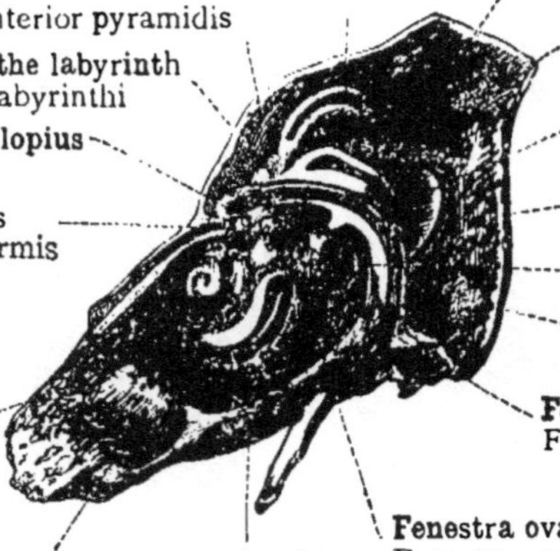

FIG. 139.—THE BONY LABYRINTH, LABYRINTHUS OSSEUS, SHOWN IN THE LEFT PETROUS PORTION. SEEN OBLIQUELY FROM IN FRONT AND BELOW. THE OSSEOUS SEMICIRCULAR CANALS AND ALSO THE CANAL OF THE COCHLEA HAVE BEEN PARTLY OPENED. THE RELATIONS BETWEEN THE AQUEDUCT OF FALLOPIUS AND THE OSSEOUS LABYRINTH ARE CLEARLY SHOWN

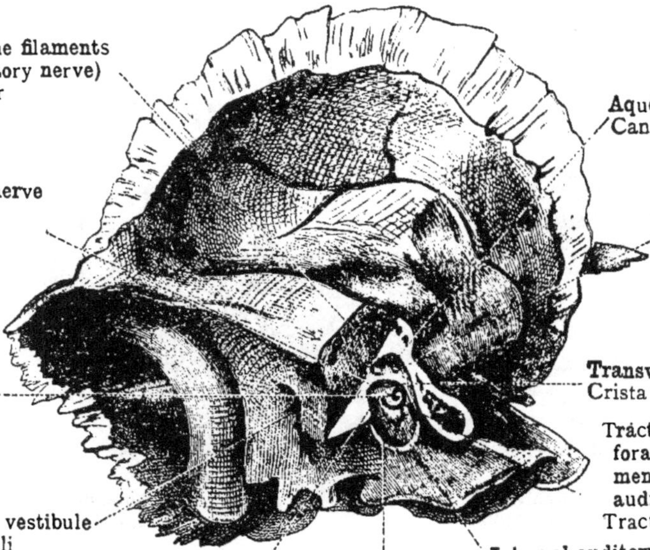

[1] The helicoid depression of the tractus spiralis foraminulentus corresponds with the base of the cochlea, and at the centre of the helix is the foramen centrale cochleæ, the orifice of the central canal of the modiolus. On the significance of this term *Area of the Cochlea*, see also note [534], p. 956*y*, in the Appendix to Part VI.; and on the significance of the term *Area of the Facial Nerve*, see note [538] on the same page.

FIG. 140.—THE INTERNAL AUDITORY MEATUS, MEATUS ACUSTICUS INTERNUS, EXPOSED FROM ABOVE BY THE REMOVAL OF A RIGHT-ANGLED WEDGE FROM THE PETROUS PORTION OF THE LEFT TEMPORAL BONE, DISPLAYING THE FUNDUS OF THE INTERNAL AUDITORY MEATUS, OR RENIFORM FOSSA, DIVIDED BY THE TRANSVERSE CREST, OR CRISTA FALCIFORMIS, INTO SUPERIOR AND INFERIOR FOSSÆ. SEEN FROM BEHIND AND ABOVE.

Os temporale—Temporal bone.

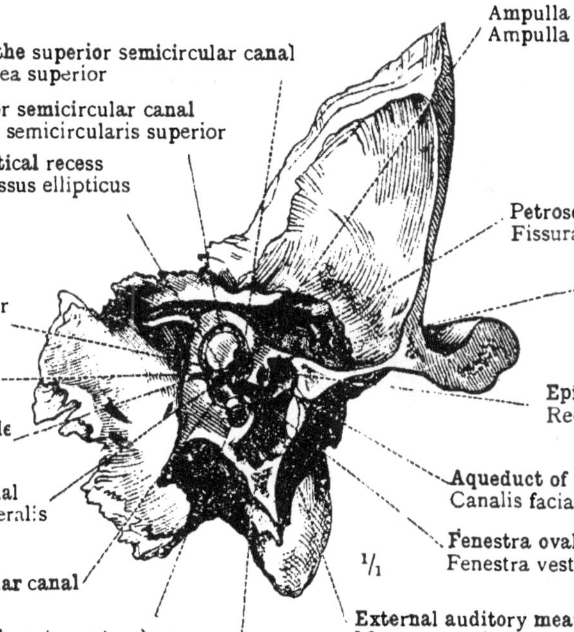

[1] Regarding the signification of the terms *crus simplex* and *crus commune*, see Appendix to Part VI., p. 956y, note [529]

FIG. 141.—PORTIONS OF THE OSSEOUS LABYRINTH AND THE TYMPANUM, SHOWN IN THE LEFT TEMPORAL BONE BY A VERTICAL SECTION THROUGH THE PETROUS PORTION IN THE PLANE OF THE SUPERIOR SEMICIRCULAR CANAL. SEEN OBLIQUELY FROM IN FRONT AND WITHIN.

The fenestra ovalis is divided vertically

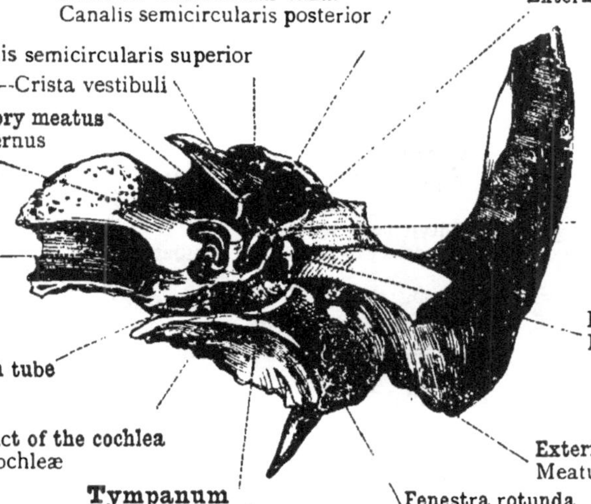

FIG. 142.—PORTIONS OF THE OSSEOUS LABYRINTH AND THE TYMPANUM, SHOWN IN THE LEFT TEMPORAL BONE BY A HORIZONTAL SECTION THROUGH THE PETROUS PORTION ALONG THE INTERNAL AND THE EXTERNAL AUDITORY MEATUS. SEEN FROM ABOVE.

Os temporale—Temporal bone

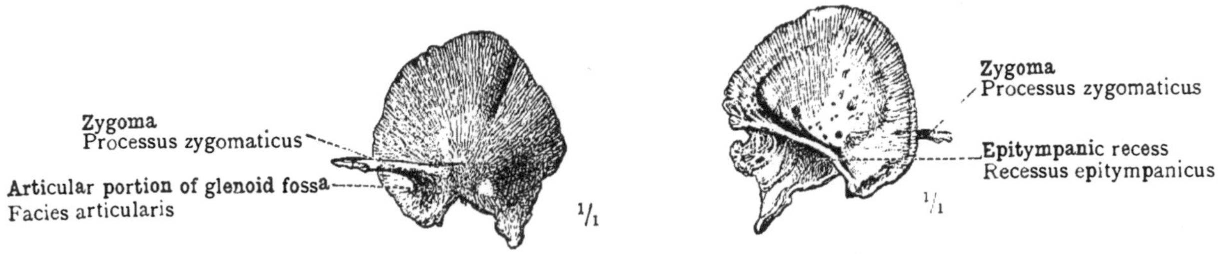

SQUAMOUS PORTION OF TEMPORAL BONE—SQUAMA TEMPORALIS.

TYMPANIC RING—ANNULUS TYMPANICUS.

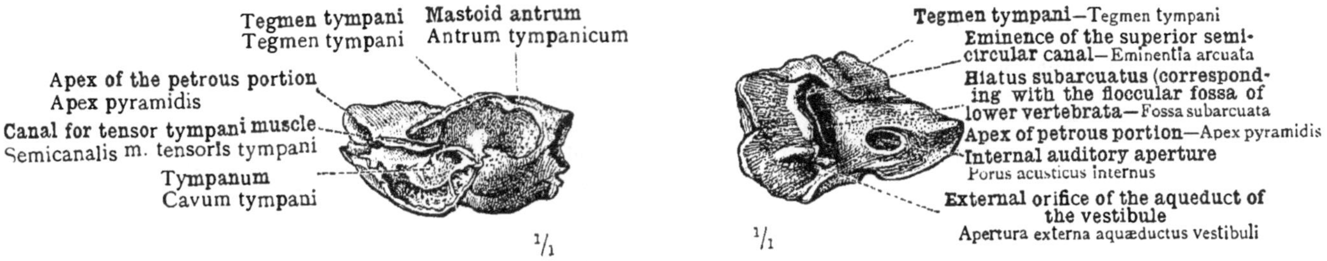

PETROUS PORTION OF TEMPORAL BONE—PARS PETROSA (PYRAMIS).

FIG. 143.—SEEN FROM WITHOUT. FIG. 144.—SEEN FROM WITHIN.

THE THREE PARTS OF THE LEFT TEMPORAL BONE FROM AN EIGHT-MONTHS FŒTUS (MONTHS OF FOUR WEEKS EACH)

Body-length, 15½ inches.

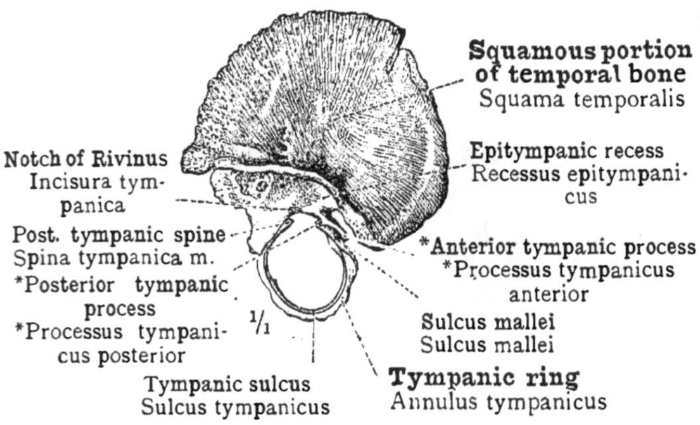

FIG. 145.—THE SQUAMOUS PORTION OF THE TEMPORAL BONE AND THE TYMPANIC RING UNITED. SEEN FROM WITHIN.

From a fœtus at term (body-length, 19 inches).

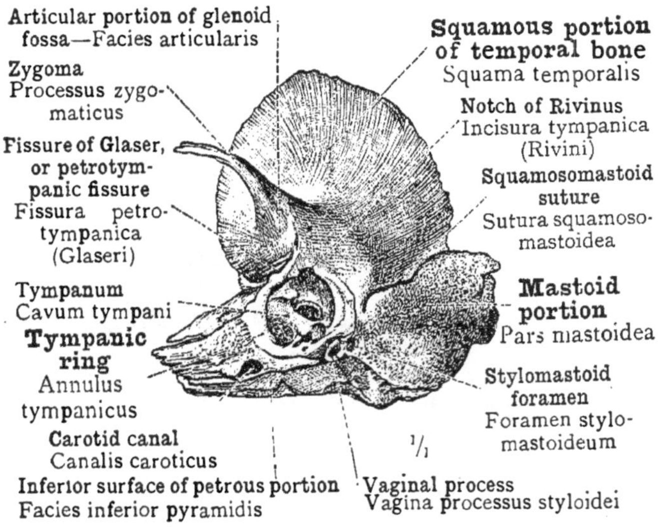

FIG. 146.—THE THREE PORTIONS OF THE LEFT TEMPORAL BONE UNITED. SEEN FROM WITHOUT AND BELOW.

From a new-born male infant (body-length, 21 inches).

Development of the Temporal Bones.

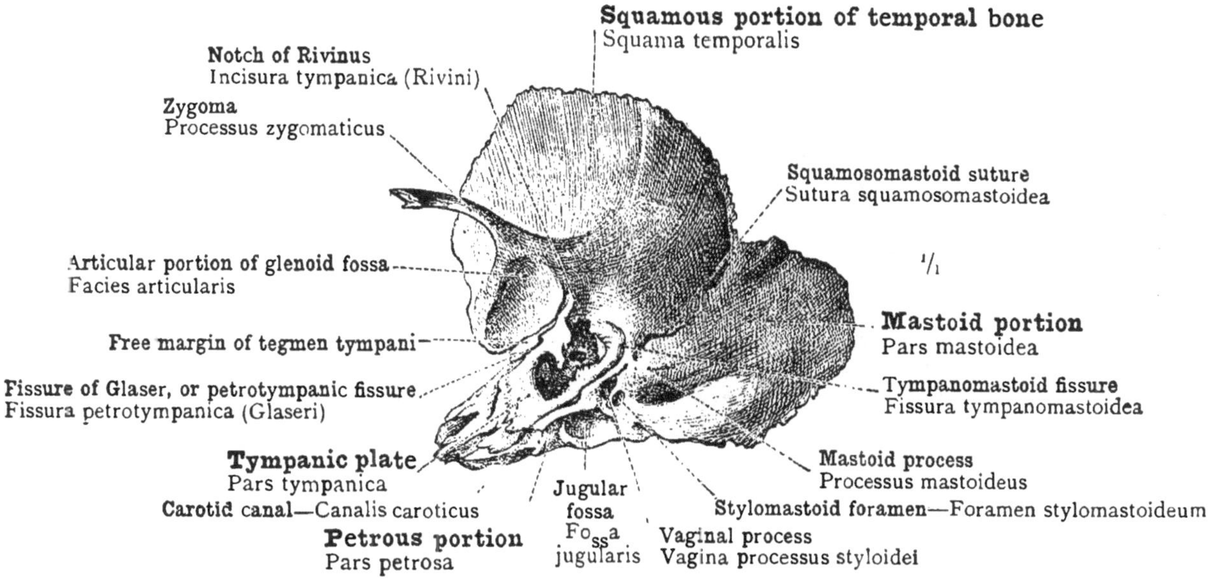

FIG. 147.—THE LEFT TEMPORAL BONE OF A BOY AT THE AGE OF EIGHT MONTHS: FORMATION OF THE TYMPANIC PLATE AND OF THE EXTERNAL AUDITORY MEATUS. SEEN OBLIQUELY FROM WITHOUT AND BELOW

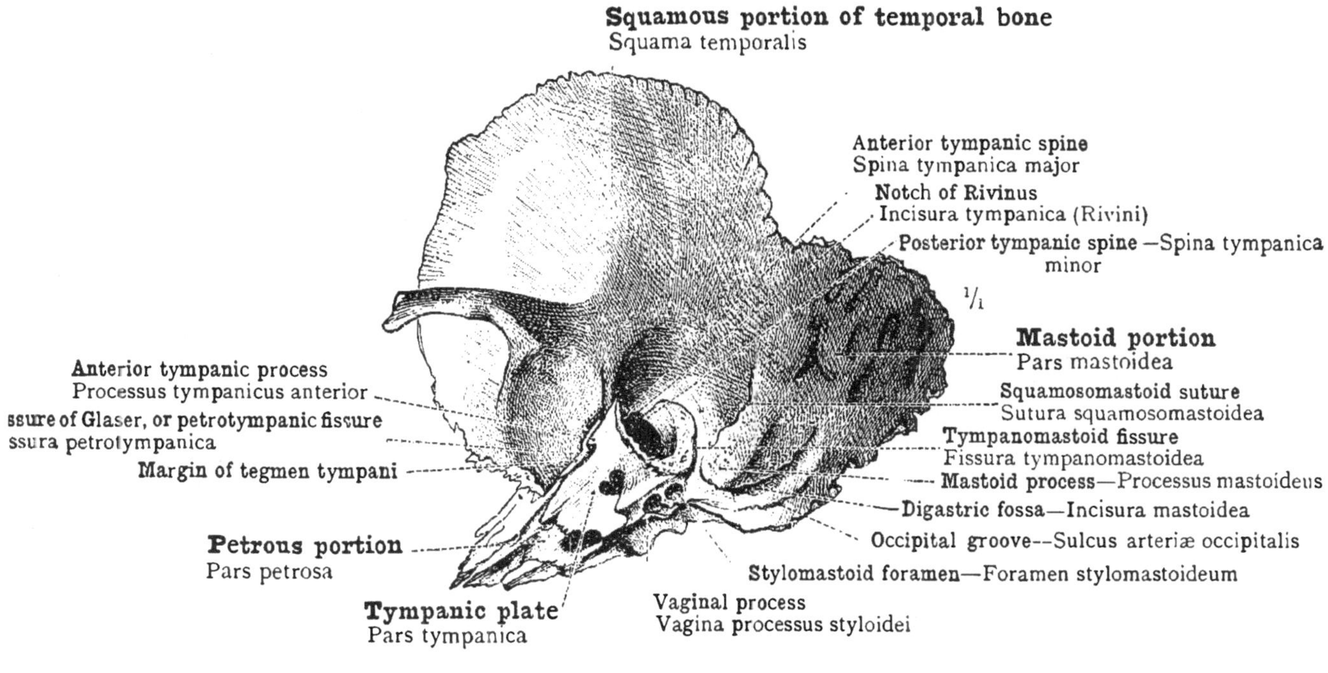

IG. 148.—THE LEFT TEMPORAL BONE OF A GIRL AT THE AGE OF THREE YEARS: FORMATION OF THE TYMPANIC PLATE AND OF THE EXTERNAL AUDITORY MEATUS. SEEN OBLIQUELY FROM WITHOUT AND BELOW.

Development of the Temporal Bones.

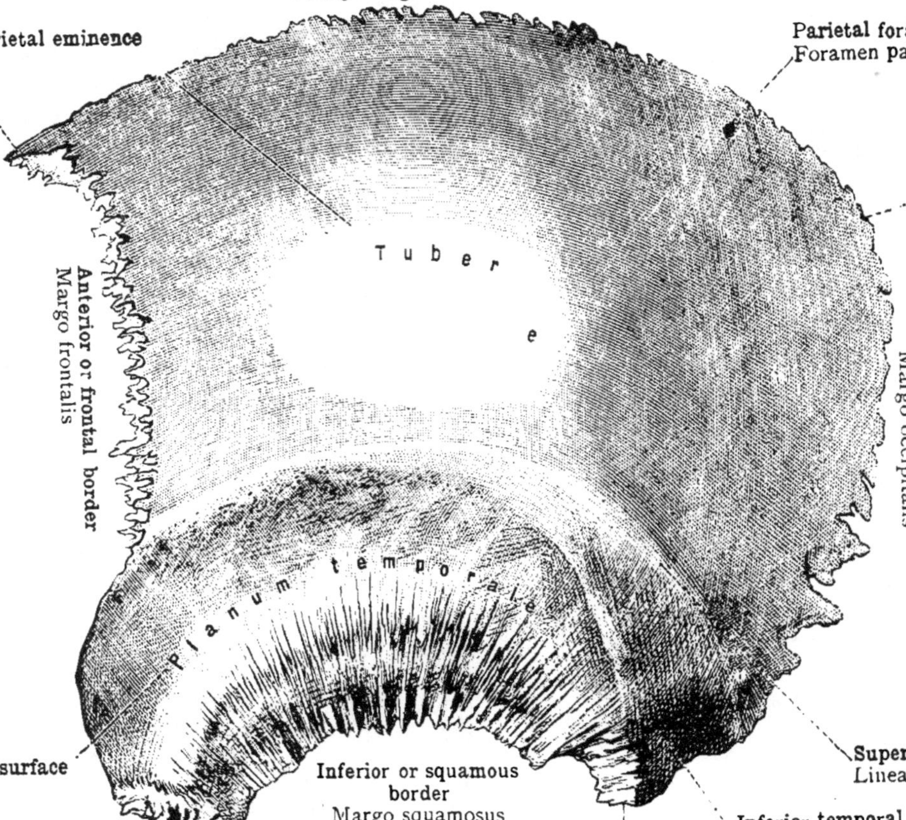

FIG. 149.—THE LEFT PARIETAL BONE SEEN FROM WITHOUT. EXTERNAL SURFACE: FACIES PARIETALIS.

Os parietale—Parietal bone.

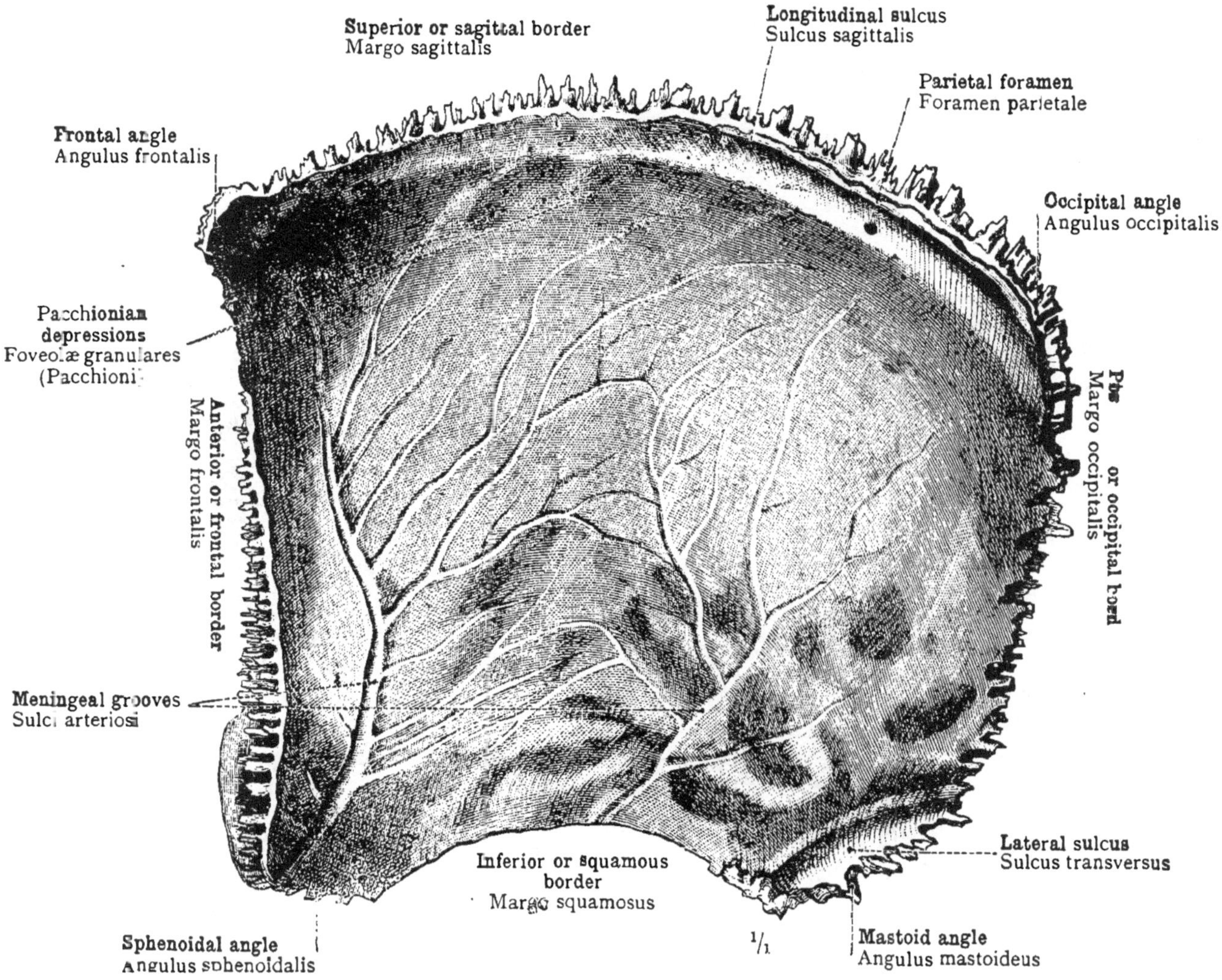

Fig. 150.—The Right Parietal Bone seen from Without. Internal Surface · Facies Cerebralis.

Os parietale—Parietal bone.

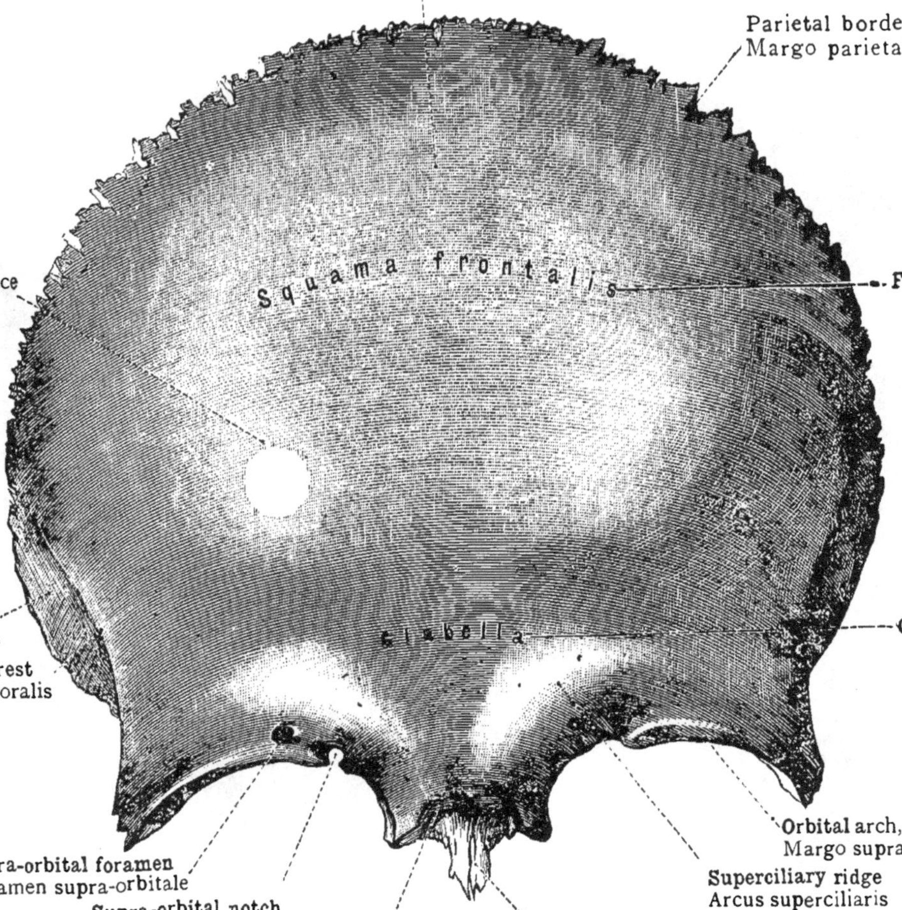

FIG. 151.—THE FRONTAL BONE SEEN FROM BEFORE. EXTERNAL SURFACE: FACIES FRONTALIS.

Os frontale—Frontal bone.

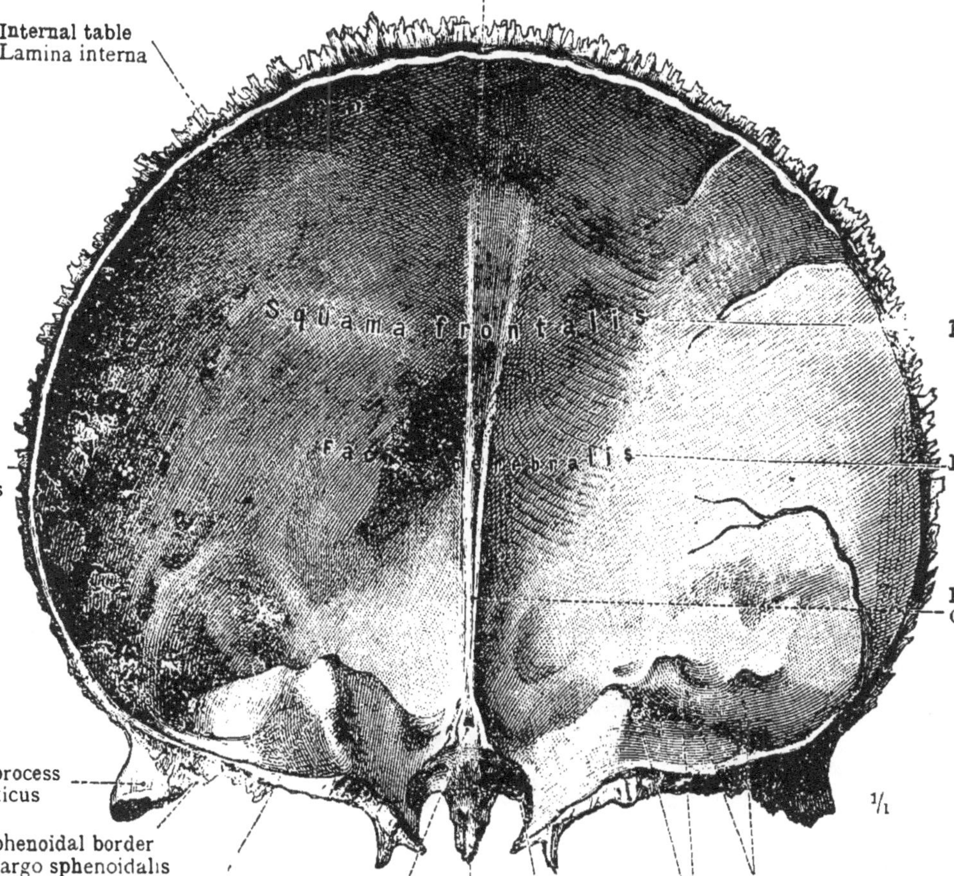

[1] Ridges (juga cerebralia) and sulci (impressiones digitatæ) corresponding respectively to the sulci and convolutions of the superjacent portion of the frontal lobes of the cerebrum.—TR.

FIG. 152.—THE FRONTAL BONE SEEN FROM BEHIND. INTERNAL SURFACE: FACIES CEREBRALIS.

Os frontale—Frontal bone.

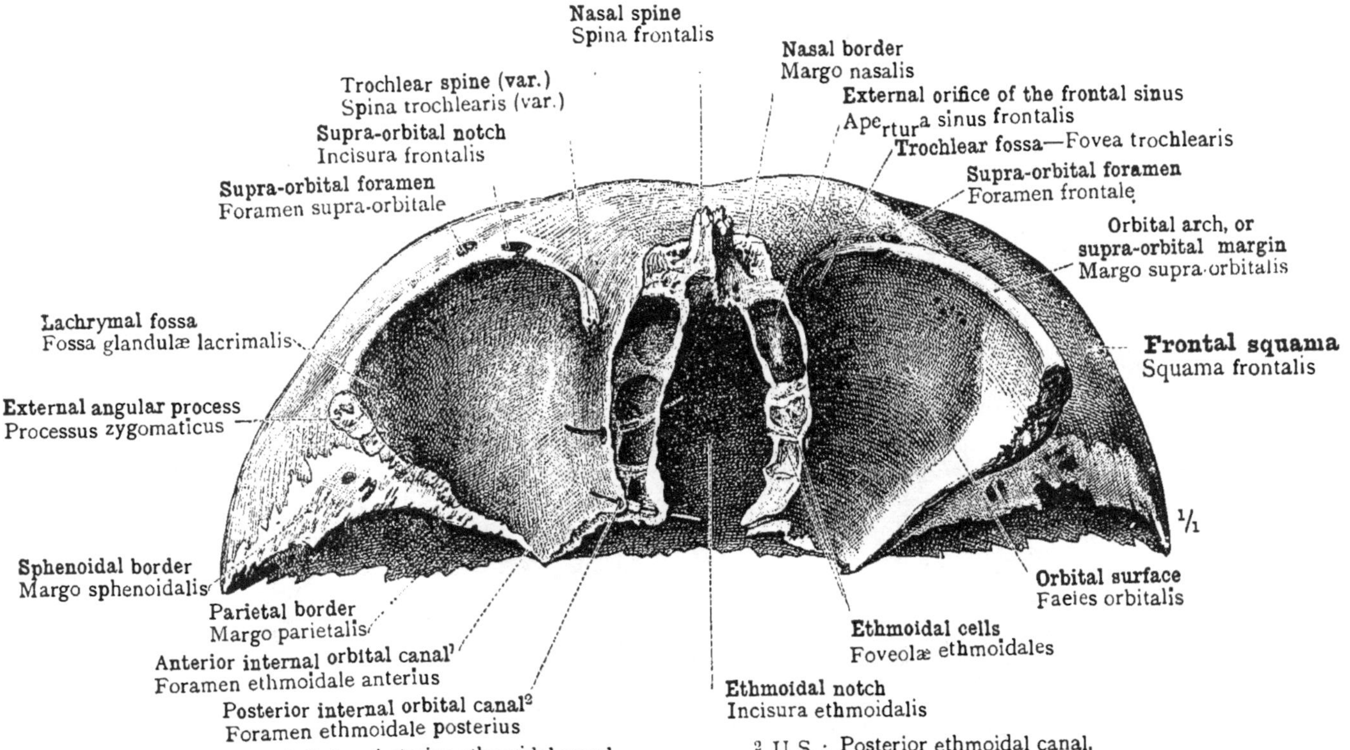

1 U.S.: Anterior ethmoidal canal. 2 U.S.: Posterior ethmoidal canal.

FIG. 153.—THE FRONTAL BONE SEEN FROM BELOW.

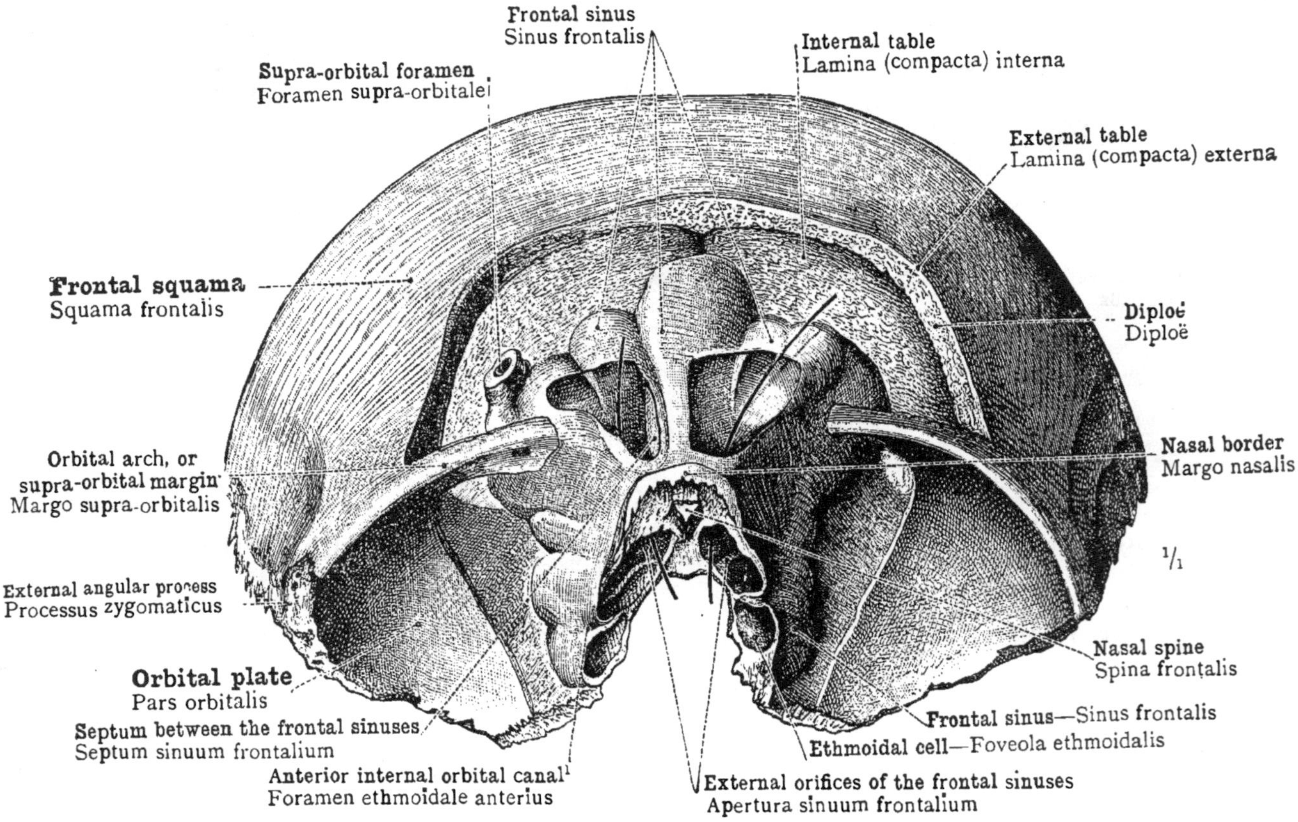

1 U.S.: Anterior ethmoidal canal.

FIG. 154.—THE FRONTAL SINUSES, SINUS FRONTALES, SHOWN BY THE REMOVAL OF THE EXTERNAL TABLE AND THE DIPLOË, AND PARTLY OPENED UP. SEEN FROM BEFORE AND BELOW.

Os frontale—Frontal bone.

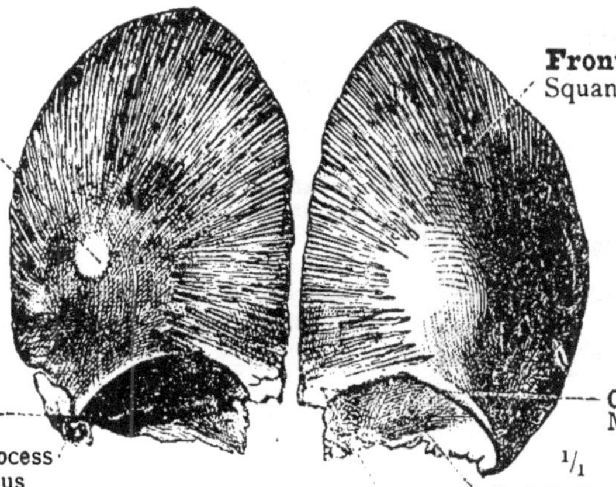

FIG. 155.—THE TWO HALVES OF THE FRONTAL BONE FROM A HUMAN FŒTUS IN THE EIGHTH MONTH (MONTHS OF FOUR WEEKS EACH). SEEN FROM BEFORE.

Body-length of fœtus 15 inches.

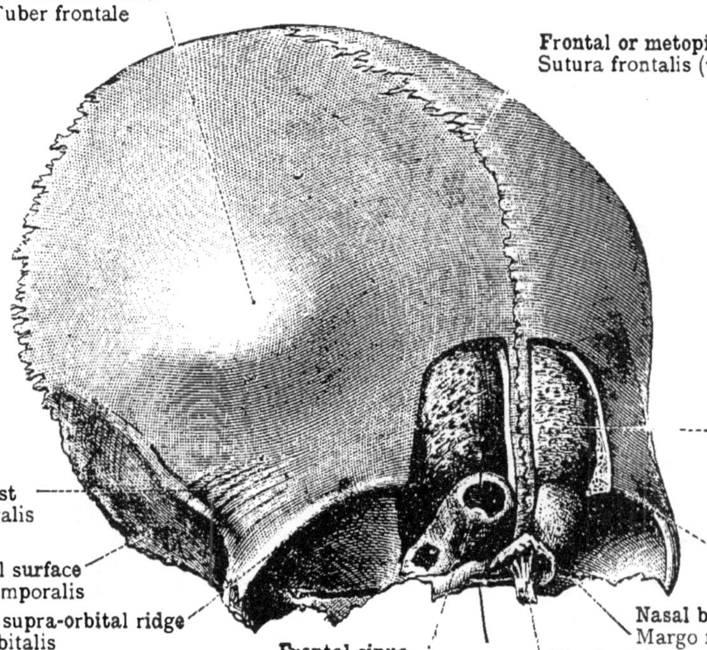

FIG. 156.—THE FRONTAL BONE OF A GIRL AGED SEVEN YEARS IN WHICH THE FRONTAL SINUSES HAVE BEEN EXPOSED. SEEN OBLIQUELY FROM BEFORE AND FROM THE RIGHT SIDE.

Development of the Frontal Bones.

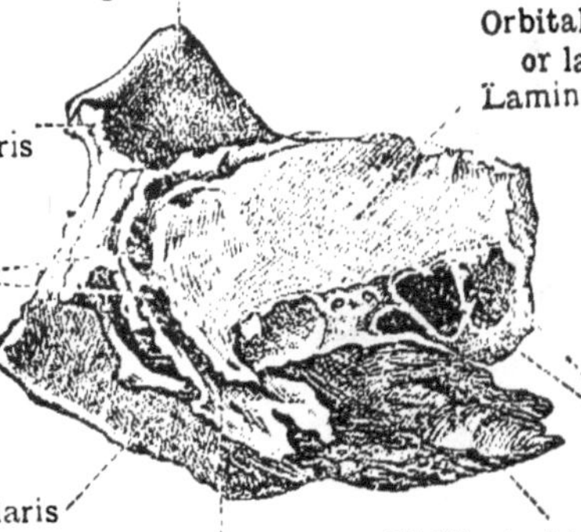

FIG. 157.—THE ETHMOID BONE SEEN FROM THE LEFT SIDE

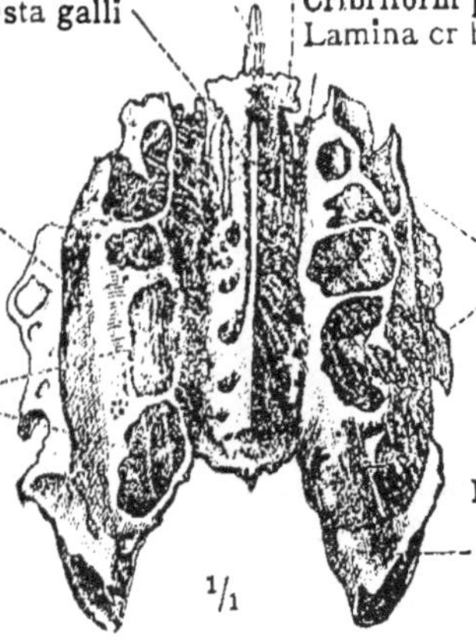

FIG. 158.—THE ETHMOID BONE SEEN FROM ABOVE.

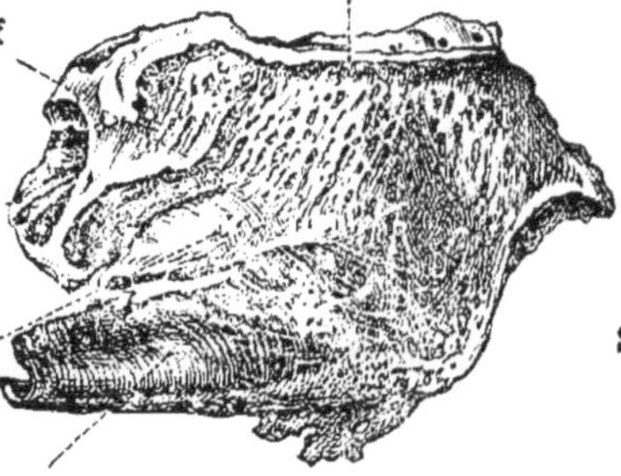

FIG. 159.—THE LEFT HALF OF THE ETHMOID BONE SEEN FROM WITHIN. SUPERIOR AND MIDDLE TURBINATE BONES.

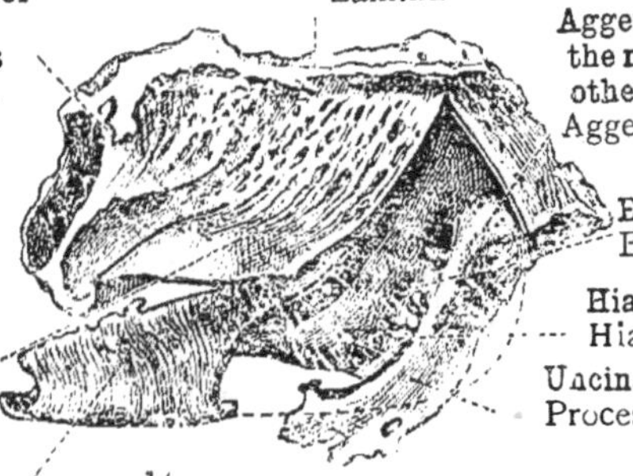

FIG. 160.—THE LEFT HALF OF THE ETHMOID BONE SEEN FROM WITHIN.

The anterior portion of the middle turbinate bone of the nose has been removed. The free border of the removed portion is indicated by a dotted line.

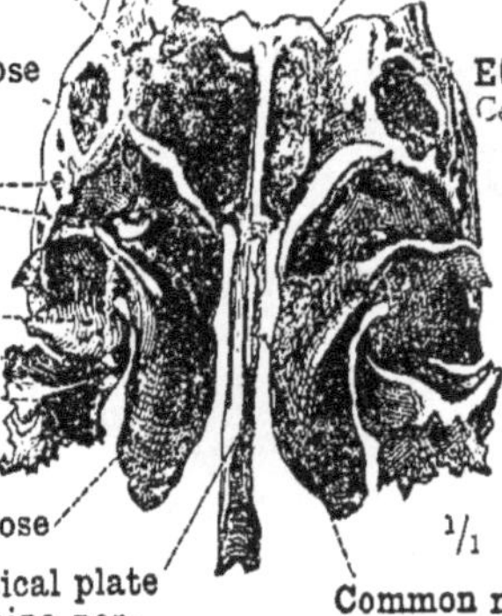

FIG. 161.—THE ETHMOID BONE SEEN FROM BEHIND AND BELOW. VERTICAL PLATE OF THE ETHMOID AS UPPER PART OF THE BONY SEPTUM OF THE NOSE.

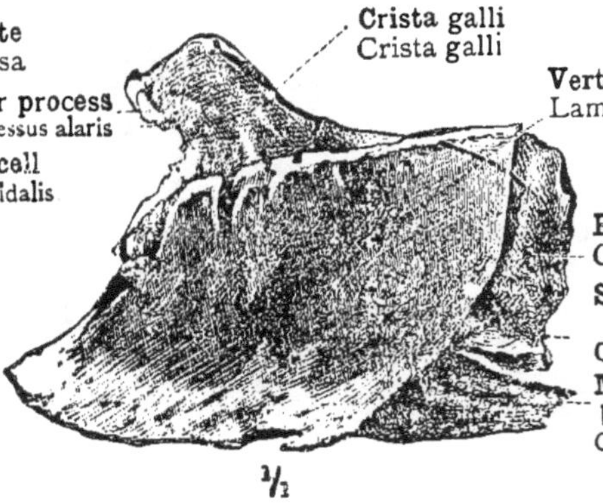

FIG. 162.—AN ETHMOID BONE THE LEFT LATERAL MASS OF WHICH HAS BEEN REMOVED.

The entire surface of the vertical plate is exposed.

Os ethmoidale—Ethmoid bone.

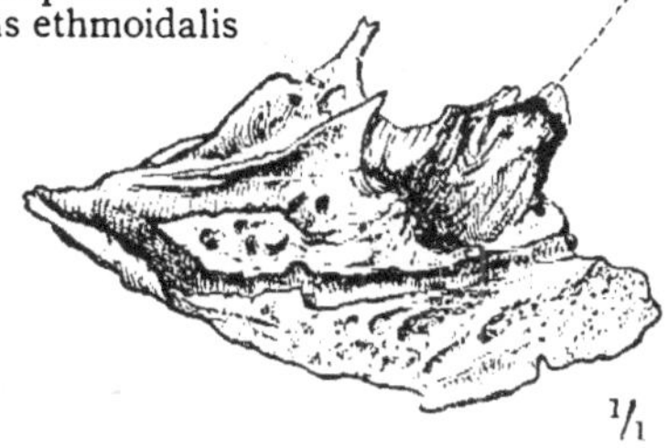

FIG. 163.—INNER SURFACE,

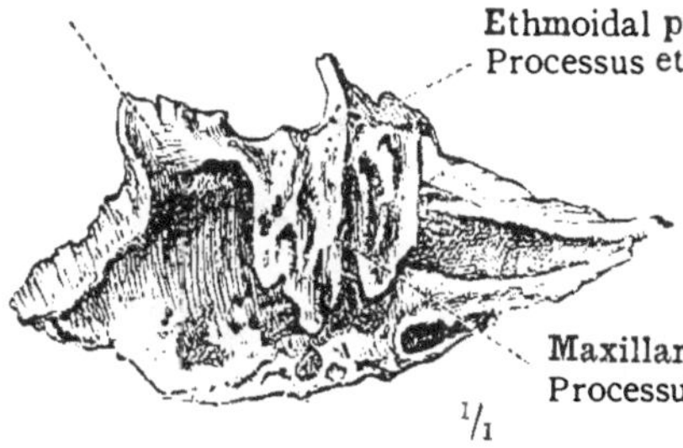

FIG. 164.—OUTER SURFACE.

CONCHA NASALIS INFERIOR—THE INFERIOR TURBINATE BONE OF THE LEFT SIDE.

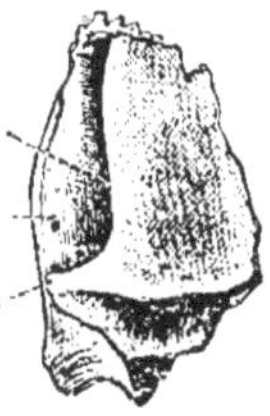

FIG. 165.—EXTERNAL SURFACE.

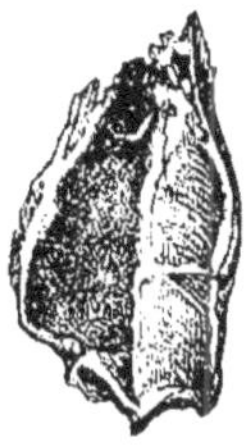

FIG. 166.—INTERNAL SURFACE.

OS LACRIMALE: LACHRYMAL BONE OF THE LEFT SIDE.

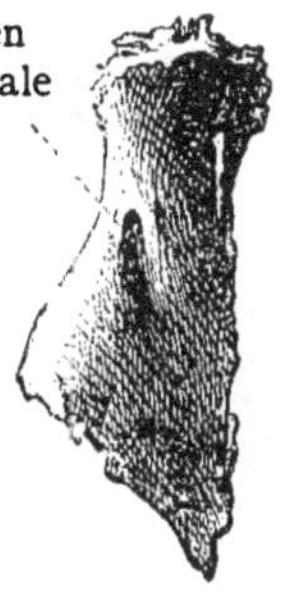

FIG. 167.—ANTERIOR SURFACE.

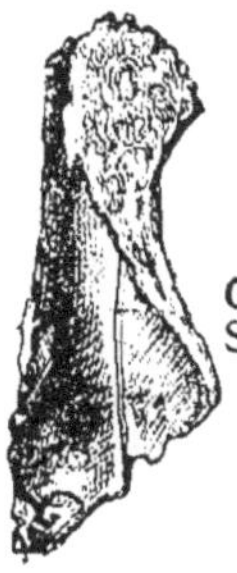

FIG. 168.—POSTERIOR SURFACE.

OS NASALE: NASAL BONE OF THE LEFT SIDE.

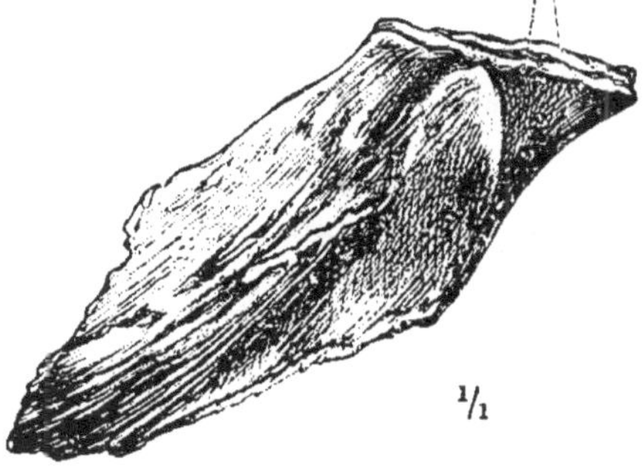

FIG. 169.—SEEN FROM THE LEFT SIDE.

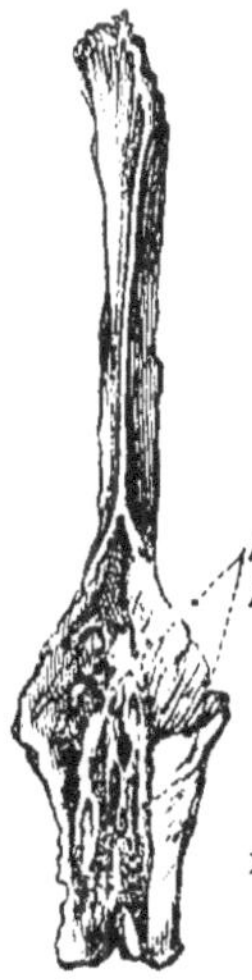

FIG. 170.—SEEN FROM ABOVE.

VOMER—THE VOMER.

Bones of the Nasal Region.

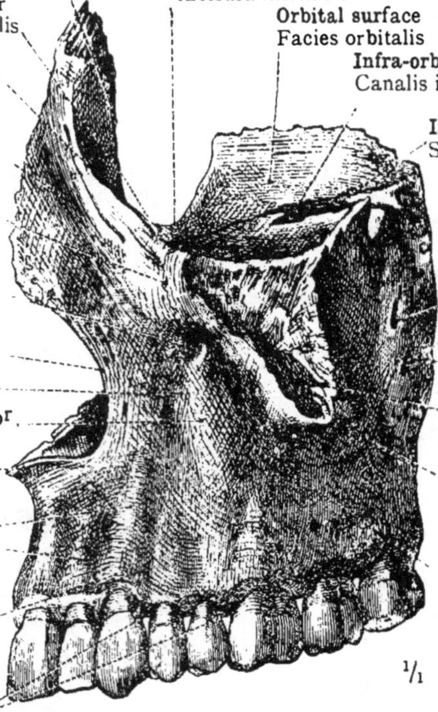

[1] Eminences corresponding in position to the fangs of the teeth

FIG. 171.—LEFT SUPERIOR MAXILLARY BONE: EXTERNAL SURFACE.

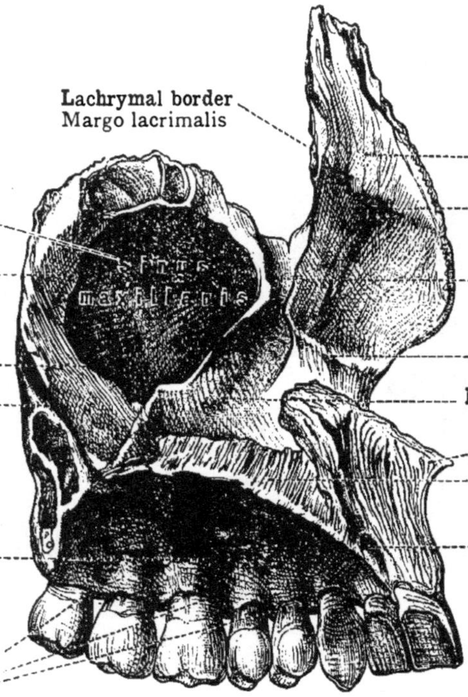

FIG. 172.—LEFT SUPERIOR MAXILLARY BONE: INTERNAL SURFACE. VIEW INTO THE MAXILLARY SINUS, OR ANTRUM OF HIGHMORE.

Maxilla—Superior maxilla.

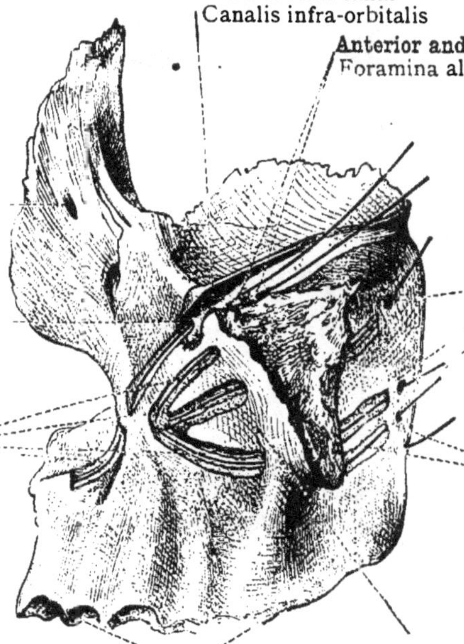

FIG. 173.—THE LEFT SUPERIOR MAXILLARY BONE. EXTERNAL SURFACE.

The dental canals are exposed by partial removal of the superficial plate of bone, and their course is shown by means of bristles passed through them.

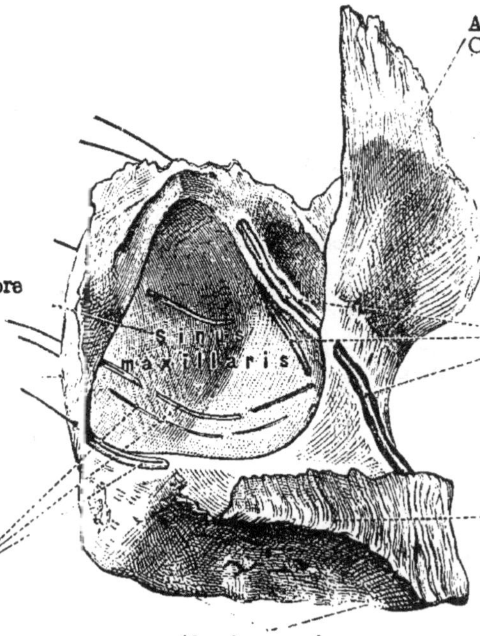

FIG. 174.—THE LEFT SUPERIOR MAXILLARY BONE. INTERNAL SURFACE.

The foremost and the hindmost of the dental canals have been exposed by the removal of the superficial plate of bone. By means of bristles passed through the canals the situation of the respective dental foramina is indicated. Most of the inner wall of the antrum of Highmore has been cut away.

Maxilla—Superior maxillary bone.

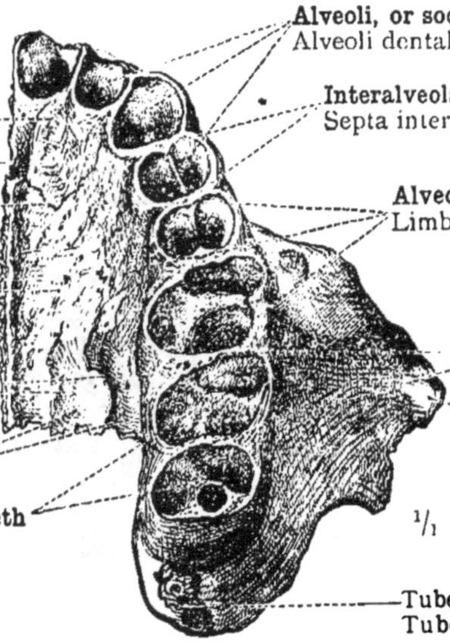

FIG. 175.—THE LEFT SUPERIOR MAXILLARY BONE. SEEN FROM BELOW.

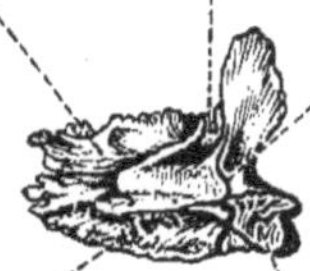

FIG. 176.—SEEN FROM THE INNER SIDE.

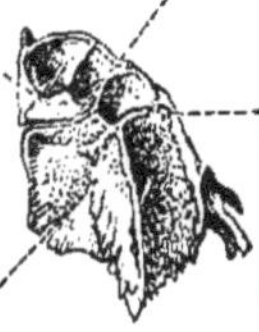

FIG. 177.—SEEN FROM BELOW.

THE LEFT SUPERIOR MAXILLARY BONE OF A FŒTUS AT THE END OF THE SIXTH MONTH (MONTHS OF FOUR WEEKS EACH).

Body-length, 12 inches.

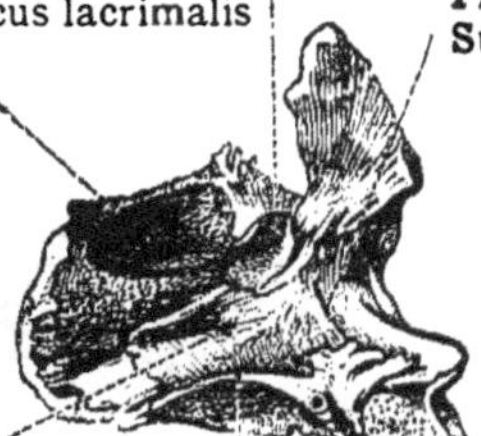

FIG. 178.—SEEN FROM THE INNER SIDE.

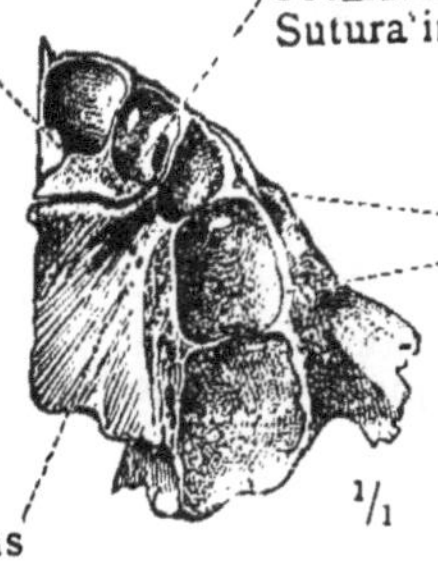

FIG. 179. SEEN FROM BELOW.

THE LEFT SUPERIOR MAXILLARY BONE OF A BOY BORN AT FULL TERM.

Body-length, 21 inches.

Maxilla—Superior maxillary bone.

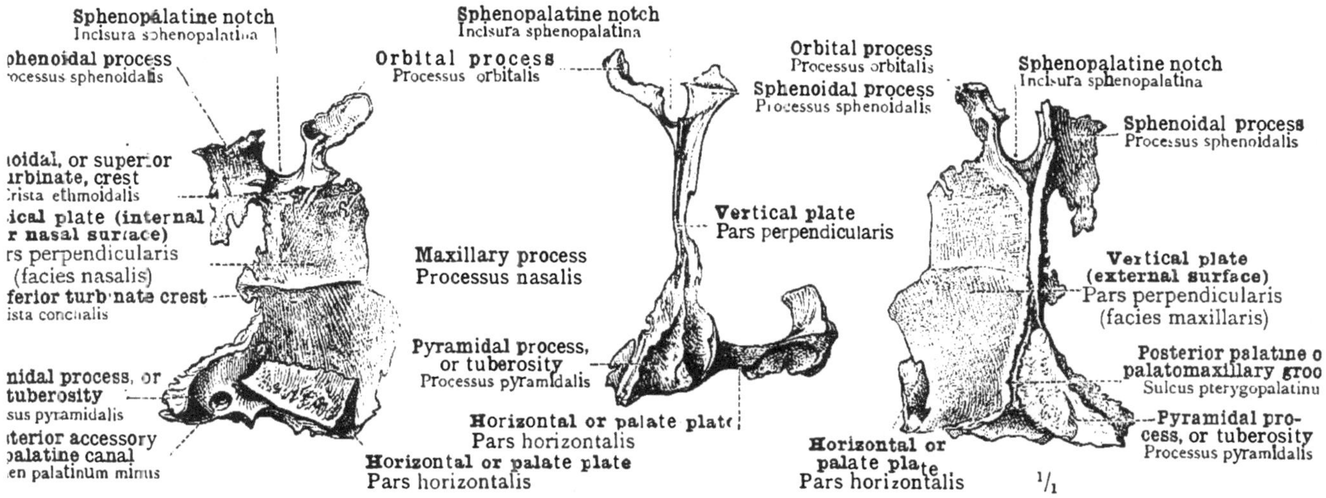

FIG. 180.—INNER SURFACE. FIG. 181.—SEEN FROM BEHIND. FIG. 182.—OUTER SURFACE.

OS PALATINUM.—THE PALATE-BONE (OF THE LEFT SIDE).

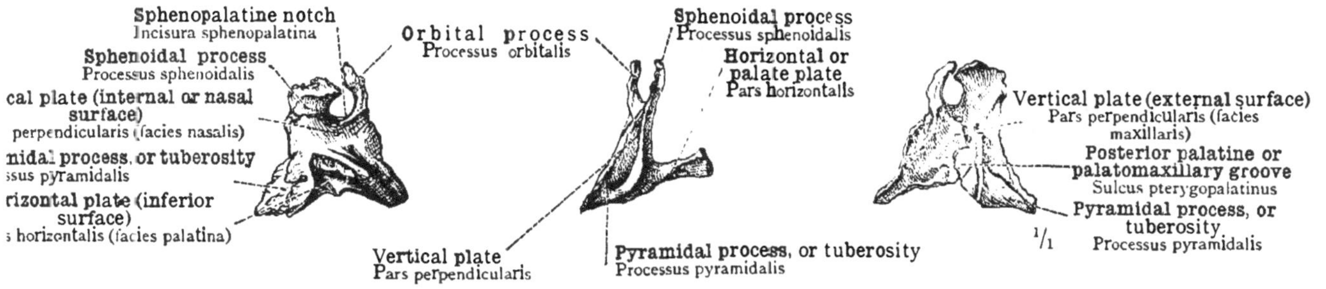

FIG. 183.—INNER SURFACE. FIG. 184.—SEEN FROM BEHIND. FIG. 185.—OUTER SURFACE.

THE LEFT PALATE-BONE OF A BOY BORN AT FULL TERM.

Body-length, 21 inches.

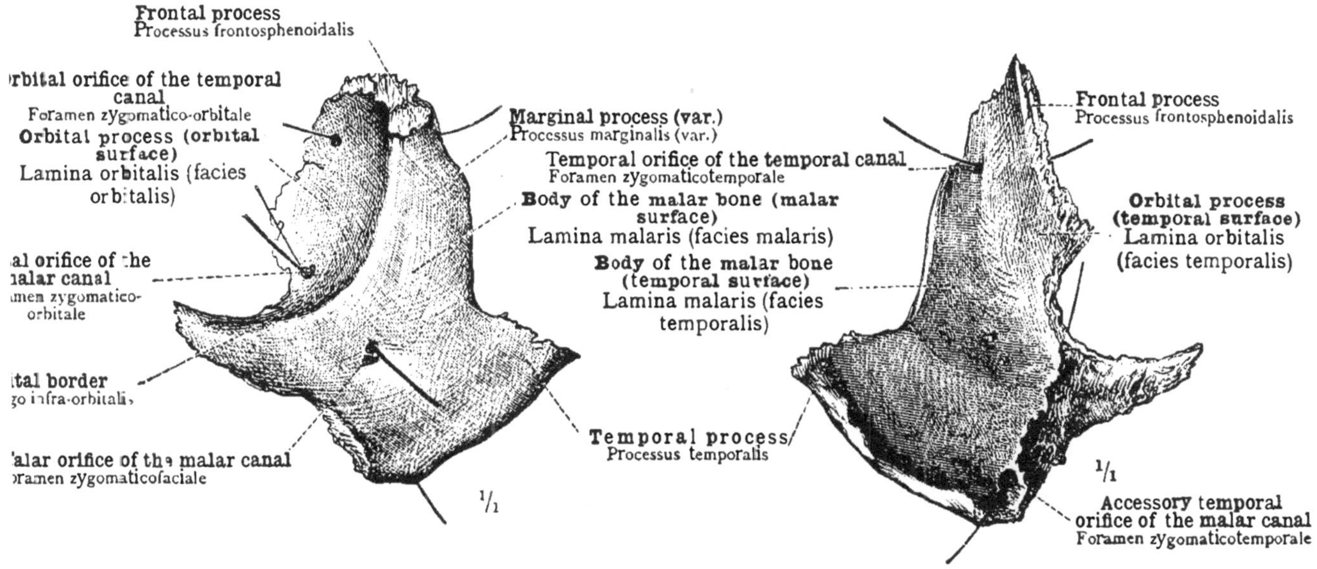

FIG. 186.—SEEN FROM BEFORE. FIG. 187.—SEEN FROM BEHIND.

OS ZYGOMATICUM—MALAR BONE (OF THE LEFT SIDE).

Supplementary Bones of the Upper Jaw.

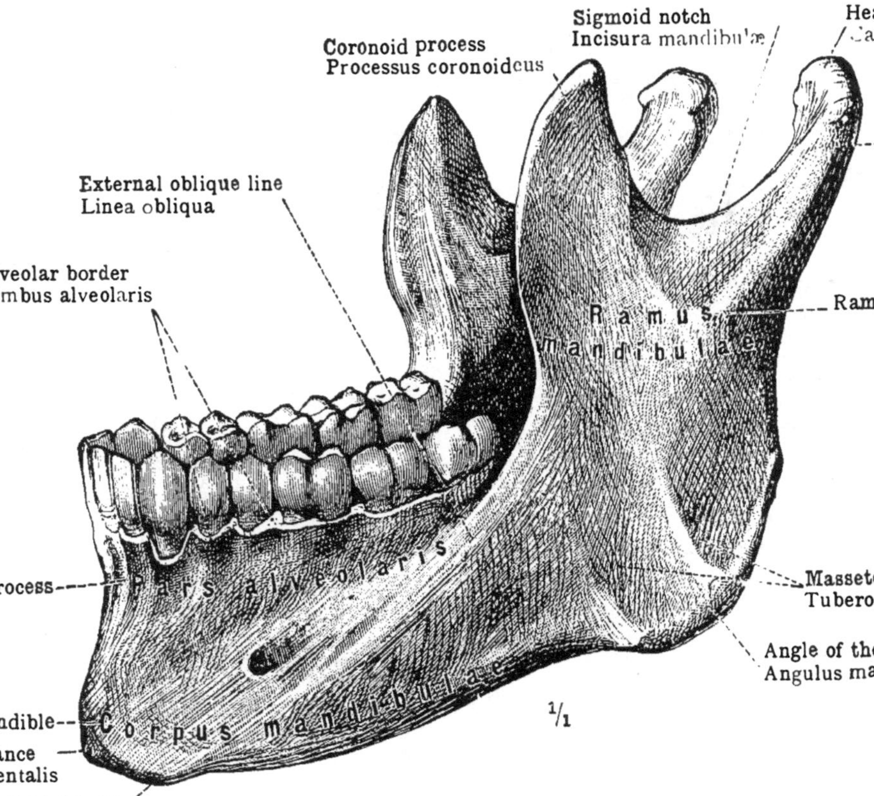

FIG. 188.—THE INFERIOR MAXILLARY BONE SEEN FROM THE LEFT SIDE.

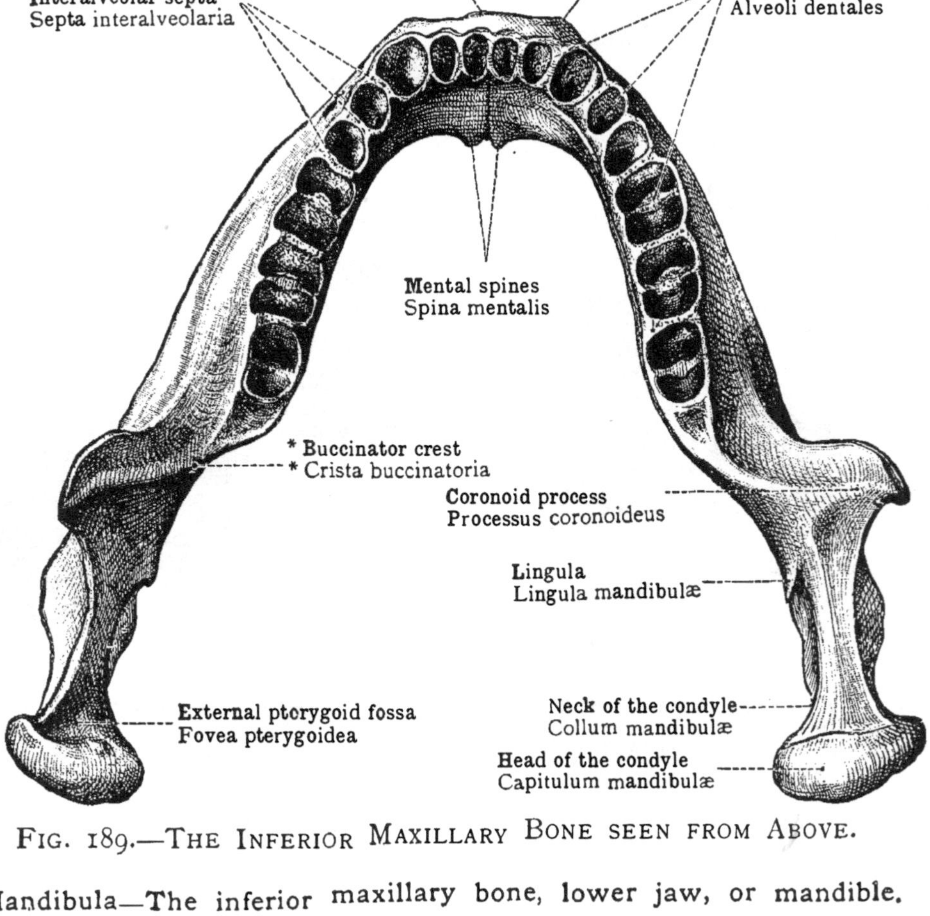

FIG. 189.—THE INFERIOR MAXILLARY BONE SEEN FROM ABOVE.

Mandibula—The inferior maxillary bone, lower jaw, or mandible.

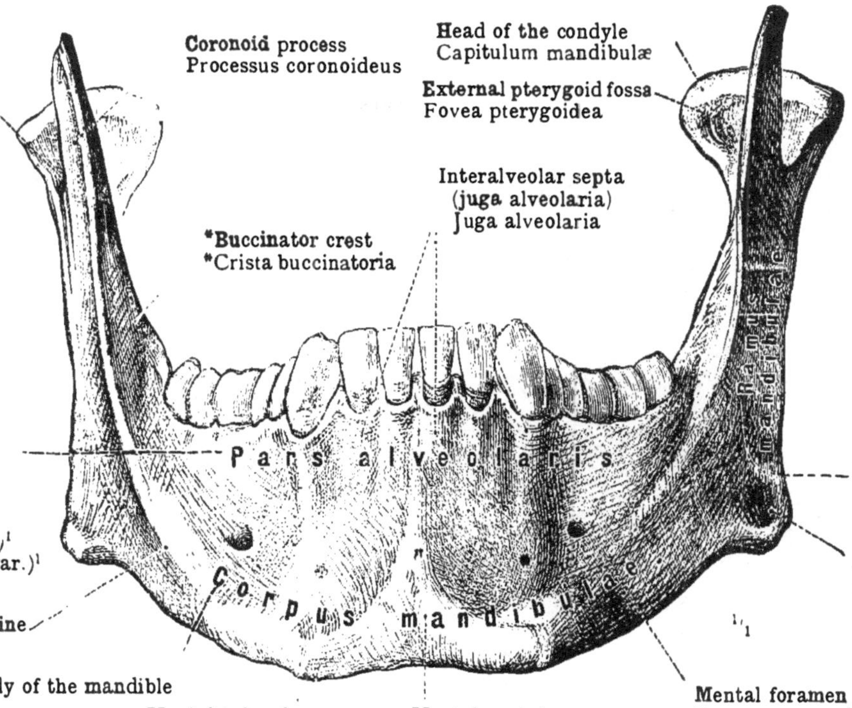

FIG. 190.—THE INFERIOR MAXILLARY BONE SEEN FROM BEFORE.

[1] "The angle of the jaw," writes Quain, ". . . is more or less rounded off." The specimen from which Fig. 190 was drawn has, however, an abnormal projection at each angle, to which in the German nomenclature the name *processus angularis* (*var*) is given. This variety is not described by Quain or by Macalister.—TR.

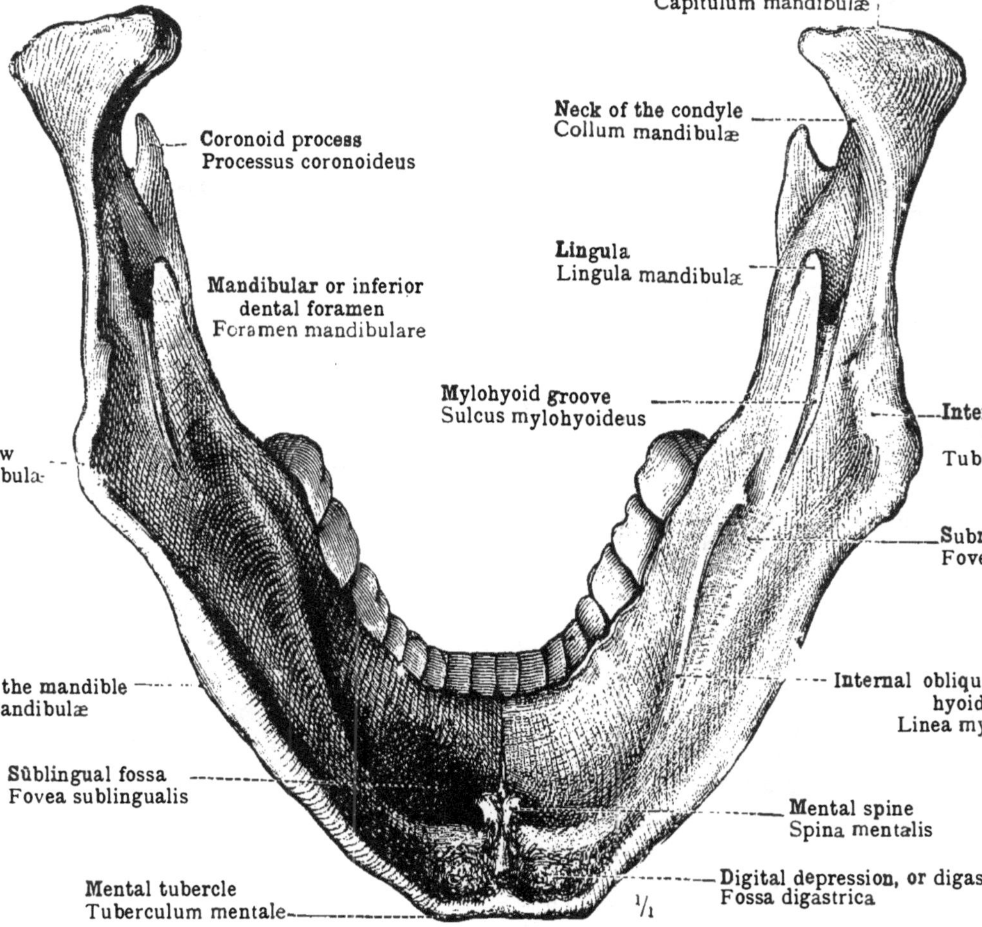

FIG. 191.—THE INFERIOR MAXILLARY BONE SEEN FROM BEHIND.

Mandibula—The inferior maxillar

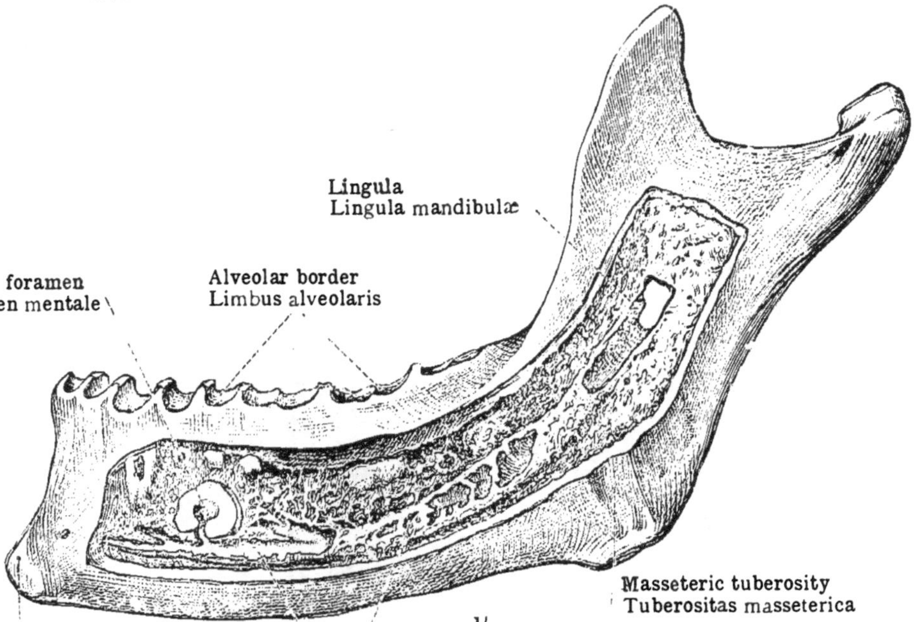

FIG. 192.—THE INFERIOR MAXILLARY BONE SEEN FROM THE LEFT SIDE.
The mandibular or inferior dental canal has been exposed by the removal of a portion of the superficial plate of bone.

FIG. 193.—THE LEFT HALF OF THE INFERIOR MAXILLARY BONE OF A HUMAN EMBRYO AT THE END OF THE FIFTH MONTH (MONTHS OF FOUR WEEKS EACH).
Body-length, 7½ inches.

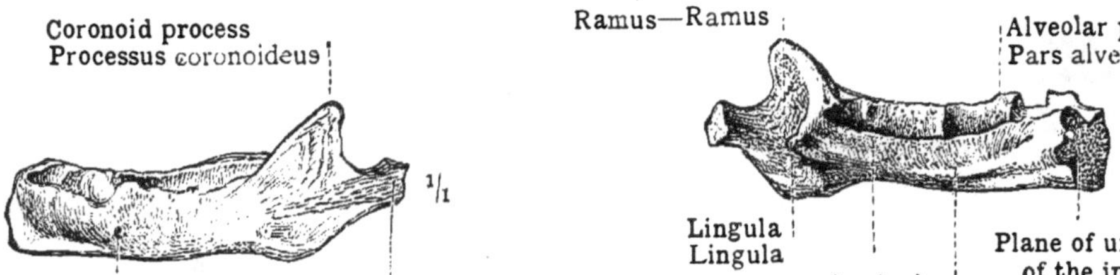

FIG. 194.—THE LEFT HALF OF THE INFERIOR MAXILLARY BONE OF A HUMAN EMBRYO IN THE MIDDLE OF THE EIGHTH MONTH (MONTHS OF FOUR WEEKS EACH).
Body-length, 15 inches.

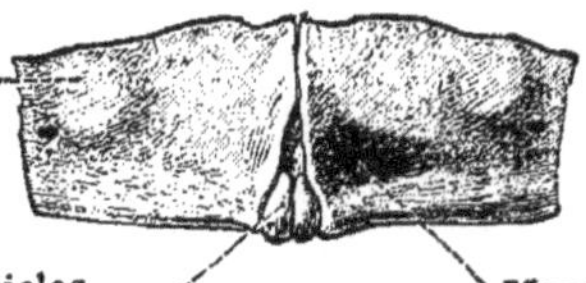

FIG. 195.—MENTAL REGION OF A NEW-BORN BOY. THE LATERAL HALVES OF THE INFERIOR MAXILLARY BONE HAVE NOT YET UNITED; BETWEEN THEM ARE THE MENTAL OSSICLES. SEEN FROM BEFORE.

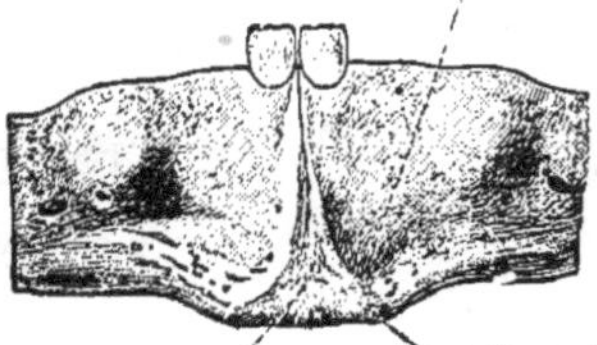

FIG. 196.—THE FULLY DEVELOPED MENTAL PROTUBERANCE, IN A CHILD AGED SIX AND A HALF MONTHS. THE MENTAL OSSICLES HAVE UNITED WITH EACH OTHER AND WITH THE LATERAL HALVES OF THE INFERIOR MAXILLARY BONE.

r mandible:

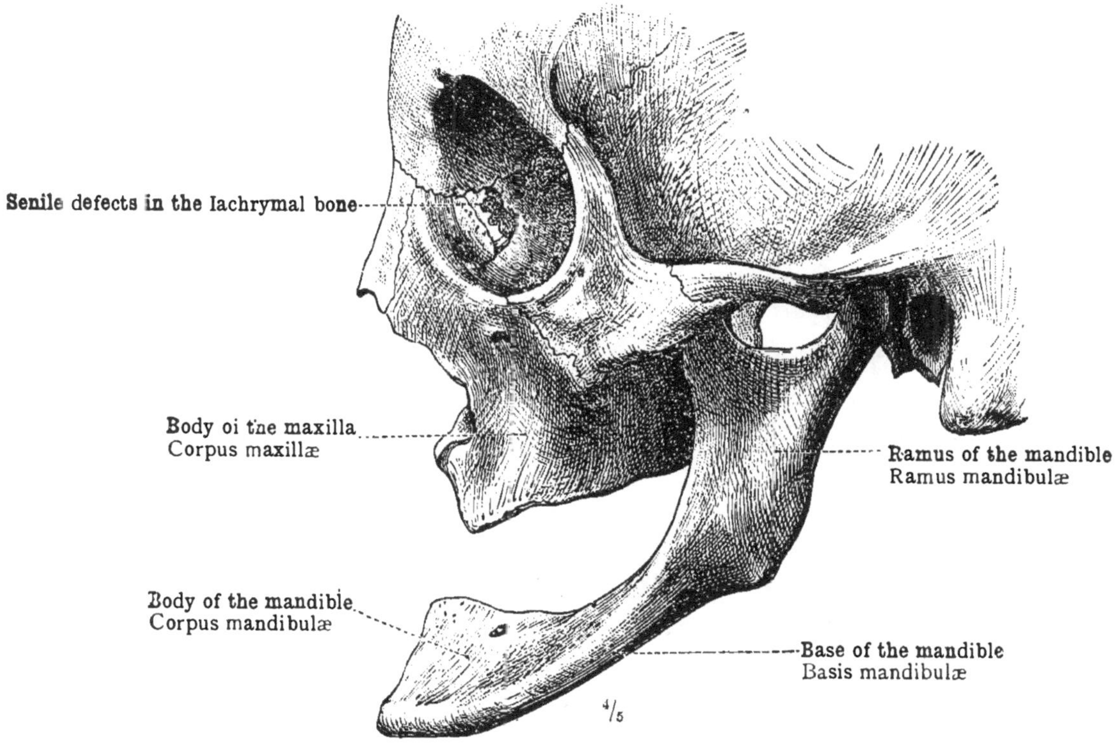

FIG. 197.—FACIAL PORTION OF THE SKULL OF A WOMAN AGED EIGHTY-FOUR YEARS, SHOWING ATROPHY OF THE ALVEOLAR PROCESSES OF THE SUPERIOR AND INFERIOR MAXILLARY BONES (NUTCRACKER FACE).

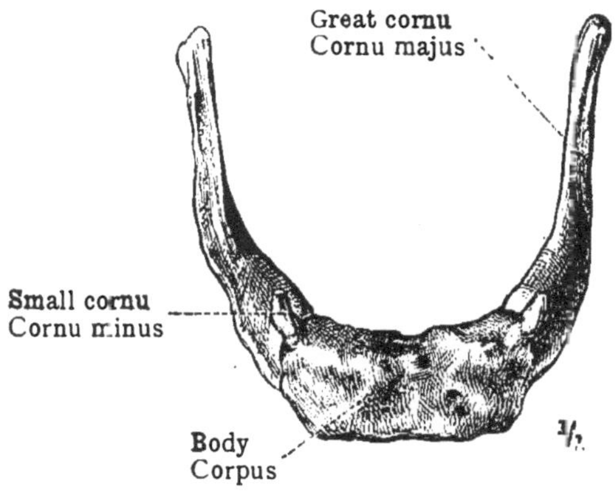

FIG. 198.—SEEN FROM ABOVE.

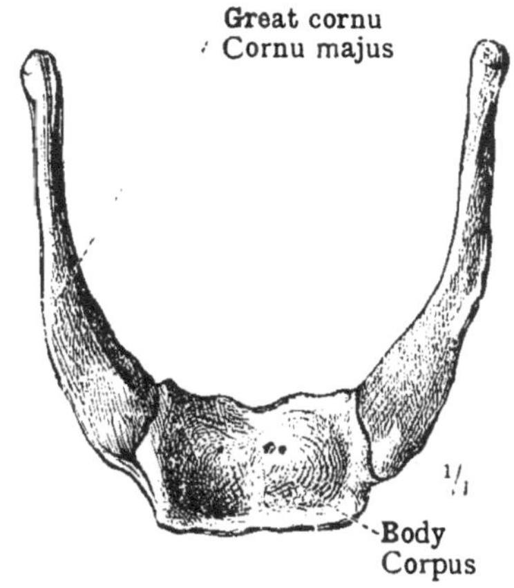

FIG. 199.—SEEN FROM BELOW

OS HYOIDEUM—THE HYOID BONE.

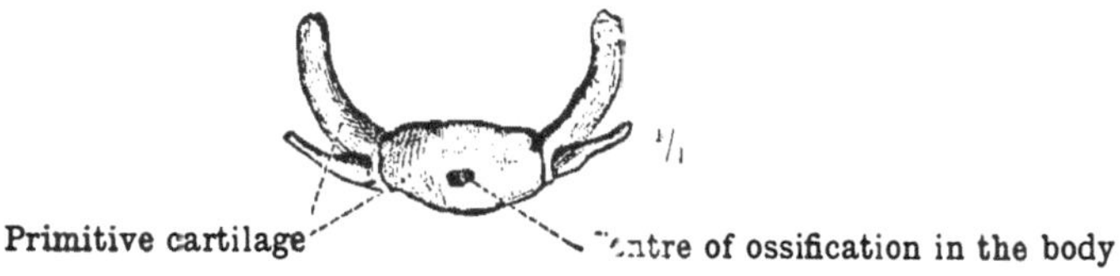

FIG. 200.—THE HYOID BONE OF A BOY, STILL-BORN AT FULL TERM.
Body-length, 21 inches.

Senile atrophy of the jaws: Os hyoideum—the hyoid bone.

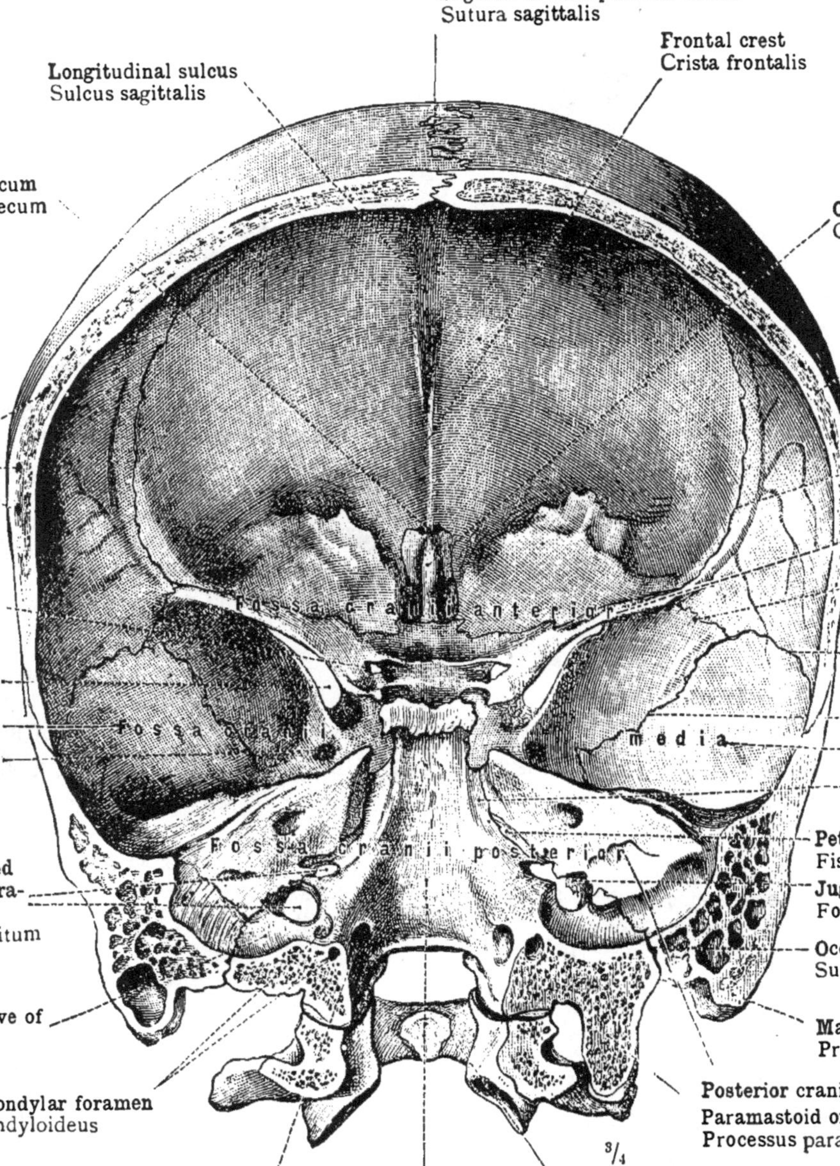

FIG. 201.—SKULL DIVIDED INTO AN ANTERIOR AND A POSTERIOR PORTION BY A FRONTAL SECTION PASSING THROUGH THE MASTOID PROCESSES. THE FIRST CERVICAL VERTEBRA HAS ALSO BEEN DIVIDED BY THE SECTION, AND LEFT ATTACHED TO THE SKULL.

VIEW OF THE ANTERIOR PORTION OF THE CRANIAL CAVITY. THE ANTERIOR AND MIDDLE CRANIAL FOSSÆ, AS WELL AS THE ANTERIOR PORTION OF THE POSTERIOR CRANIAL FOSSA, SEEN FROM BEHIND. ON THE RIGHT SIDE IS A PARAMASTOID PROCESS ARTICULATING WITH THE ATLAS.

Cavum cranii cerebralis—Cranial cavity.

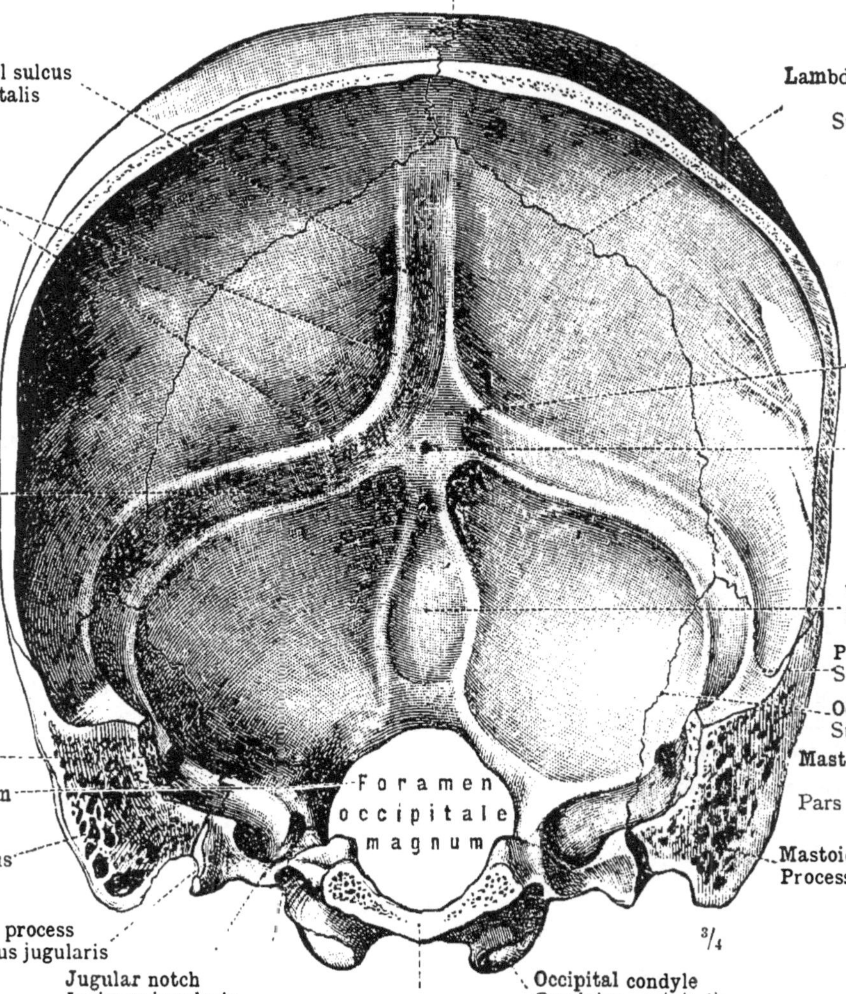

FIG. 202.—SKULL DIVIDED INTO AN ANTERIOR AND A POSTERIOR PORTION BY A FRONTAL SECTION PASSING THROUGH THE MASTOID PROCESSES AND THE BASILAR PORTION OF THE OCCIPITAL BONE. VIEW OF THE POSTERIOR PORTION OF THE CRANIAL CAVITY. THE DIVISION OF THE LONGITUDINAL SULCUS INTC RIGHT LATERAL AND LEFT LATERAL SULCUS IS SHOWN THE LATERAL SULCUS PASSES CN EITHER SIDE INTO THE SIGMOID SULCUS, WHICH TERMINATES IN THE JUGULAR FORAMEN.

Cavum cranii cerebralis—Cranial cavitv.

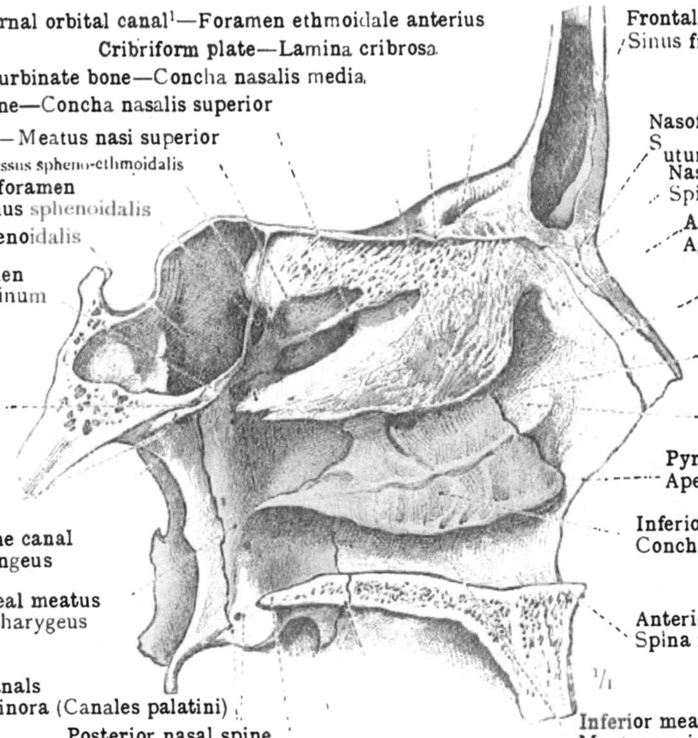

¹ U.S.: Anterior ethmoidal canal. ² See note to p. 48.

FIG. 203.—THE EXTERNAL WALL OF THE NASAL CAVITY WITH THE TURBINATE BONES AND THE NASAL MEATUS: MEDIAN SAGITTAL SECTION. LEFT SIDE.

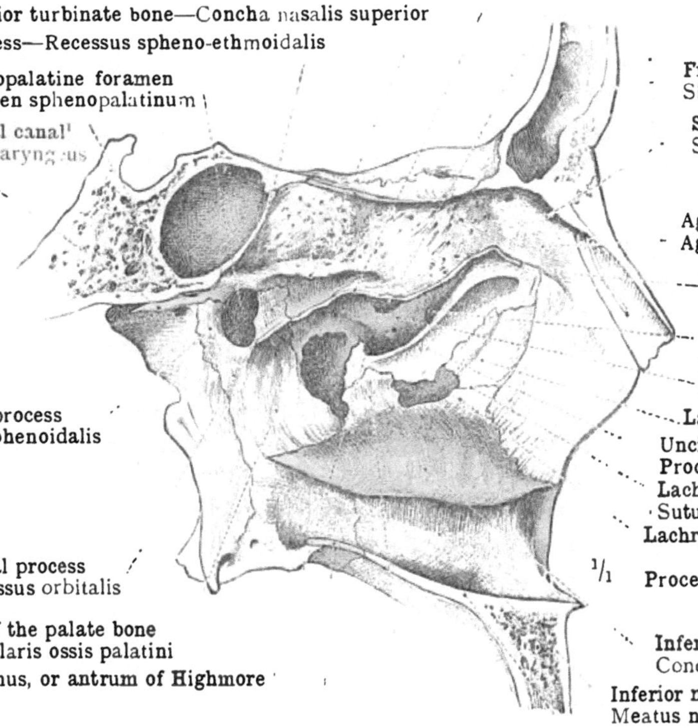

¹ See note to p. 48.

FIG. 204.—THE EXTERNAL WALL OF THE NASAL CAVITY: MEDIAN SAGITTAL SECTION. LEFT SIDE.

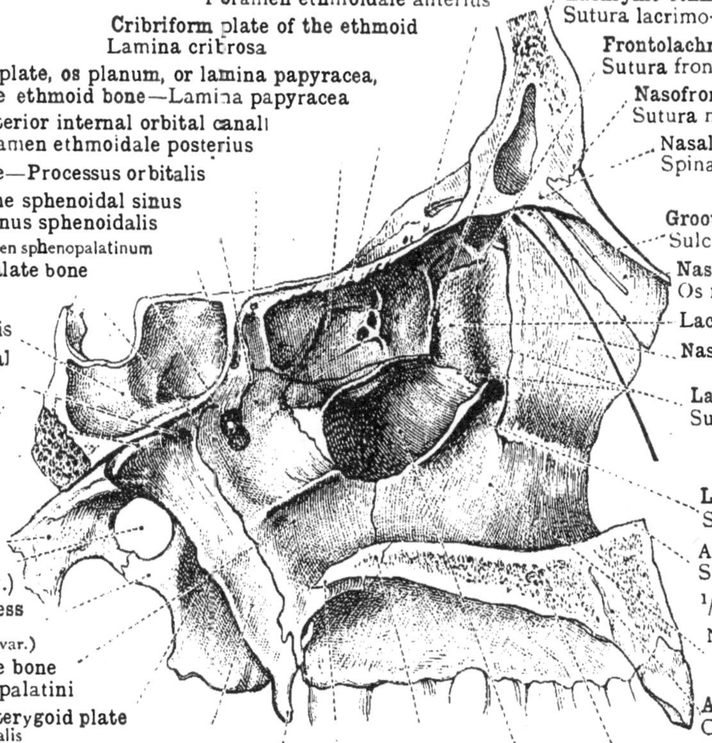

[1] U.S.: Posterior ethmoidal canal. [2] U.S.: Anterior ethmoidal canal.

FIG. 205.—THE EXTERNAL WALL OF THE *NASAL* CAVITY AFTER REMOVAL OF THE THREE TURBINATE BONES AND THE LATERAL MASS OF THE ETHMOID: MEDIAN SAGITTAL SECTION. LEFT SIDE.

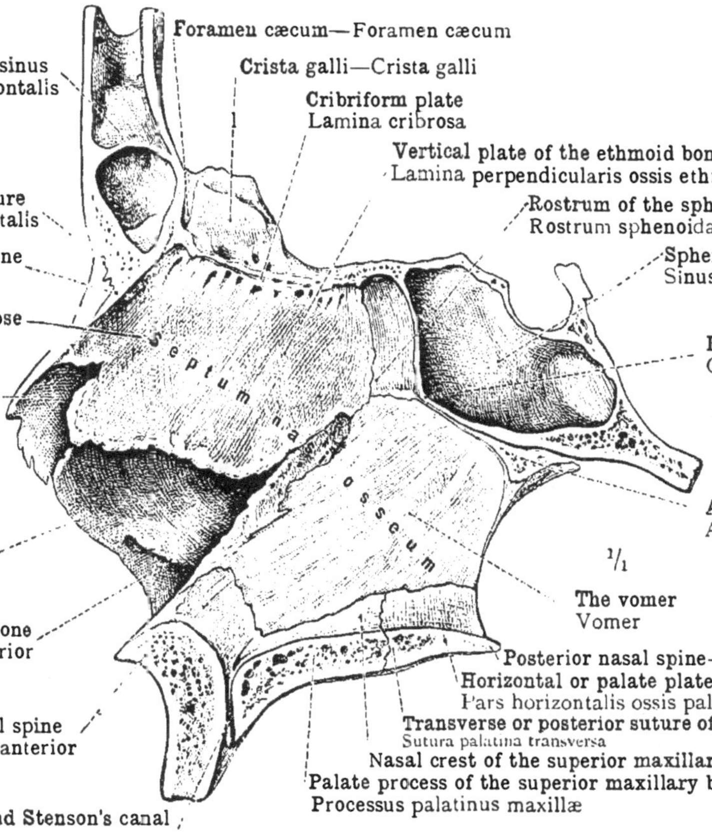

FIG. 206.—THE BONY SEPTUM OF THE *NOSE* SEEN FROM THE LEFT SIDE: SAGITTAL SECTION

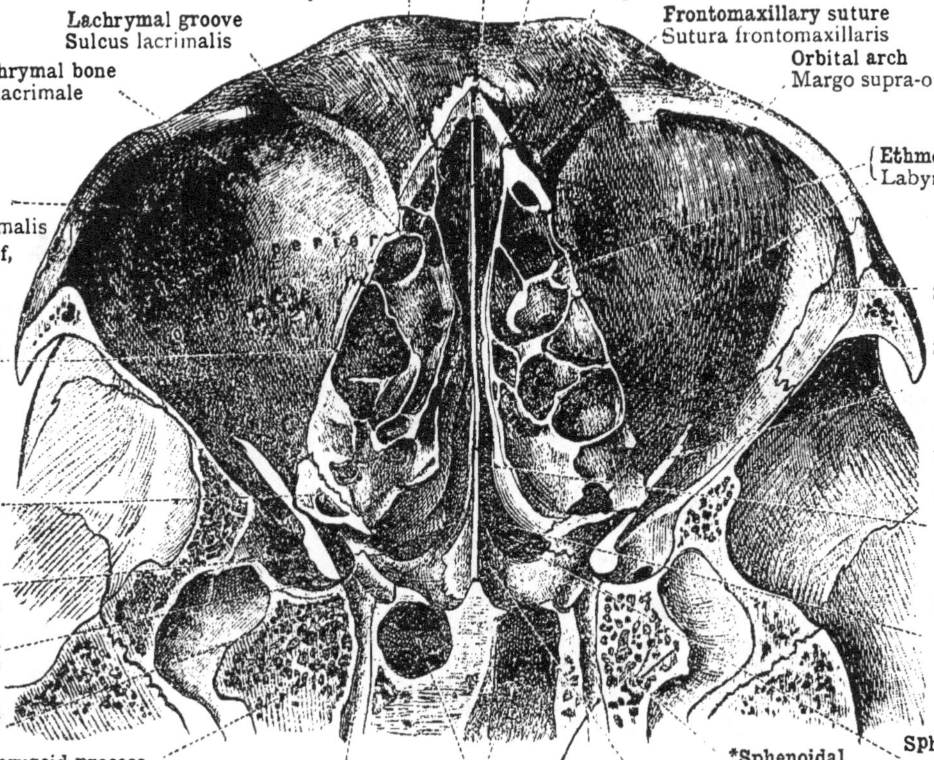

[1] I am indebted to Professor Toldt for the following account of the **Sphenoidal canaliculus*, which is accurately described neither by Quain nor by Macalister: "It begins in the scaphoid fossa and divides as it ascends into two branches, the inner of which opens into the Vidian canal, while the outer opens on the cerebral surface of the great wing of the sphenoid bone, between the lingula of the sphenoid bone and the foramen ovale." The outer branch is termed by English anatomists the *foramen of Vesalius*, and transmits an emissary vein: the inner branch gives passage to the *sphenoidal branch* of the otic ganglion, by means of which this ganglion communicates with the Vidian nerve.—Tr.

Fig. 207.—By Means of a nearly Horizontal Section passing through the Centre of the Entrance to the Orbit, the Upper Parts of the Nasal Fossæ and of the Orbits are displayed. Seen from Below.

Posteriorly the section passes through the body of the sphenoid bone and the root of the pterygoid process, opening up the Vidian canal through its whole length. A bristle has been passed into the *sphenoidal canaliculus[1] from the Vidian canal. The lateral masses of the ethmoid bone (ethmoidal labyrinths) are divided in the horizontal plane.

Cavum nasi et orbita—The nasal fossæ and the orbits.

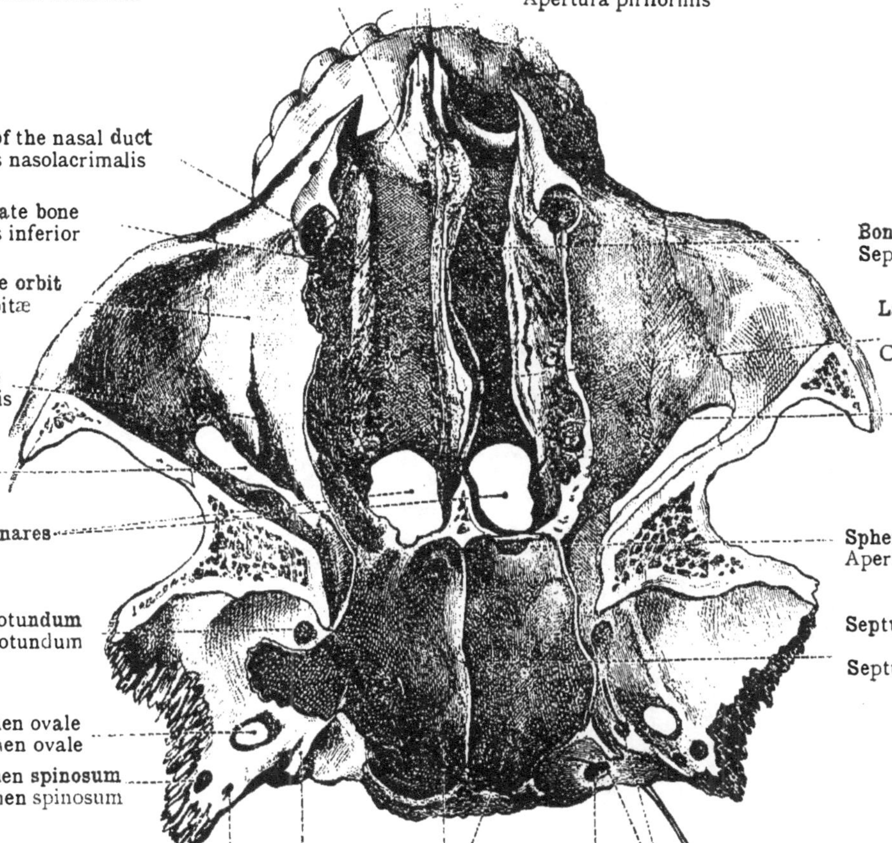

[1] See note to p. 92.

FIG. 208.—BY MEANS OF A NEARLY HORIZONTAL SECTION IN A PLANE A LITTLE ABOVE THAT OF THE INFERIOR WALLS OF THE ORBITS, THE LOWER PORTIONS OF THE NASAL FOSSÆ AND OF THE ORBITS HAVE BEEN EXPOSED. SEEN FROM ABOVE.

Posteriorly the section passes through the sphenoidal sinuses, in this specimen exceptionally capacious. The upper orifices of the *sphenoidal canaliculus (*see note to p.* 92) are indicated by bristles.

Cavum nasi et orbita—Nasal cavity and orbits.

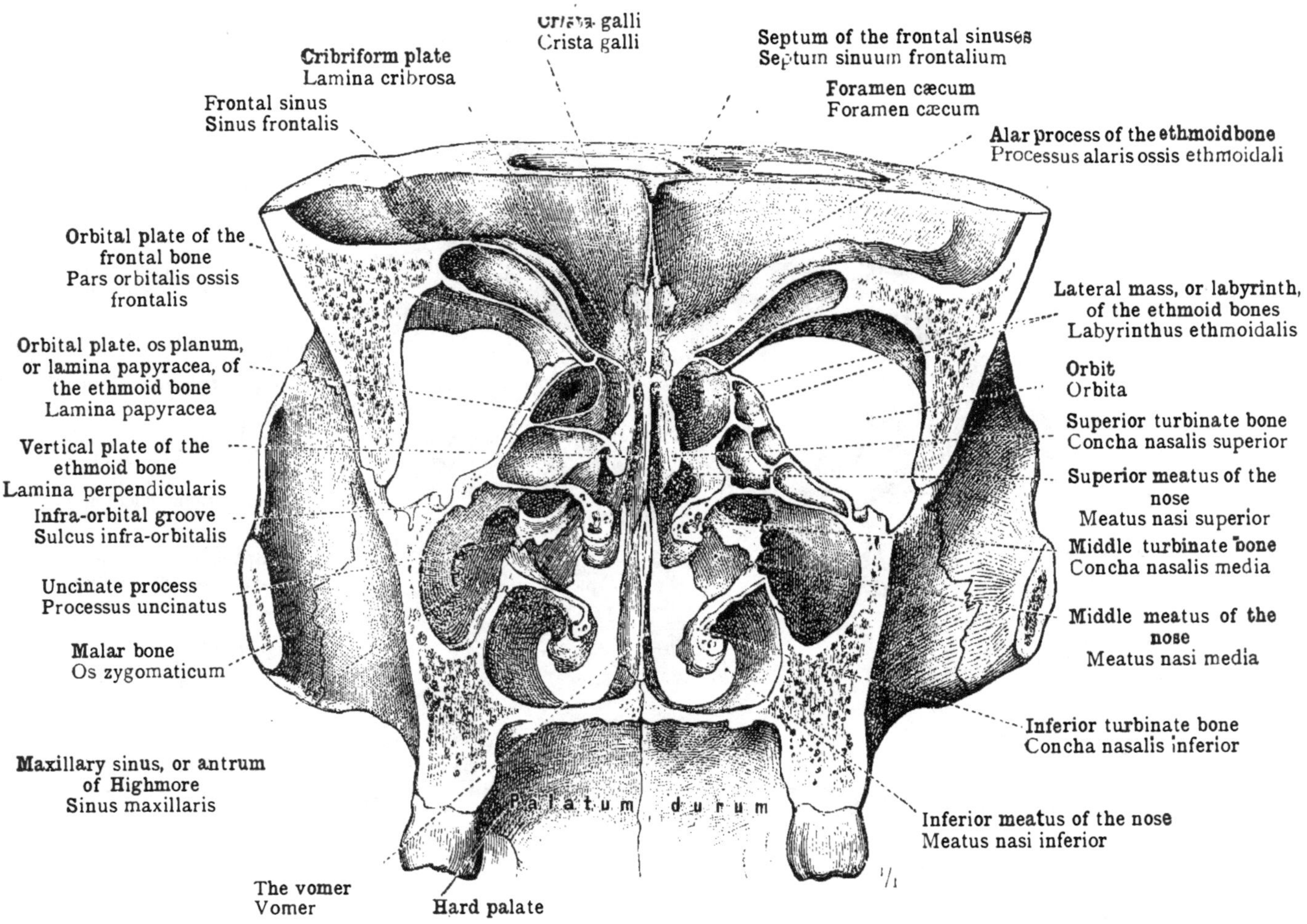

FIG. 209.—BY MEANS OF A SECTION PASSING THROUGH THE MOST ANTERIOR PORTIONS OF BOTH ZYGOMATIC ARCHES, THE NASAL CAVITY AND THE ORBITS ARE DIVIDED TOWARDS THEIR POSTERIOR EXTREMITIES IN THE FRONTAL PLANE.

The anterior portion of the skull thus divided is figured from behind. The three turbinate bones of the nose and the three nasal meatus, as well as the bony septum of the nose, are seen in frontal section. The maxillary sinuses are also opened up, and the communication of these sinuses with the general cavity of the nose is to be seen above the uncinate process.

Cavum nasi et orbita—Nasal cavity and orbits.

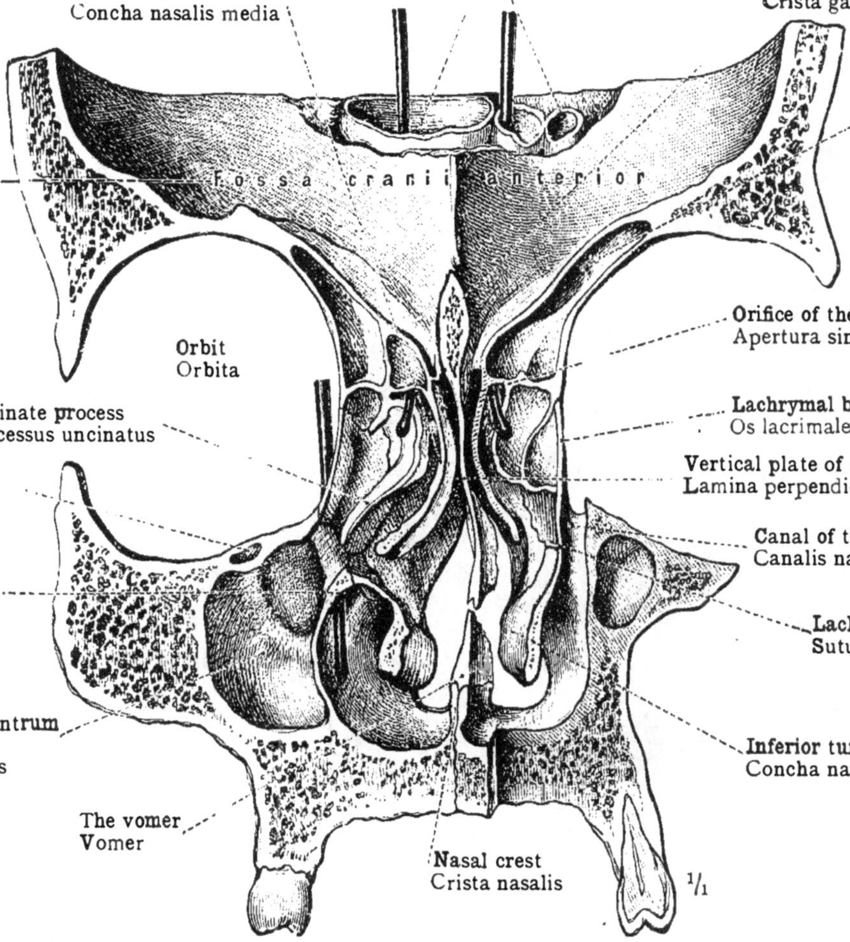

FIG. 210.—BY MEANS OF A SECTION PASSING VERTICALLY THROUGH THE POSTERIOR PORTIONS OF BOTH LACHRYMAL BONES, THE ANTERIOR PORTION OF THE NASAL CAVITY AND OF THE ORBITS IS DISPLAYED IN FRONTAL SECTION. SEEN FROM BEHIND.

From the right side of the anterior portion of the skull thus divided, a layer of bone a quarter of an inch in thickness has been removed by a section in a plane parallel with the first section, so as to open up the canal of the nasal duct, canalis nasolacrimalis, in its entire length. The sounds passed into the two frontal sinuses indicate the orifices of these sinuses in the nasal fossæ. A third sound has been passed through the left canal of the nasal duct from the orbit into the nasal cavity.

Cavum nasi et orbita—Nasal cavity and orbits.

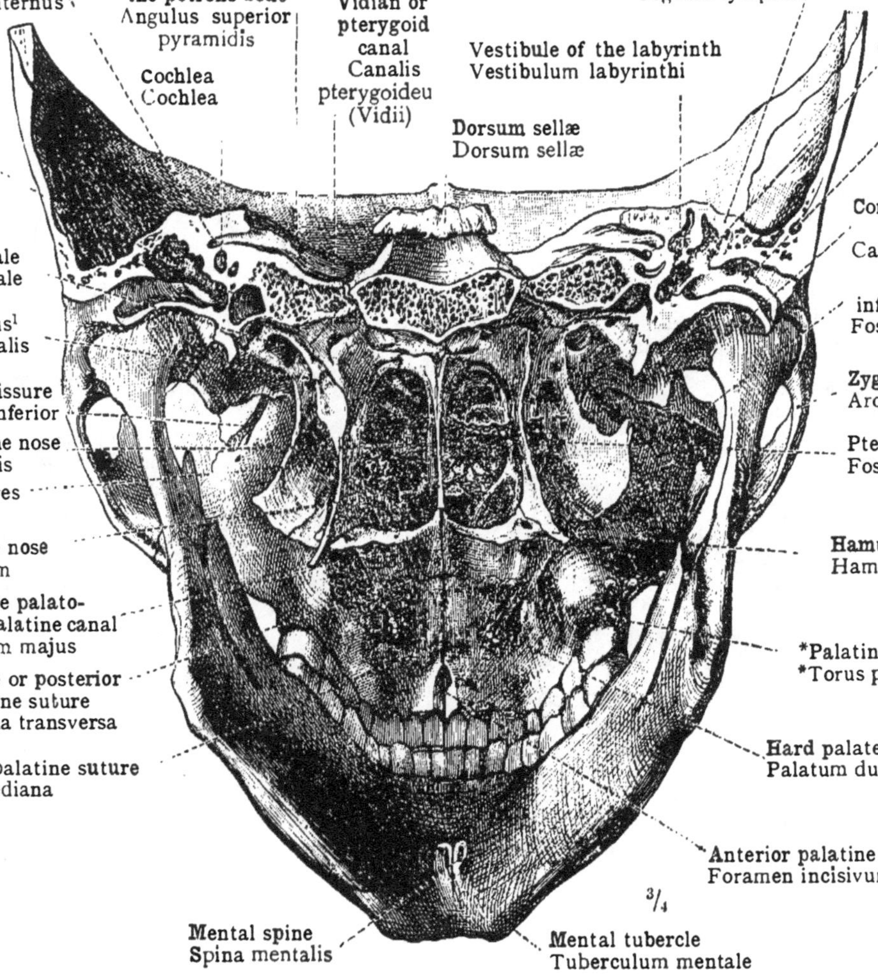

[1] See note to p. 92.

FIG. 211.—ANTERIOR PORTION OF THE SKULL, SEPARATED FROM THE POSTERIOR PORTION BY A FRONTAL SECTION PASSING THROUGH THE TWO EXTERNAL AUDITORY MEATUS.

The view from behind shows the posterior nares with the posterior border of the bony septum of the nose, the bony framework of the oral cavity, and the zygomatic fossæ ; further, in frontal section, the tympanic cavities, with portions of the bony labyrinths and the internal auditory meatus.

Cranium viscerale—Facial portion of the skull.

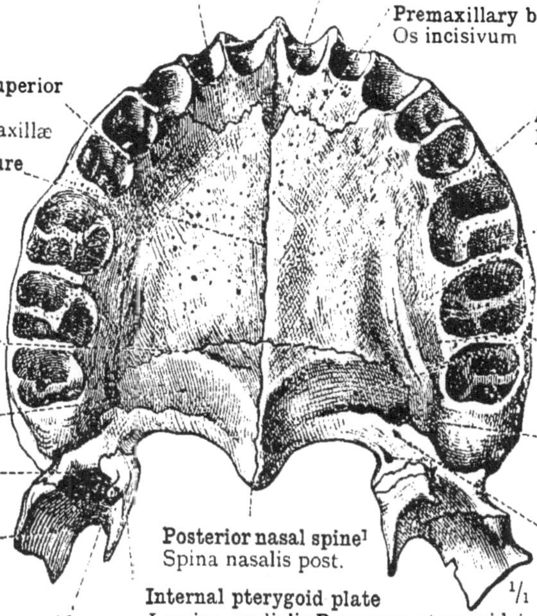

[1] In the English nomenclature *palatine spine* is an alternative name for the *posterior nasal spine*.—TR.
[2] The English nomenclature recognises one *palatine groove* only, that running forwards on the under surface of the hard palate from the inferior orifice of the posterior palatine canal, lodging the large palatine nerve and vessels.—TR.

FIG. 212.—THE HARD PALATE, PALATUM DURUM, WITH THE ALVEOLAR PROCESS OF THE SUPERIOR MAXILLARY BONE, REMOVED BY A SECTION PASSING HORIZONTALLY THROUGH BOTH SUPERIOR MAXILLARY BONES ABOVE THE FLOOR OF THE *NASAL* FOSSÆ. SEEN FROM BELOW.

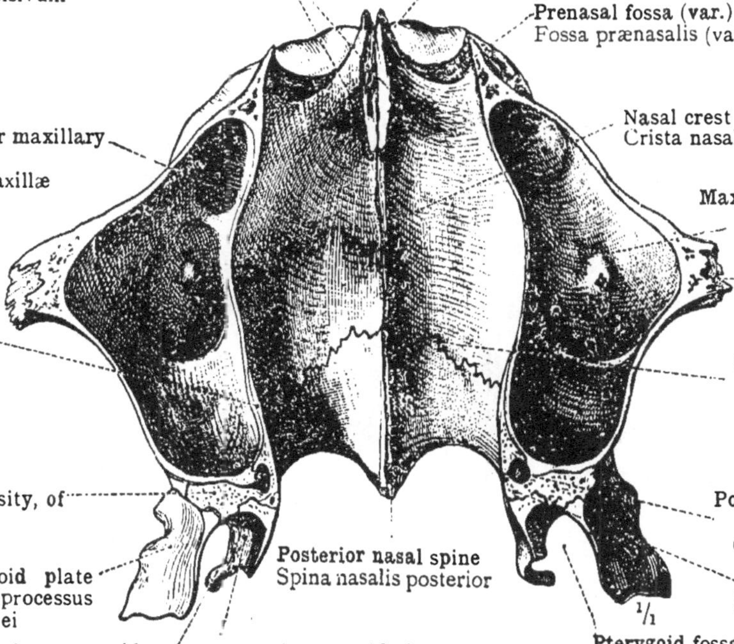

FIG. 213.—THE FLOOR (INFERIOR WALL) OF THE *NASAL* FOSSÆ WITH THE MAXILLARY SINUSES LYING ON EITHER SIDE, SHOWN BY MEANS OF A HORIZONTAL SECTION THROUGH THE SUPERIOR MAXILLARY BONES. SEEN FROM ABOVE.

Cranium viscerale—Facial portion of the skull.

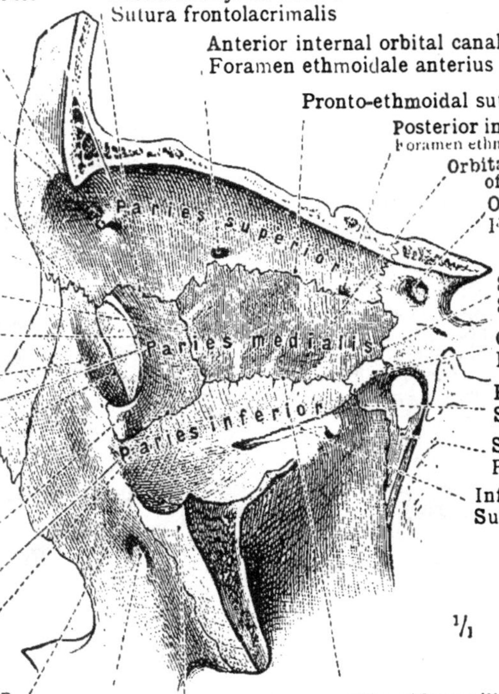

[1] U.S.: Anterior ethmoidal canal. [2] U.S.: Posterior ethmoidal canal.

FIG. 214.—INTERNAL PORTION OF THE LEFT ORBIT, SHOWN BY THE REMOVAL OF THE EXTERNAL WALL. SEEN FROM THE LEFT SIDE.

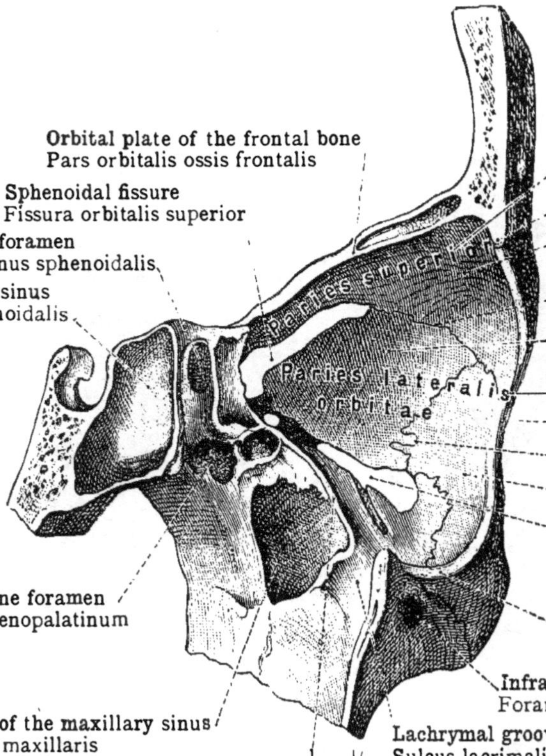

FIG. 215.—EXTERNAL PORTION OF THE LEFT ORBIT, SHOWN BY THE REMOVAL OF THE INTERNAL WALL OF THE ORBIT AND OF A PORTION OF THE SUPERIOR MAXILLARY BONE IN A LONGITUDINALLY HEMISECTED SKULL.

Orbita—The orbits.

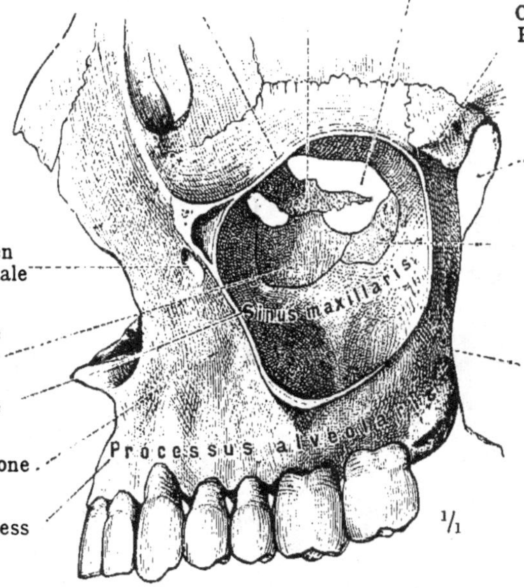

FIG. 216.—THE LEFT MAXILLARY SINUS, OR ANTRUM OF HIGHMORE, SHOWN BY THE REMOVAL OF THE EXTERNAL WALL OF THE BODY OF THE SUPERIOR MAXILLARY BONE AND THE MALAR BONE. SEEN FROM THE LEFT SIDE.

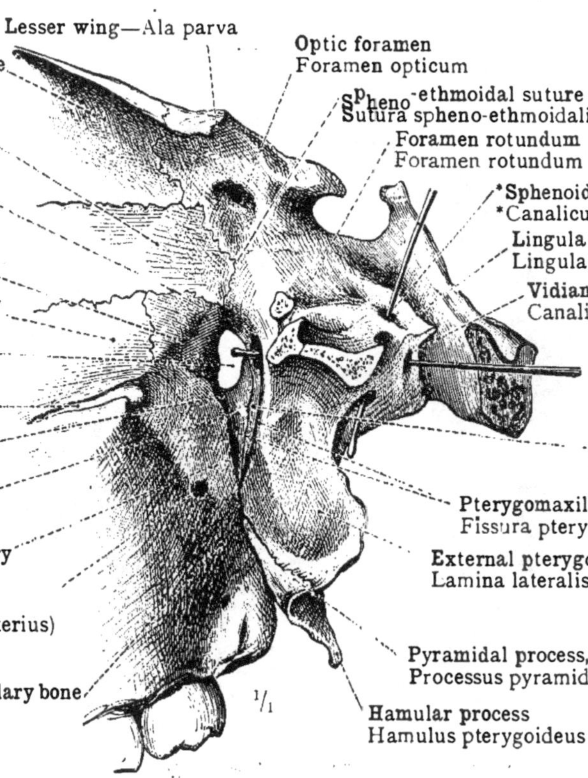

[1] See note to p. 92.

FIG. 217.—THE LEFT SPHENOMAXILLARY FOSSA, SHOWN BY REMOVAL OF THE MALAR BONE, THE TEMPORAL BONE, AND THE GREAT WING OF THE SPHENOID BONE. SEEN FROM THE LEFT SIDE.

A sound has been passed through the **Vidian** canal, and another through the *sphenoidal canaliculus[1] (exceptionally large in this specimen).

Sinus maxillaris—Maxillary sinus, or antrum of Highmore.—Fossa pterygopalatina—Sphenomaxillar fossa.

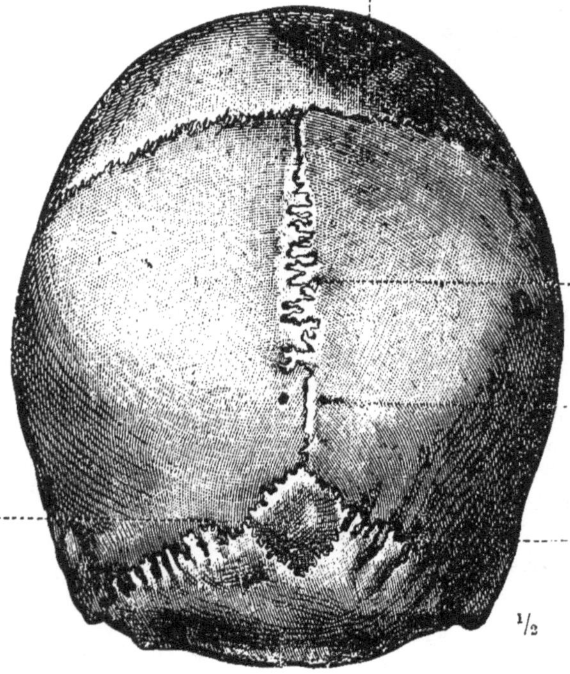

FIG. 218.—A LARGE WORMIAN BONE IN THE UPPERMOST PART OF THE LAMBDOID SUTURE.

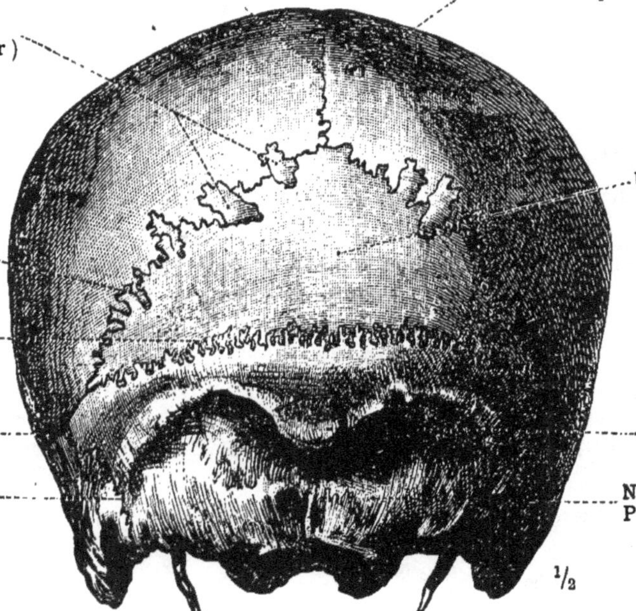

FIG. 219.—TRANSVERSE SUBDIVISION OF THE SQUAMA OCCIPITALIS. SEVERAL WORMIAN BONES IN THE LAMBDOID SUTURE.

[1] See note to p. 57.

Ossa suturarum—Wormian bones.

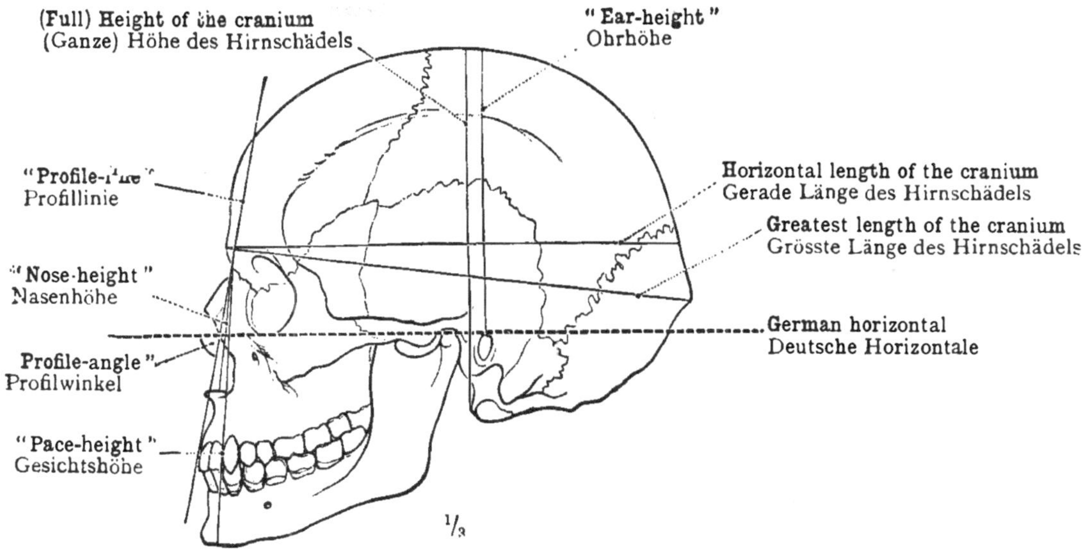

FIG. 220.—SIDE-VIEW OF THE SKULL NORMA LATERALIS.

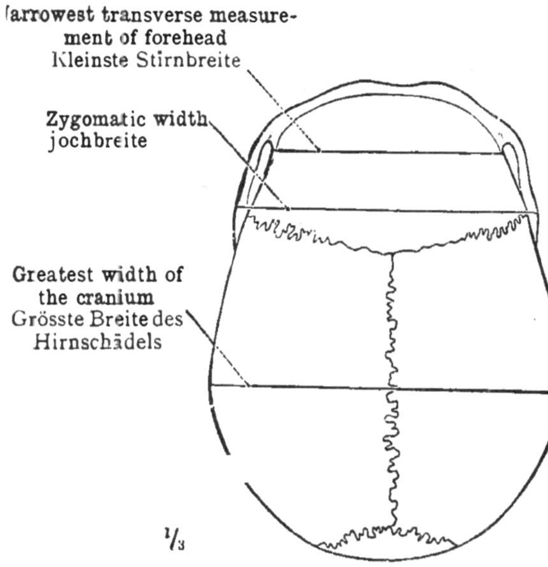

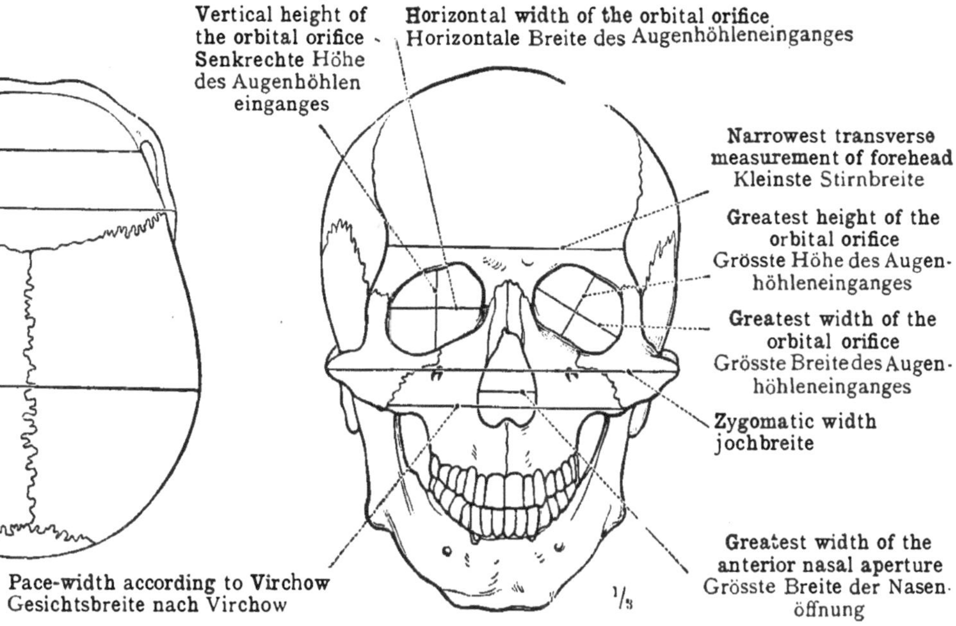

FIG. 221.—SKULL SEEN FROM ABOVE NORMA VERTICALIS.

FIG. 222.—FRONT VIEW OF THE SKULL: NORMA FRONTALIS.

TRANSLATOR'S NOTE.—The above measurements do not fully correspond with those used by English craniologists. For this reason a purely literal translation of the German terms has been given.

The Principal Measurements of the Skull.

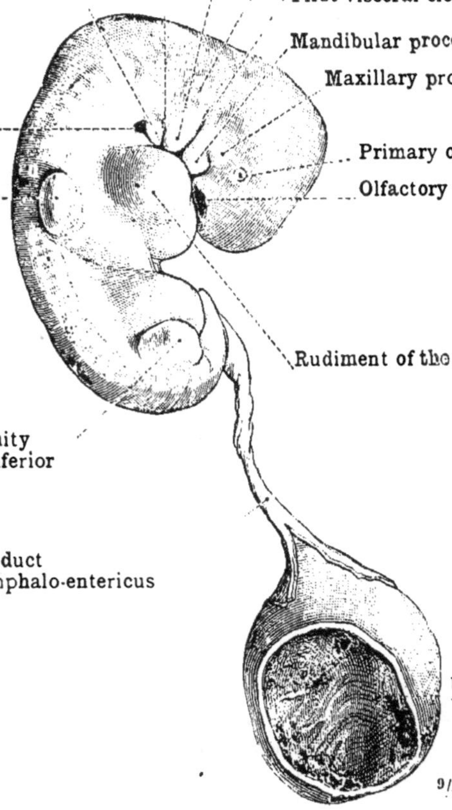

FIG. 223.—HUMAN EMBRYO, FOUR WEEKS OLD.
The umbilical vesicle has been opened.

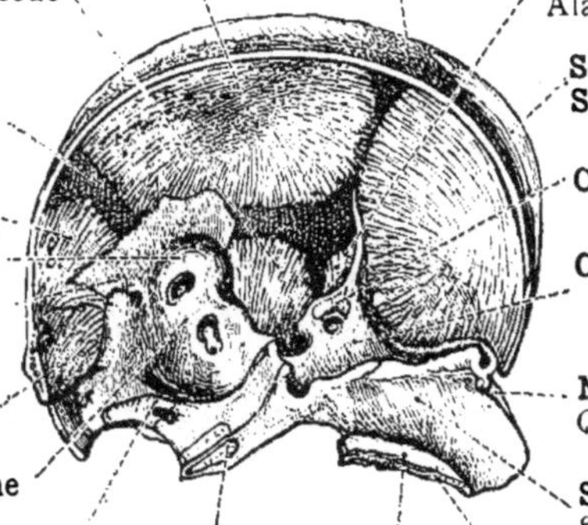

[1] See note to p. 57.

FIG. 224.—THE LEFT HALF OF THE SKULL OF A HUMAN FŒTUS AT THE END OF THE FOURTH MONTH (MONTHS OF FOUR WEEKS EACH). SEEN FROM WITHIN. THE CARTILAGINOUS PORTION OF THE PRIMORDIAL CRANIUM (CHONDROCRANIUM) IS COLOURED BLUE.
Body-length, 4½ inches.

Development of the Skull.

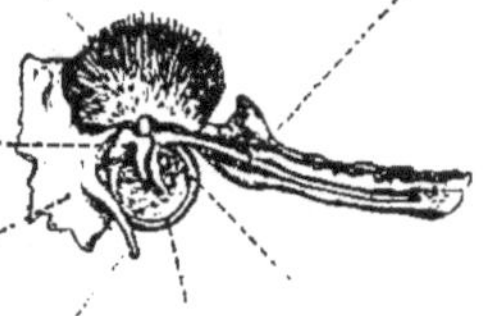

FIG. 225.—THE SQUAMOUS PORTION OF THE TEMPORAL BONE, THE TYMPANIC MEMBRANE WITH THE MALLEUS, THE INCUS, AND MECKEL'S CARTILAGE, FROM A HUMAN FŒTUS IN THE FIRST HALF OF THE FIFTH MONTH (MONTHS OF FOUR WEEKS EACH). SEEN FROM WITHIN.

Body-length, 5½ inches.

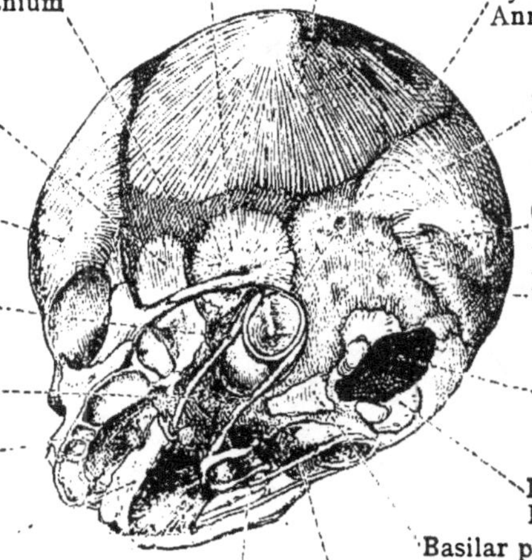

[1] See note to p. 57.

FIG. 226.—THE SKULL OF A HUMAN FŒTUS IN THE MIDDLE OF THE FIFTH MONTH (MONTHS OF FOUR WEEKS EACH). SEEN FROM THE LEFT SIDE AND BELOW.

Body length, 6½ inches. The cartilaginous bars of the visceral arches are displayed, and these, together with the cartilaginous portion of the primordial cranium, are coloured blue. Part of the cartilage of the left side of the inferior maxilla has been removed in order to lay bare a portion of Meckel's cartilage which lies beneath it.

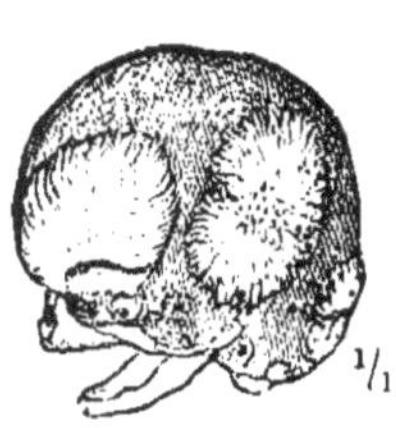

FIG. 227.—THE DRIED SKULL OF A HUMAN FŒTUS IN THE MIDDLE OF THE FOURTH MONTH (MONTHS OF FOUR WEEKS EACH).

Body-length, 3½ inches.

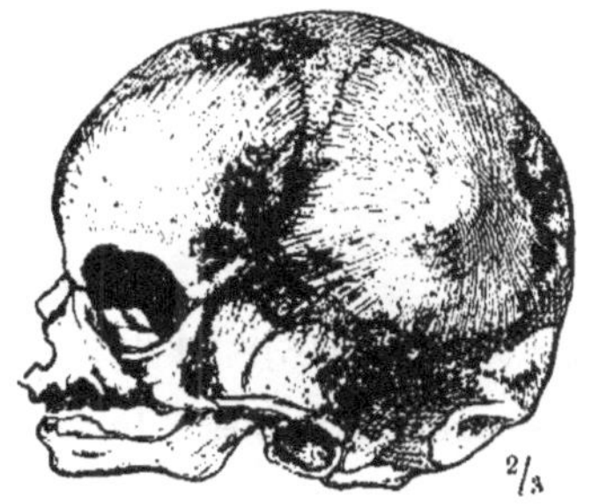

FIG. 228.—THE DRIED SKULL OF A HUMAN FŒTUS AT THE END OF THE SIXTH MONTH (MONTHS OF FOUR WEEKS EACH).

Body-length, 11⅓ inches.

Development of the Skull.

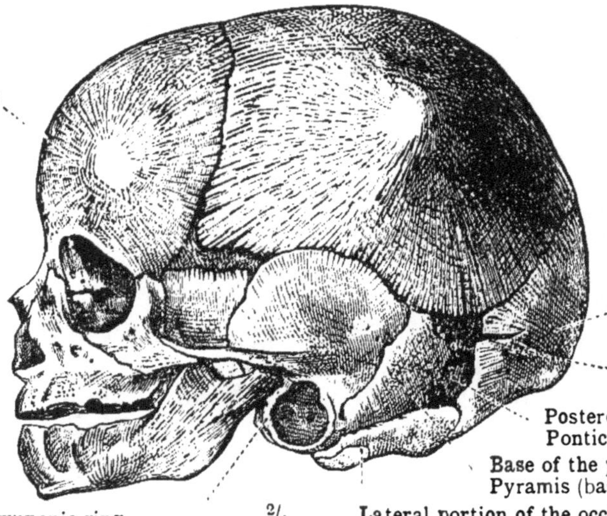

FIG. 229.—THE DRIED SKULL OF AN INFANT BORN AT FULL TERM. SEEN FROM THE LEFT SIDE.

Body-length, 20½ inches. In the anterolateral fontanelle there remains part of the membranous portion of the primordial cranium (membrane of the fontanelle); in the posterolateral fontanelle there remains part of the cartilaginous portion of the primordial cranium.

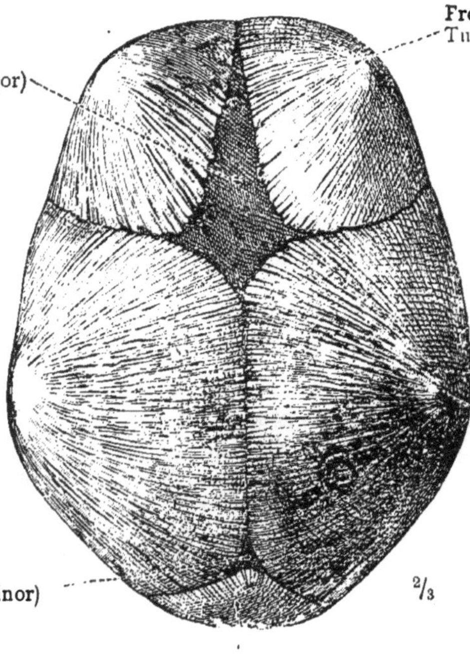

FIG. 230.—THE DRIED SKULL OF AN INFANT BORN AT FULL TERM. SEEN FROM ABOVE.

Body-length, 20½ inches. In the anterior and in the posterior fontanelle there remain parts of the membranous portion of the primordial cranium.

[1] See note to p. 57.

Development of the Skull.

SKELETON EXTREMITATUM, SUPERIORIS ET INFERIORIS

THE SKELETON OF THE UPPER AND LOWER EXTREMITIES (THE APPENDICULAR SKELETON)

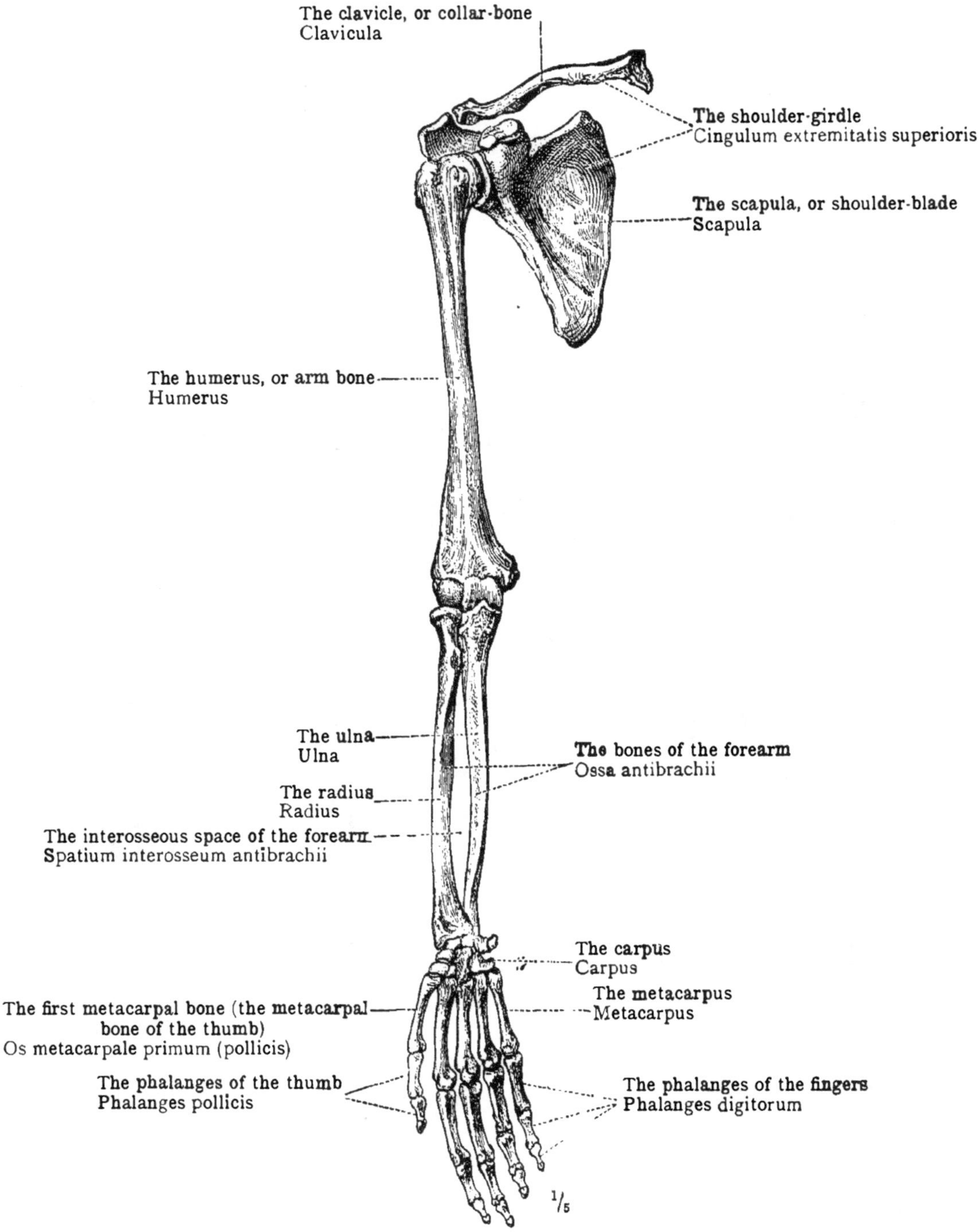

FIG. 231.—THE SKELETON OF THE UPPER EXTREMITY.

Skeleton extremitatis superioris—The skeleton of the upper extremity.

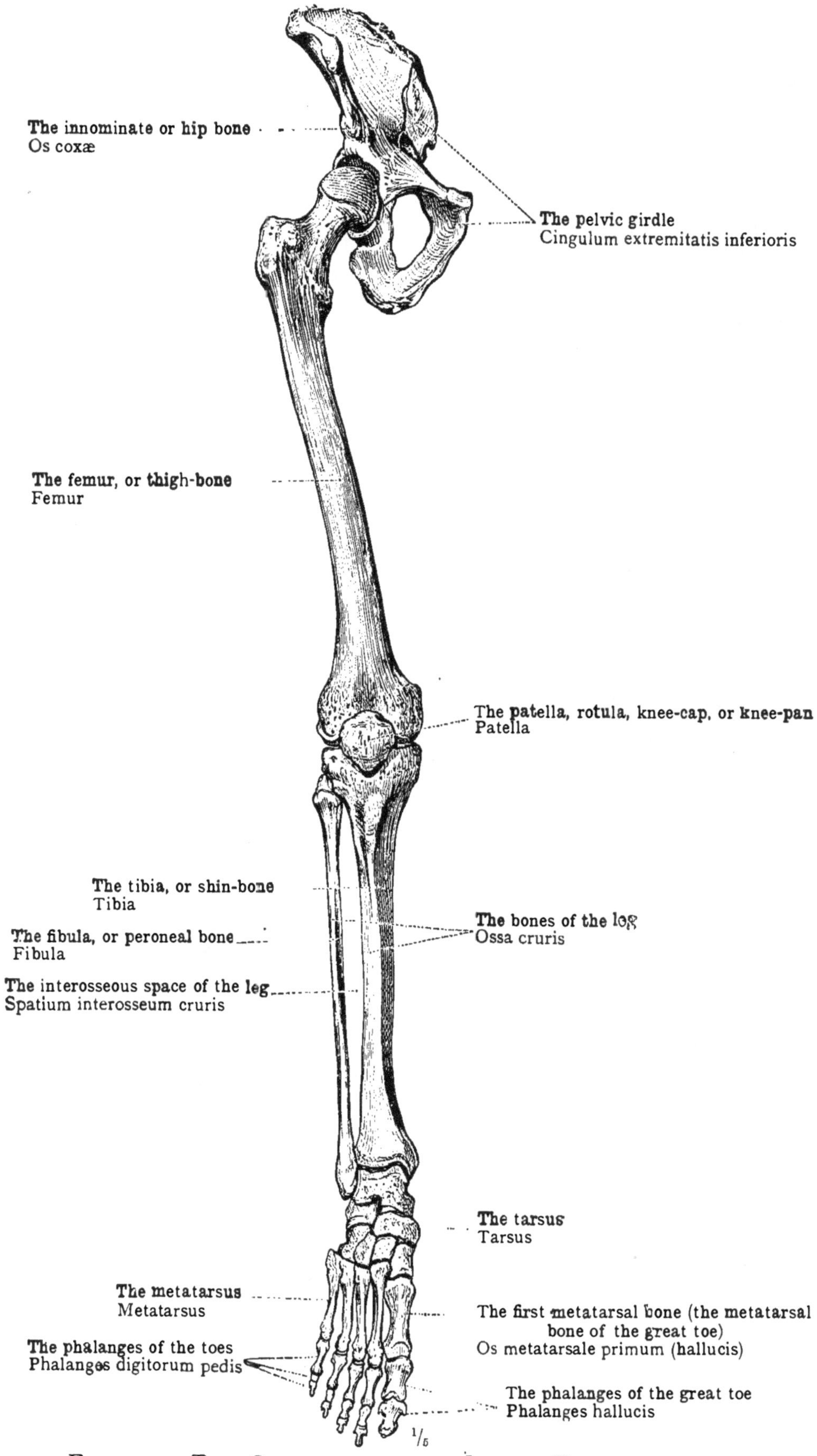

FIG. 232.—THE SKELETON OF THE LOWER EXTREMITY.

Skeleton extremitatis inferioris—The skeleton of the lower extremity.

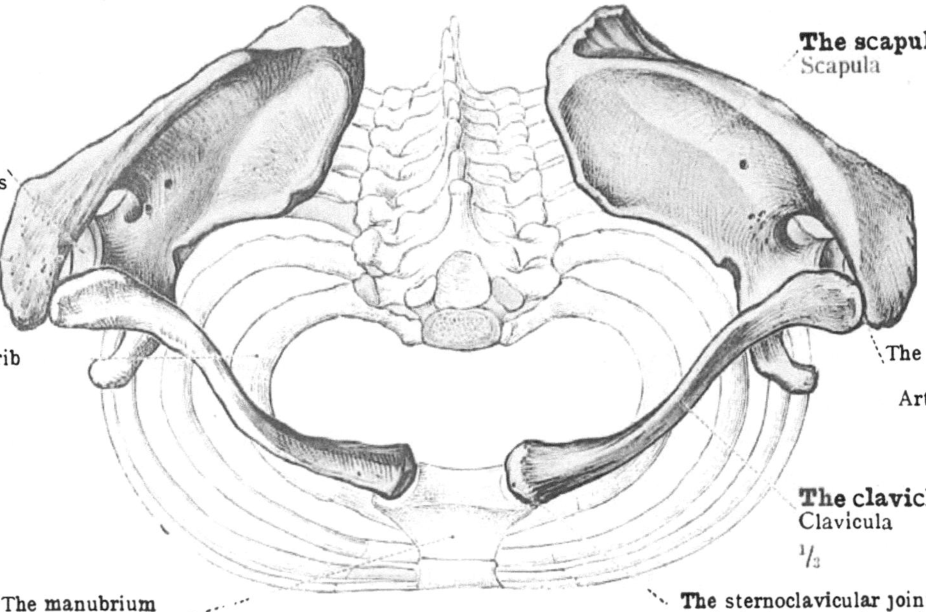

FIG. 233.—THE SHOULDER-GIRDLE AND ITS RELATION TO THE THORAX. SEEN FROM ABOVE.

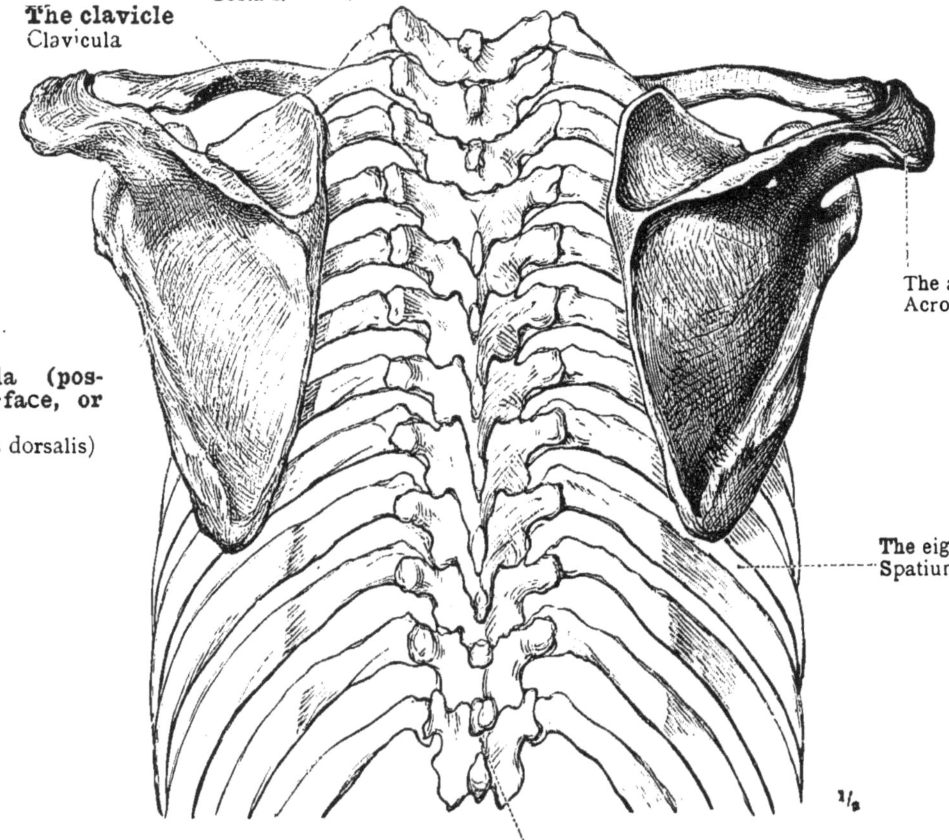

FIG. 234.—THE SHOULDER-GIRDLE AND ITS RELATION TO THE THORAX. SEEN FROM BEHIND.

Cingulum extremitatis superioris—The shoulder-girdle.

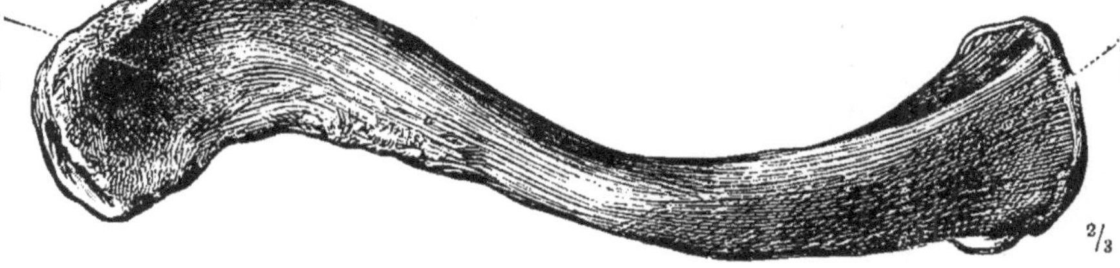

FIG. 235.—THE RIGHT CLAVICLE SEEN FROM ABOVE.

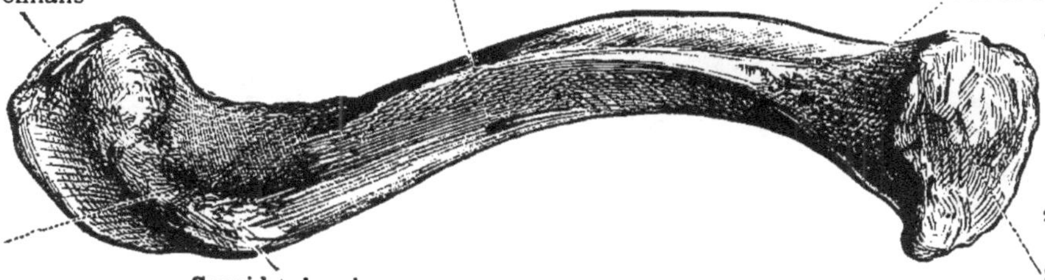

FIG. 23 .—THE RIGHT CLAVICLE SEEN FROM BELOW.

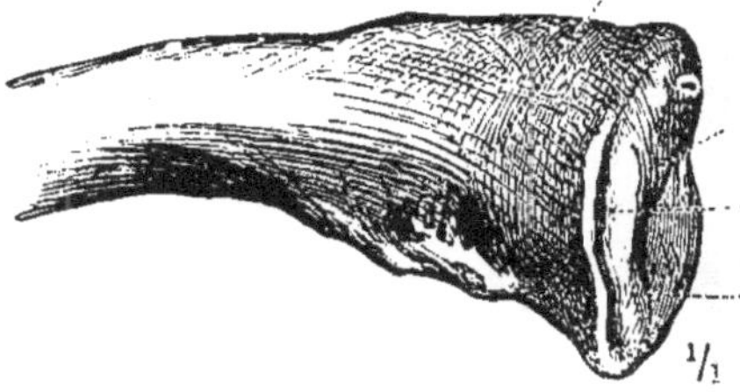

FIG. 237.—STERNAL EXTREMITY OF THE RIGHT CLAVICLE OF A FEMALE AGED TWENTY YEARS, WITH A STERNAL EPIPHYSIS. SEEN FROM BEFORE.

Clavicula—The clavicle.

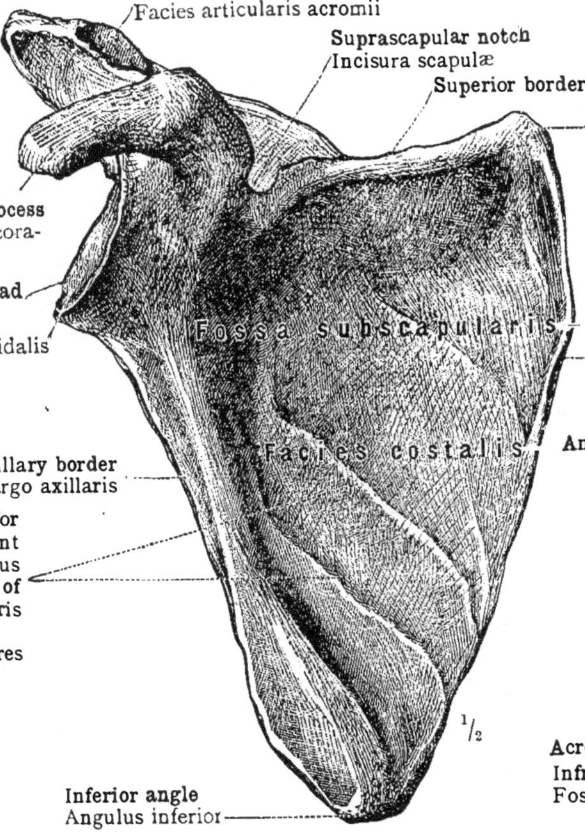

FIG. 238.—THE RIGHT SCAPULA SEEN FROM BEFORE.

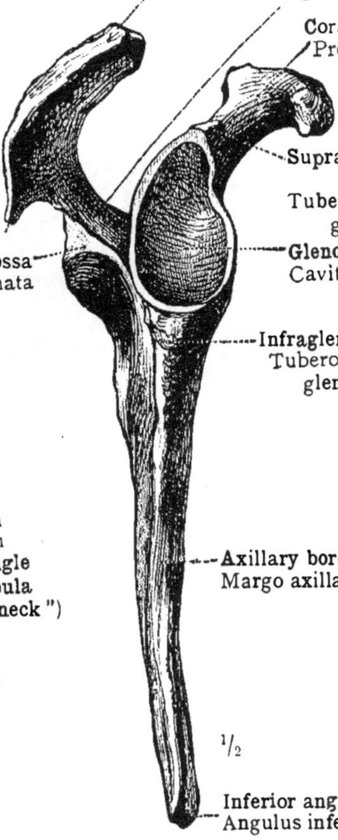

FIG. 240.—THE RIGHT SCAPULA SEEN FROM THE OUTER OR AXILLARY ASPECT.

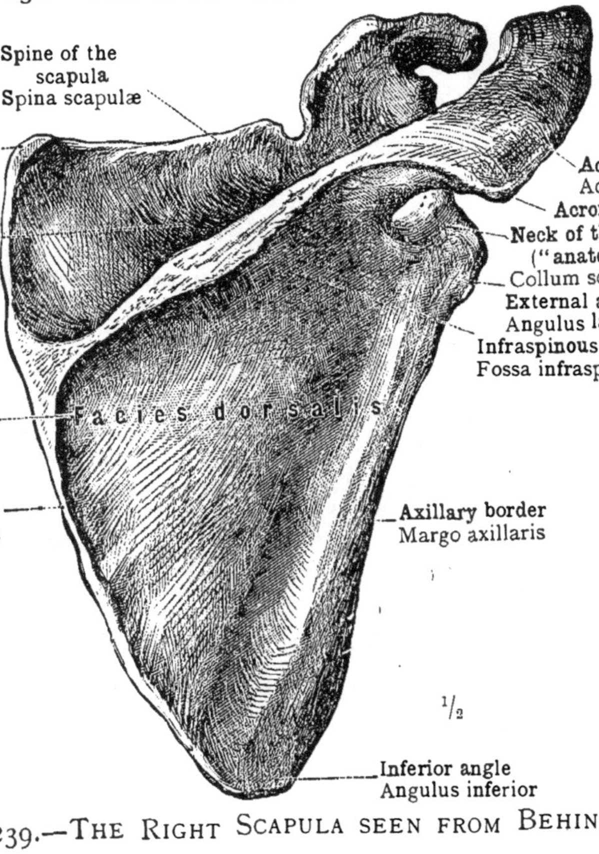

FIG. 239.—THE RIGHT SCAPULA SEEN FROM BEHIND.

Scapula—The shoulder-blade.

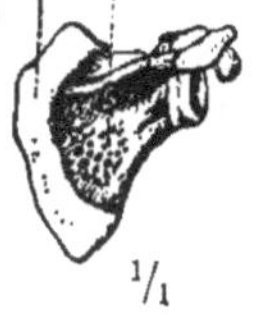

FIG. 241.—IN THE FIFTH MONTH OF INTRA-UTERINE LIFE (MONTHS OF FOUR WEEKS EACH).

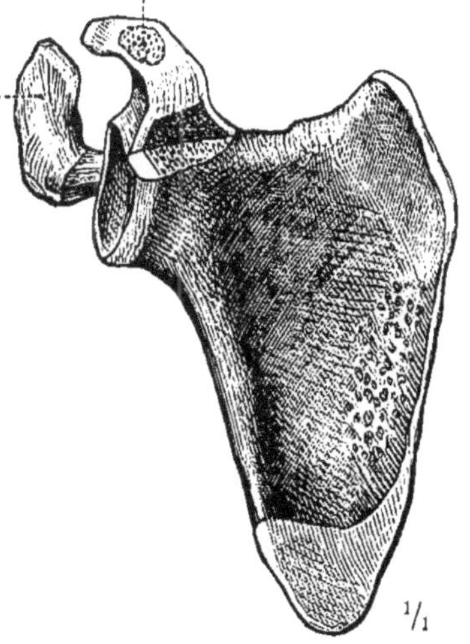

FIG. 242.—IN THE SECOND YEAR OF LIFE.

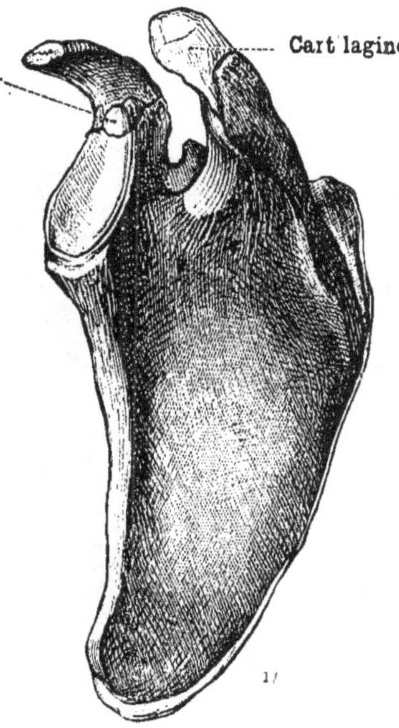

FIG. 243.—IN THE FIFTEENTH YEAR OF LIFE.

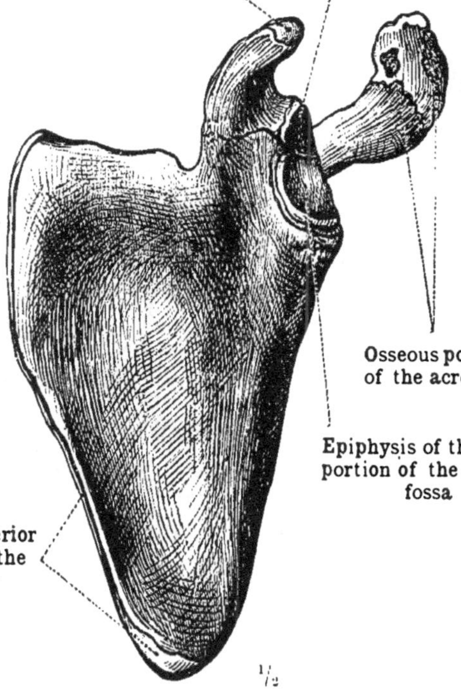

FIG. 244.—IN THE SEVENTEENTH YEAR OF LIFE.

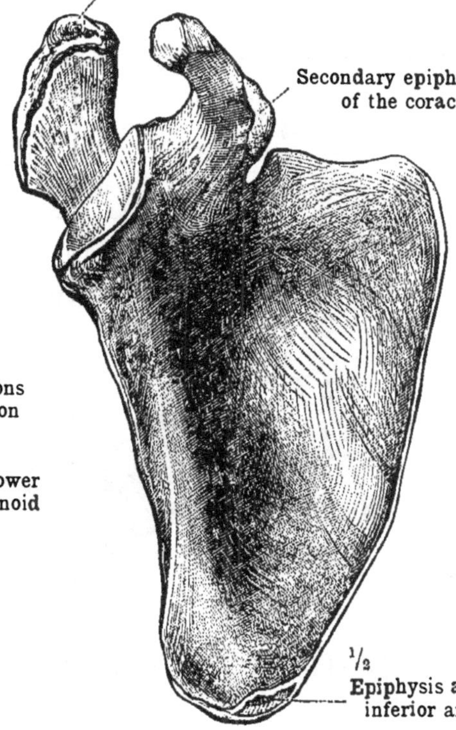

FIG. 245.—IN THE NINETEENTH YEAR OF LIFE.

Development of the Scapula.

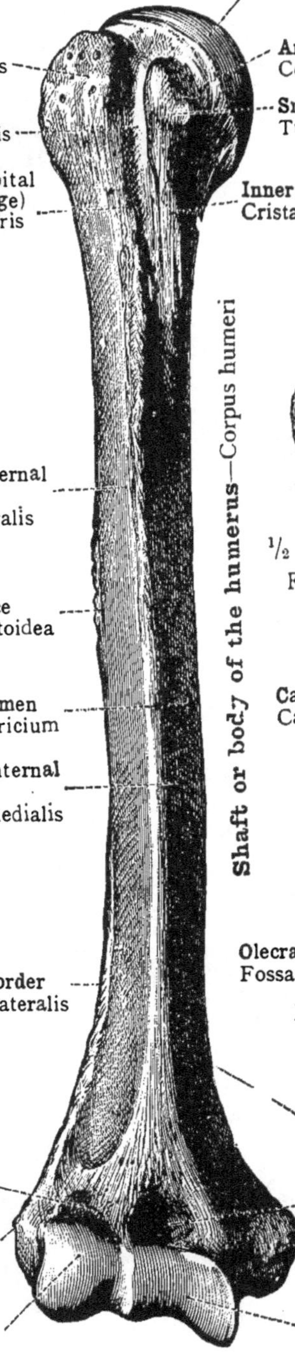

Fig. 246.—The Right Humerus seen from Before.

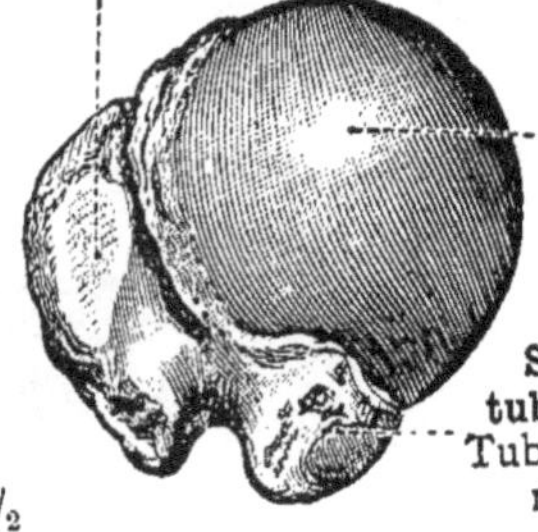

Fig. 248.—Proximal (Upper) Extremity of the Right Humerus seen from Above.

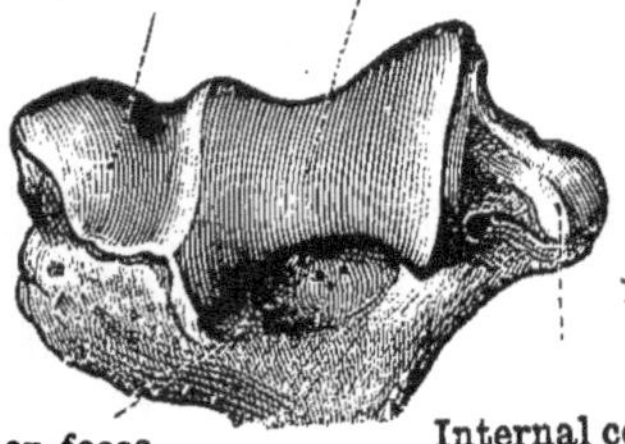

Fig. 249.—Distal (Lower) Extremity of the Right Humerus seen from Below.

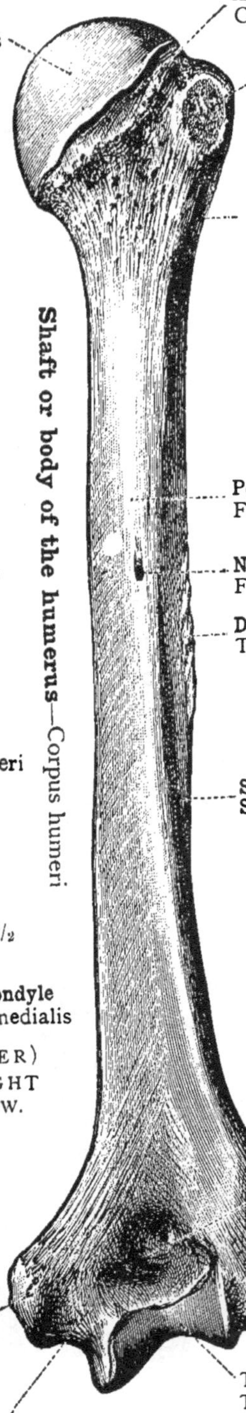

Fig. 247.—The Right Humerus seen from Behind.

Humerus—The humerus.

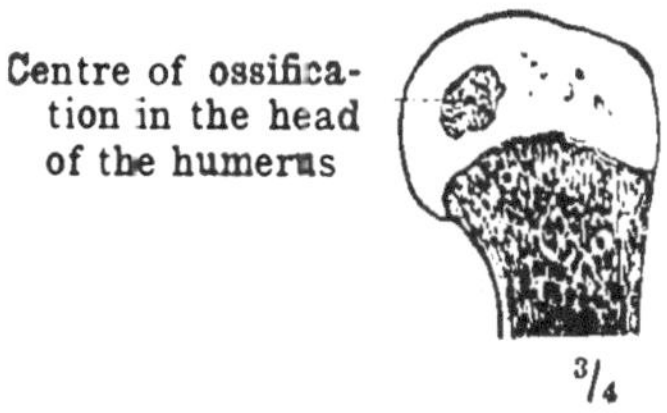

FIG. 250.—FROM A GIRL AGED FOUR MONTHS.

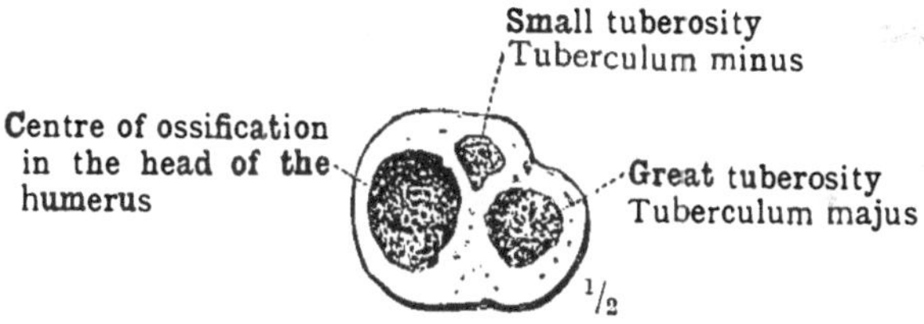

FIG. 252.—FROM A BOY AGED THREE YEARS (HORIZONTAL SECTION.)

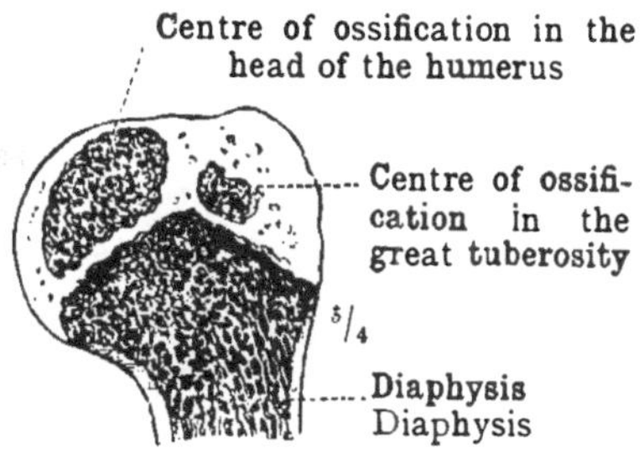

FIG. 251.—FROM A BOY AGED TWO YEARS.

THE CENTRES OF OSSIFICATION OF THE PROXIMAL EXTREMITY OF THE HUMERUS.

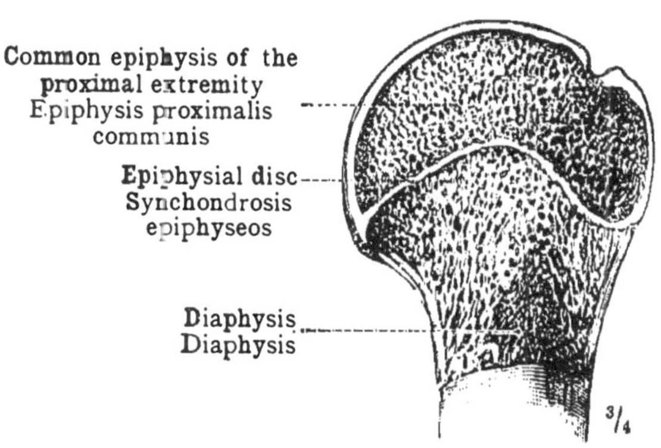

FIG. 253.—FROM A BOY AGED THIRTEEN YEARS.

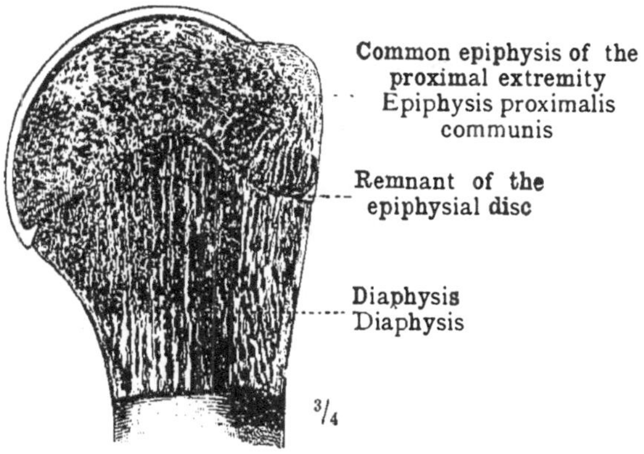

FIG. 254.—FROM A GIRL AGED NINETEEN YEARS

THE COMMON EPIPHYSIS OF THE PROXIMAL EXTREMITY OF THE HUMERUS.

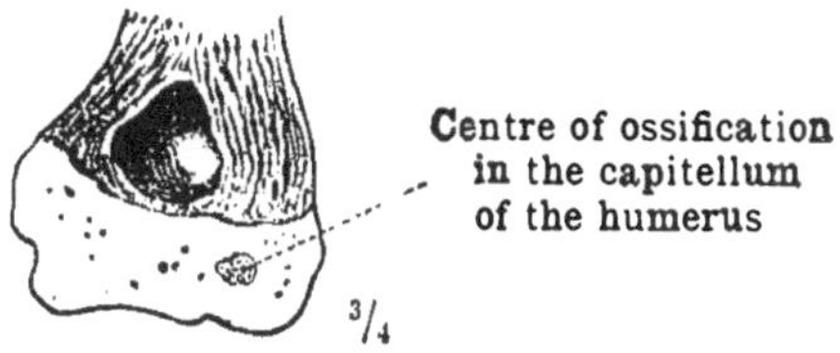

FIG. 255.—FROM A BOY AGED TWO AND A HALF YEARS.

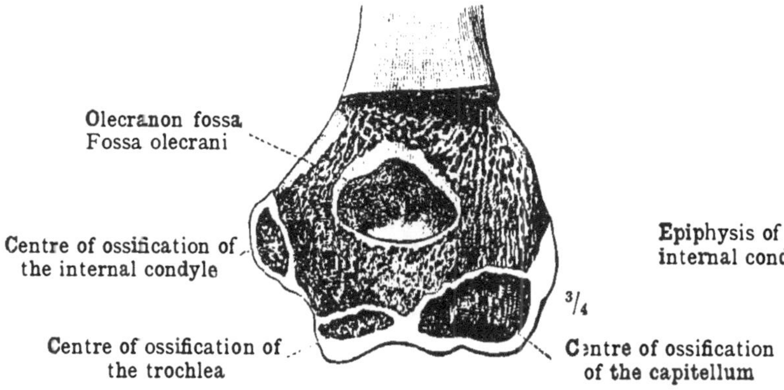

FIG. 256.—FROM A BOY AGED THIRTEEN YEARS.

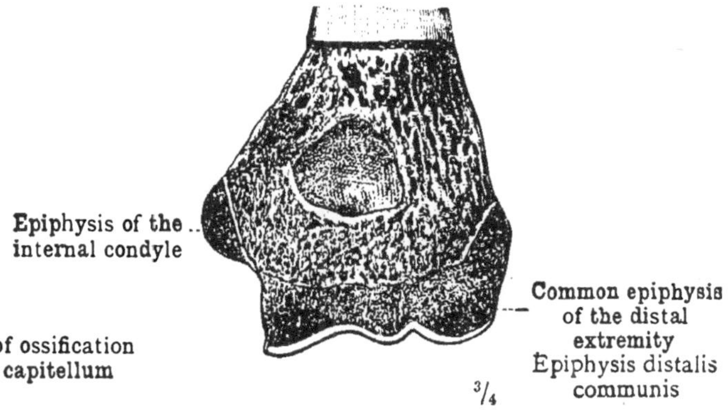

FIG. 257.—FROM A BOY AGED SEVENTEEN YEARS.

THE EPIPHYSES OF THE DISTAL EXTREMITY OF THE HUMERUS.

Development of the Humerus.

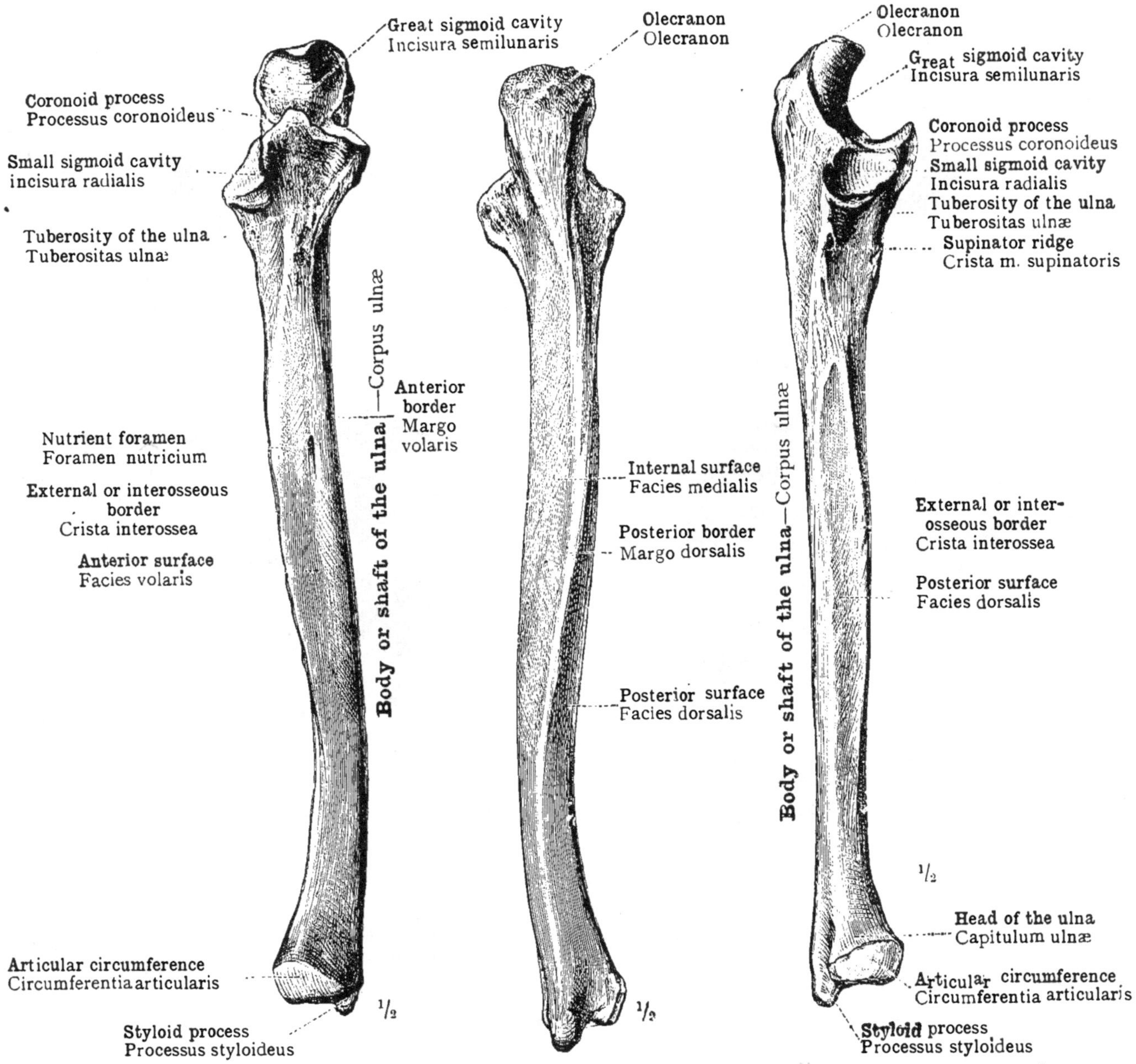

FIG. 258.—ANTERIOR ASPECT. FIG. 259.—POSTERIOR ASPECT. FIG. 260.—EXTERNAL ASPECT.

THE ULNA OF THE RIGHT SIDE.

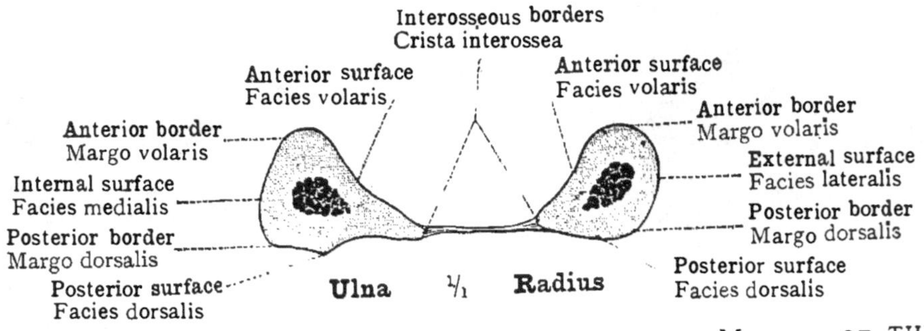

FIG. 261.—TRANSVERSE (HORIZONTAL) SECTION THROUGH THE MIDDLE OF THE ULNA AND THE RADIUS, WITH THE INTEROSSEOUS MEMBRANE, IN SUPINATION.

Ossa antibrachii—The bones of the forearm.

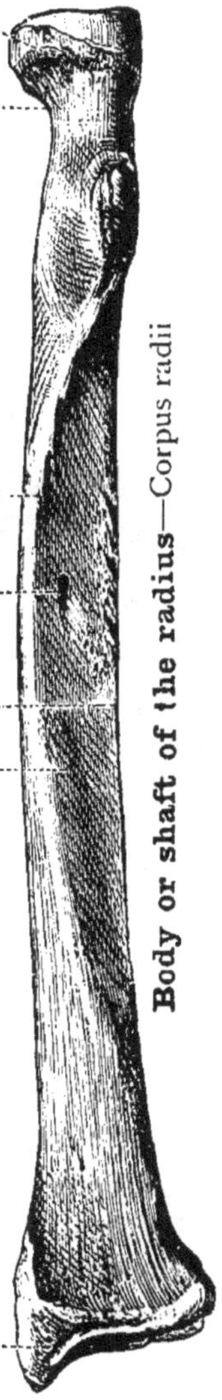

FIG. 262.—ANTERIOR ASPECT.

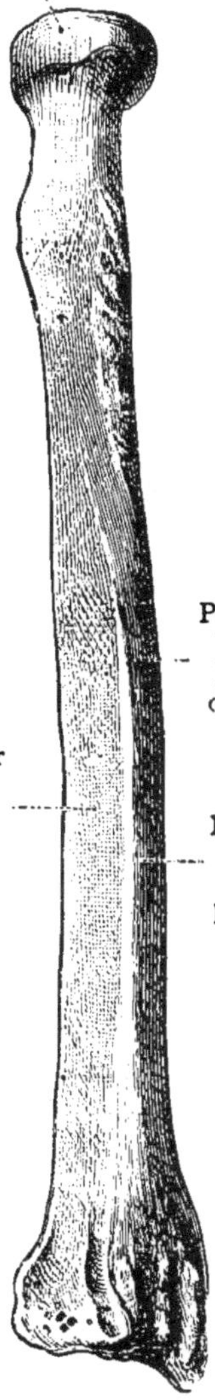

FIG. 263.—POSTERIOR ASPECT.

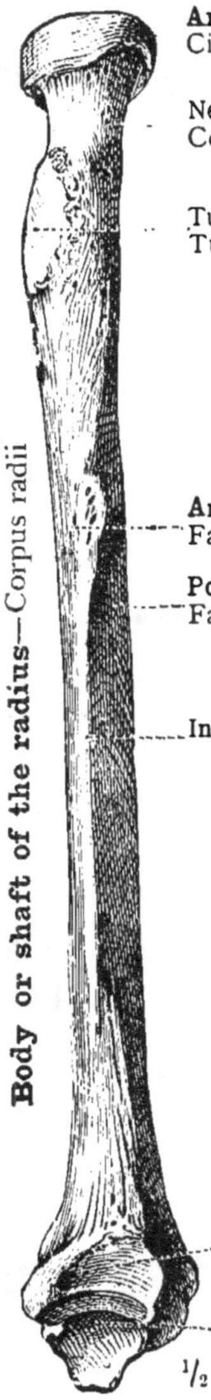

FIG. 264.—INTERNAL ASPECT.

THE RADIUS OF THE RIGHT SIDE.

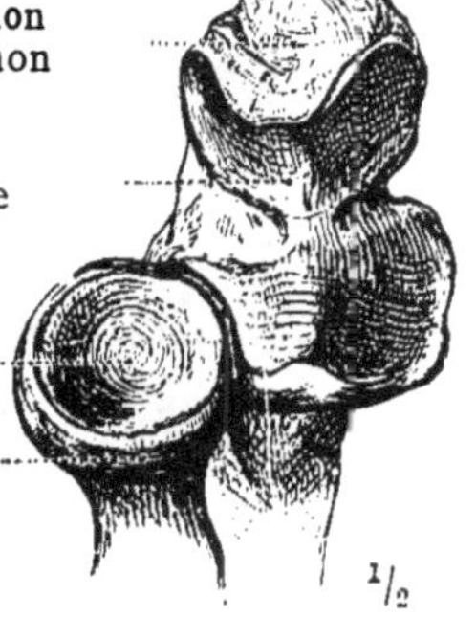

FIG. 265.—THE PROXIMAL EXTREMITIES OF THE BONES OF THE RIGHT FORE ARM SEEN FROM ABOVE.

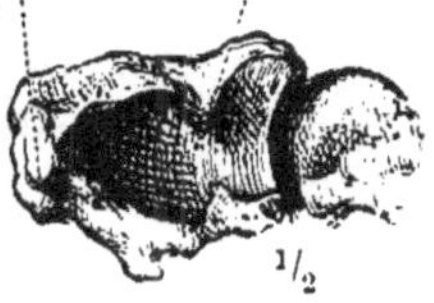

FIG. 266.—THE DISTAL EXTREMITIES OF THE BONES OF THE RIGHT FOREARM SEEN FROM BELOW.

Ossa antibrachii—The bones of the forearm.

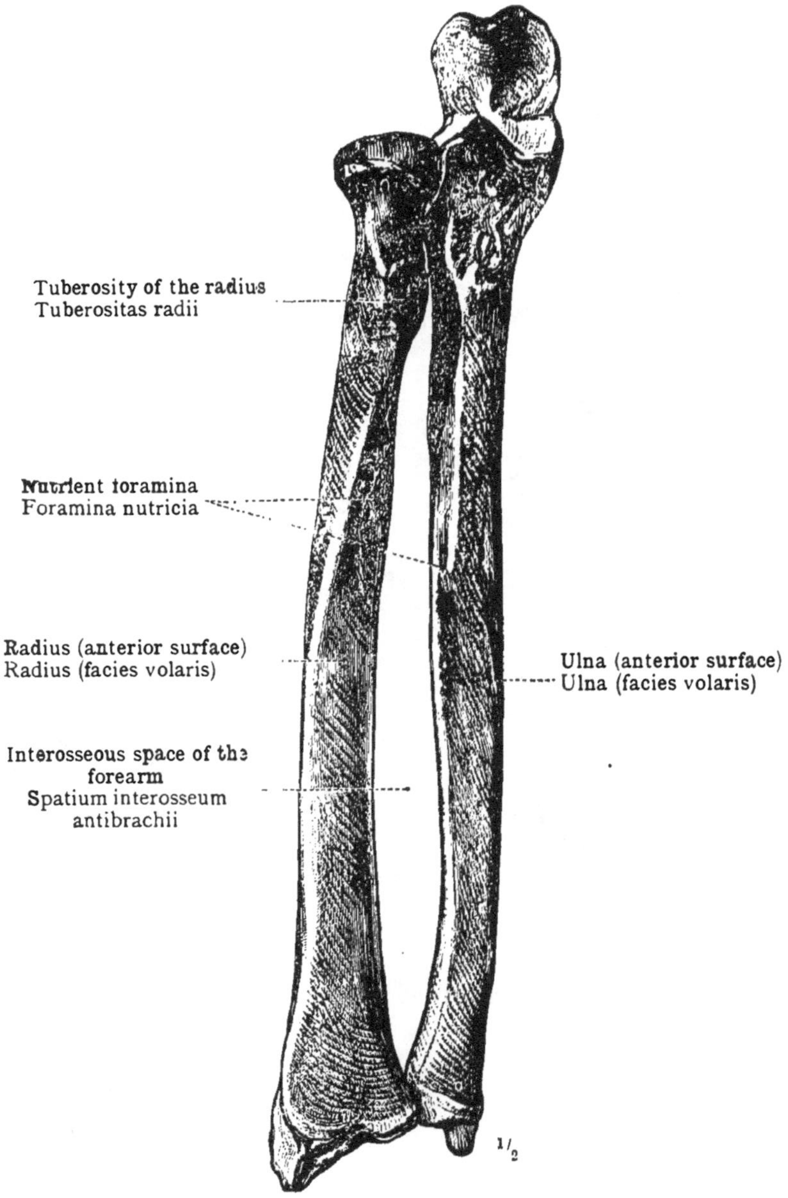

FIG. 267.—THE BONES OF THE RIGHT FOREARM, IN SUPINATION.

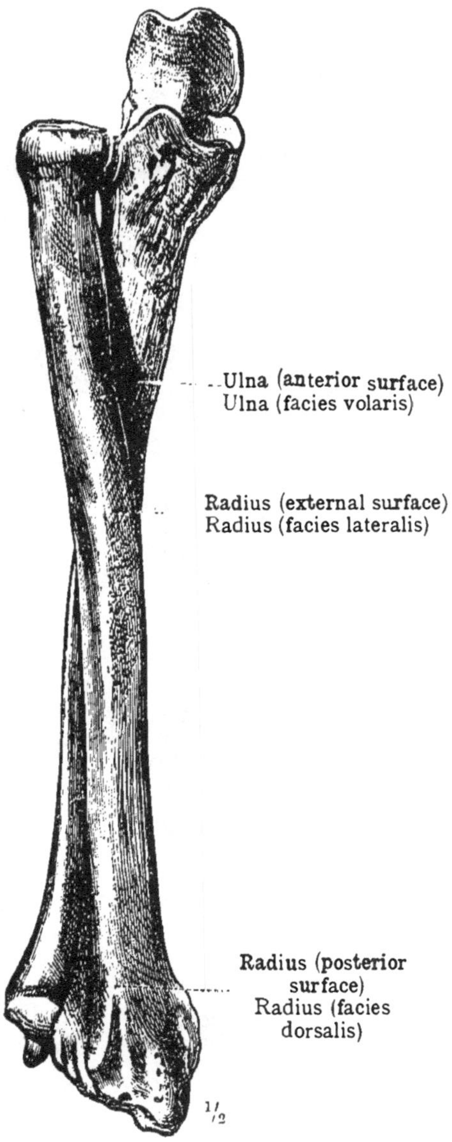

FIG. 268.—THE BONES OF THE RIGHT FOREARM, IN PRONATION.

The Bones of the Forearm in Supination and Pronation.

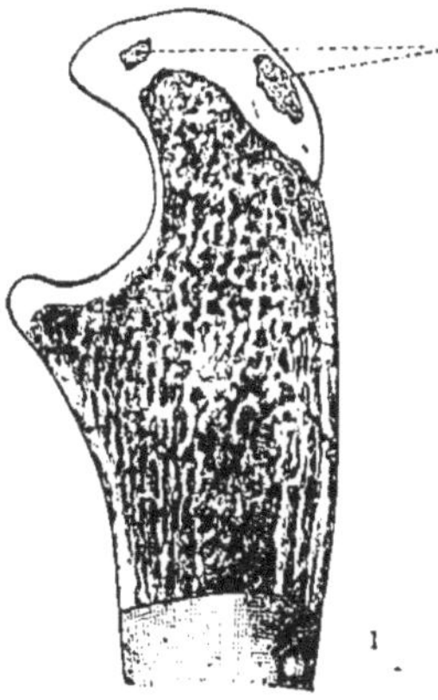

FIG 269.—FROM A BOY AGED
THIRTEEN YEARS.

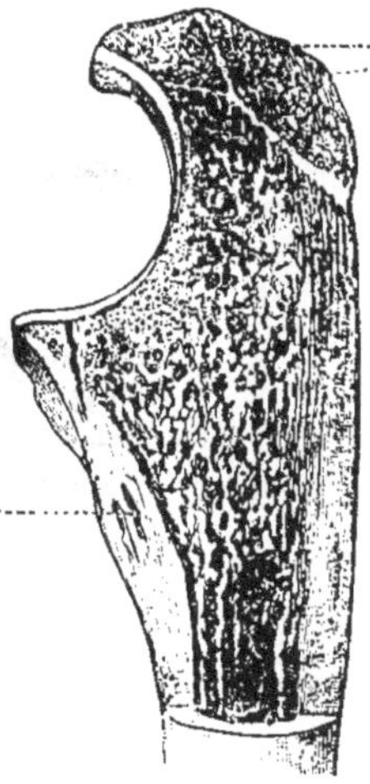

FIG. 270.—FROM A BOY AGED
SEVENTEEN YEARS.

THE DEVELOPMENT OF THE EPIPHYSIS OF THE PROXIMAL EXTREMITY OF THE ULNA.

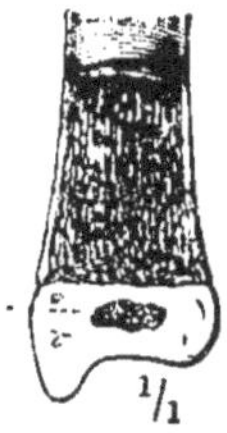

FIG. 271.—FROM A GIRL AGED
SIX YEARS.

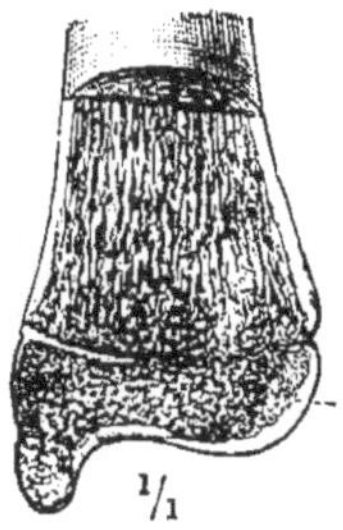

FIG. 272.—FROM A YOUNG MAN AGED
NINETEEN YEARS.

THE DEVELOPMENT OF THE EPIPHYSIS OF THE DISTAL EXTREMITY OF THE ULNA.

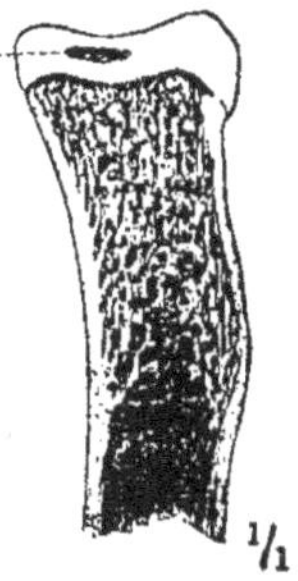

IG. 273.—FROM A BOY AGED FIVE YEARS.

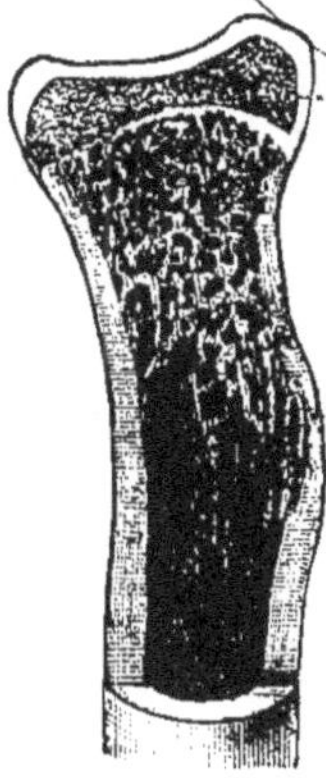

FIG. 274.—FROM A BOY AGED SEVENTEEN YEARS.

THE DEVELOPMENT OF THE EPIPHYSIS OF THE PROXIMAL EXTREMITY OF THE RADIUS.

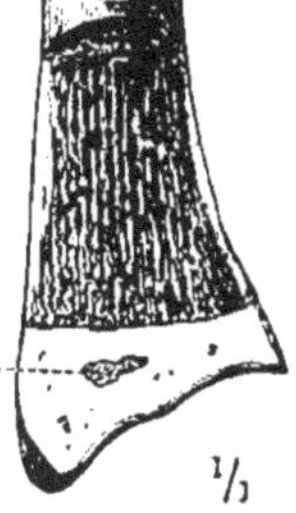

FIG. 275.—FROM A GIRL AGED
TWO YEARS.

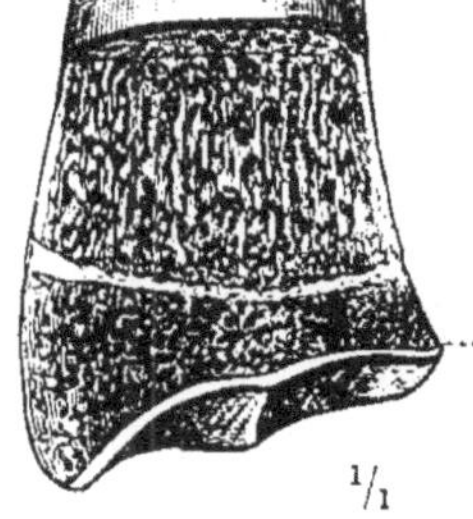

FIG. 276.—FROM A YOUNG MAN AGED
NINETEEN YEARS.

THE DEVELOPMENT OF THE EPIPHYSIS OF THE DISTAL EXTREMITY OF THE RADIUS.

Development of the Bones of the Forearm.

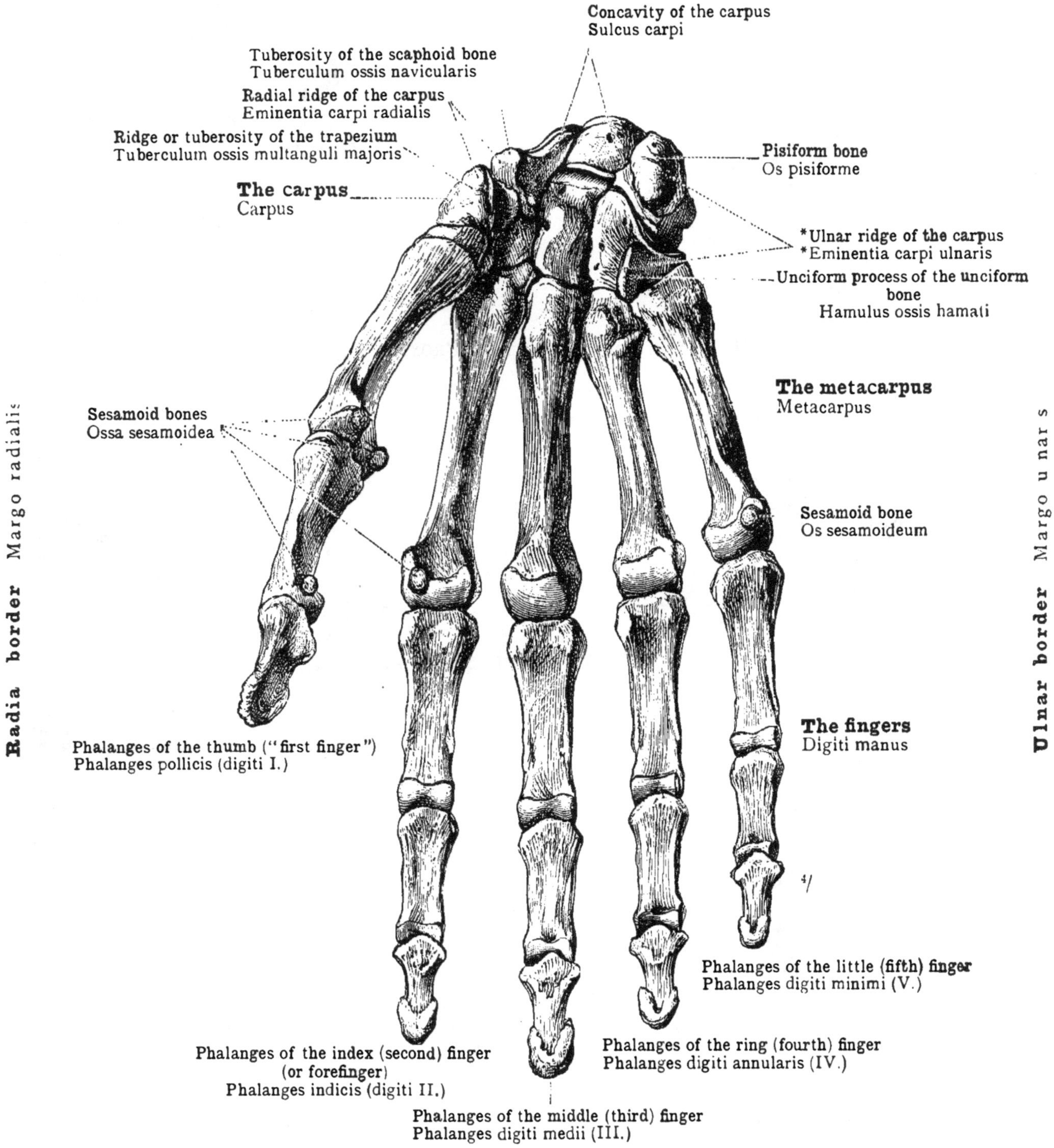

FIG. 277.—PALMAR ASPECT OF THE SKELETON OF THE RIGHT HAND (FACIES VOLARIS).

Skeleton manus—The skeleton of the hand.

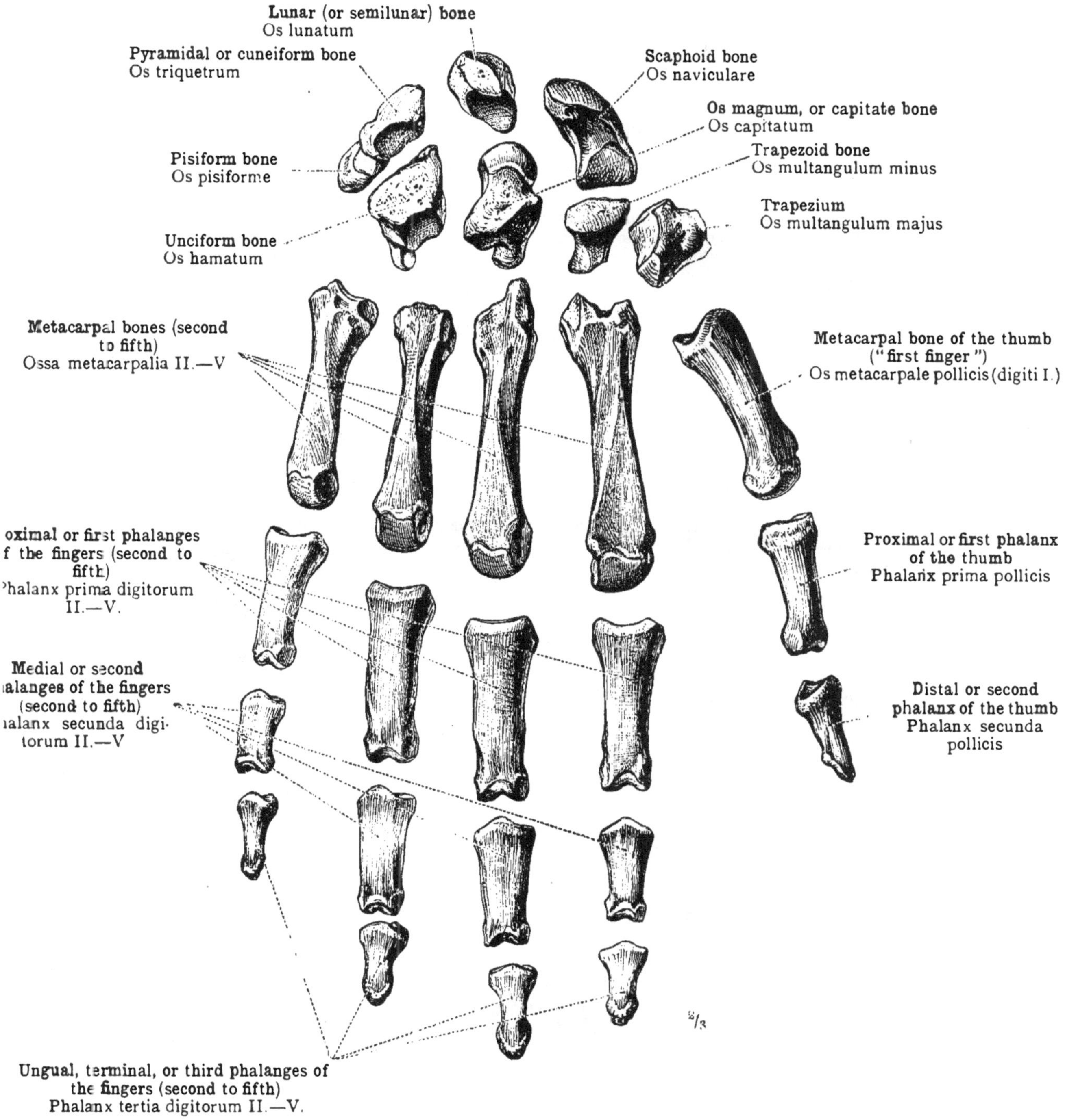

FIG. 278.—DORSAL ASPECT OF THE BONES OF THE RIGHT HAND SEEN FROM THE DORSAL SIDE (FACIES DORSALIS).

Skeleton manus—The skeleton of the hand.

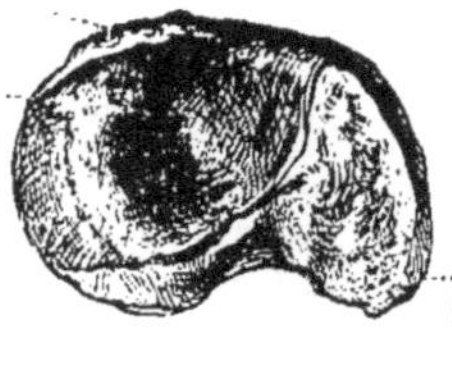

FIG. 279.—DISTAL ASPECT.

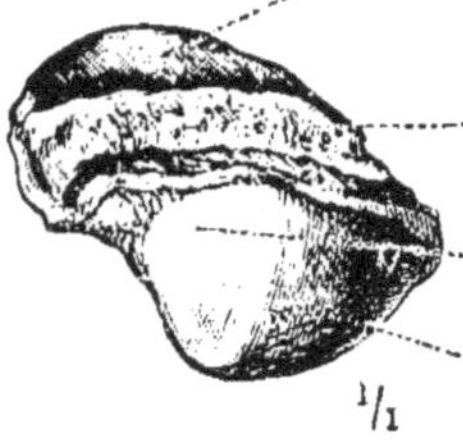

FIG. 280.—POSTERIOR ASPECT.

OS NAVICULARE MANUS—THE RIGHT SCAPHOID BONE

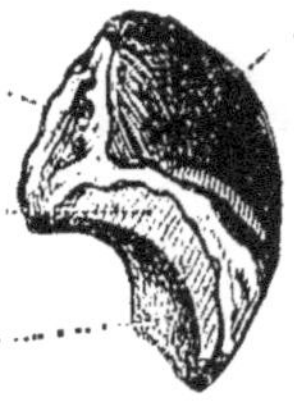

FIG. 281.—RADIAL ASPECT.

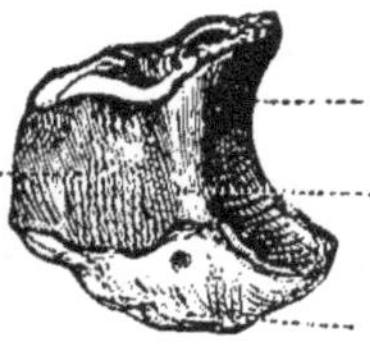

FIG. 282.—ULNAR ASPECT.

OS LUNATUM—THE RIGHT LUNAR (OR SEMILUNAR) BONE.

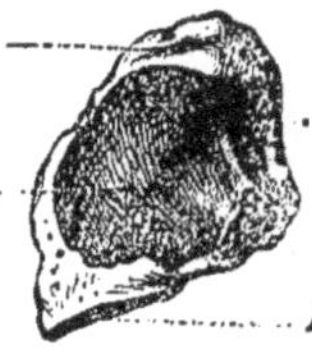

FIG. 283.—RADIAL ASPECT.

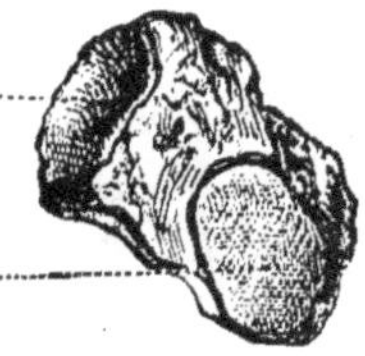

FIG. 284.—PALMAR ASPECT.

OS TRIQUETRUM—THE RIGHT PYRAMIDAL OR CUNEIFORM BONE.

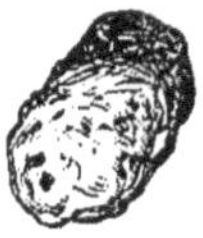

FIG. 285.—PALMAR ASPECT.

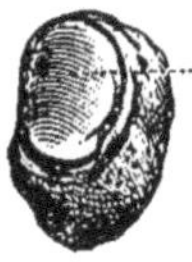

FIG. 286.—POSTERIOR ASPECT.

OS PISIFORME—THE RIGHT PISIFORM BONE.

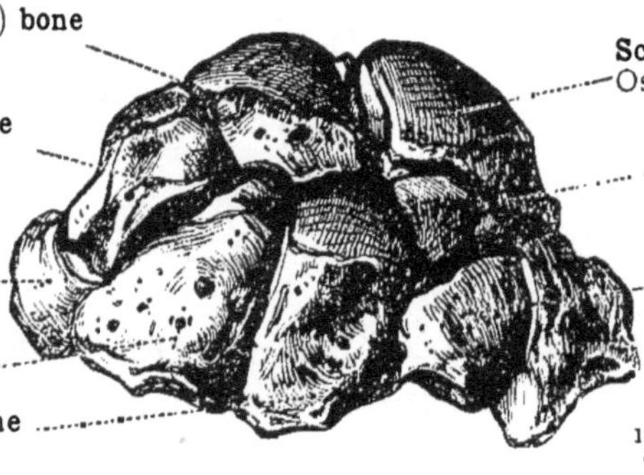

FIG. 287. THE POSTERIOR ASPECT OF THE RIGHT CARPUS, CONTAINING AN OS CENTRALE.

Ossa carpi—The bones of the carpus: first, superior, or proximal row.

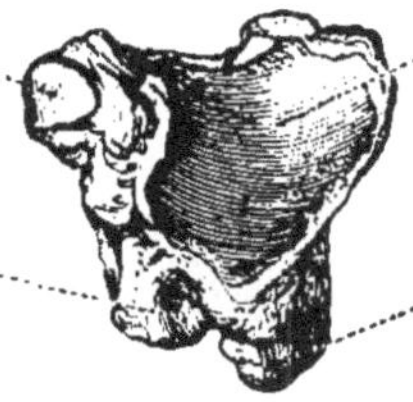

FIG. 288.—DISTAL ASPECT.

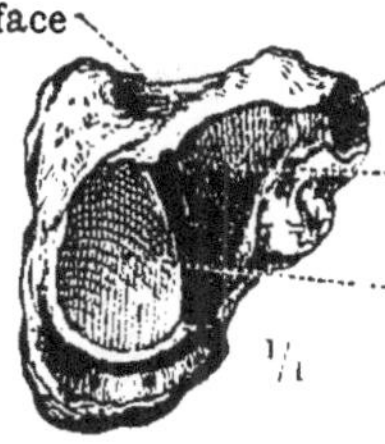

FIG. 289.—ULNAR ASPECT.

OS MULTANGULUM MAJUS—THE RIGHT TRAPEZIUM.

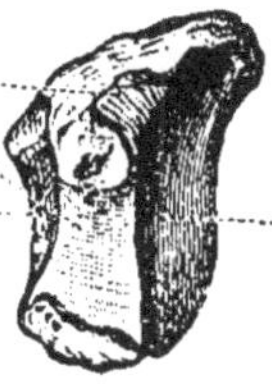

FIG. 290.—ULNAR ASPECT

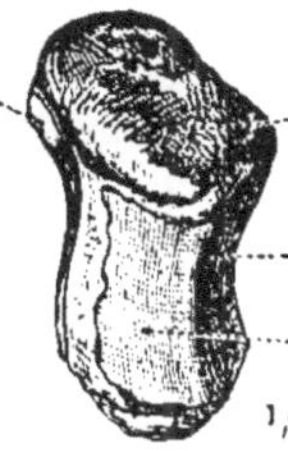

FIG. 291.—RADIAL ASPECT.

OS MULTANGULUM MINUS—THE RIGHT TRAPEZOID BONE.

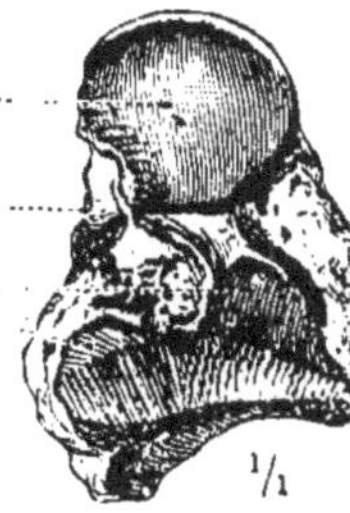

FIG. 292.—RADIAL ASPECT.

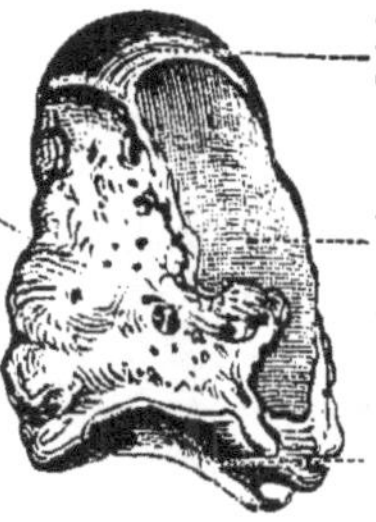

FIG. 293.—ULNAR ASPECT.

OS CAPITATUM—THE RIGHT OS MAGNUM OR CAPITATE BONE.

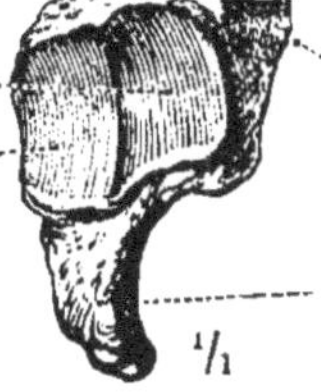

FIG. 294.—DISTAL ASPECT.

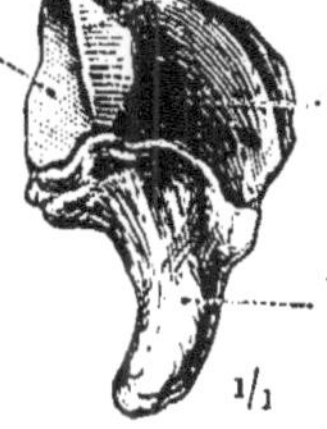

FIG. 295.—PROXIMAL ASPECT.

OS HAMATUM—THE RIGHT UNCIFORM BONE.

Ossa carpi—The bones of the carpus: second, inferior, or distal row.

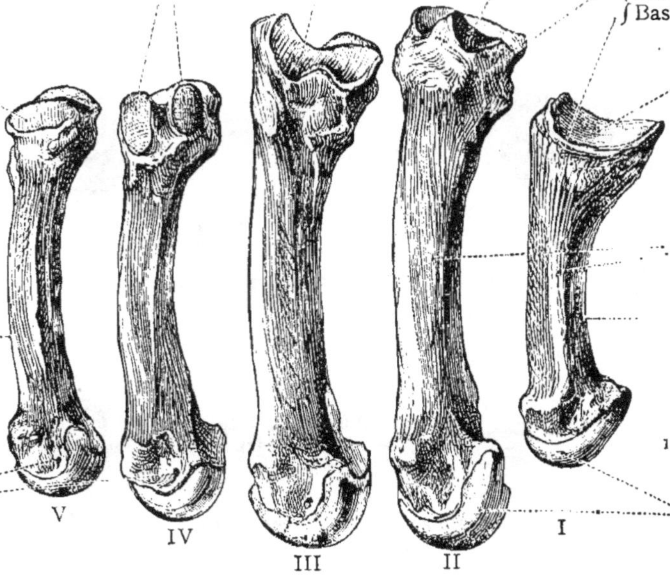

FIG. 296.—RADIAL ASPECT OF THE FIVE METACARPAL BONES OF THE RIGHT HAND.

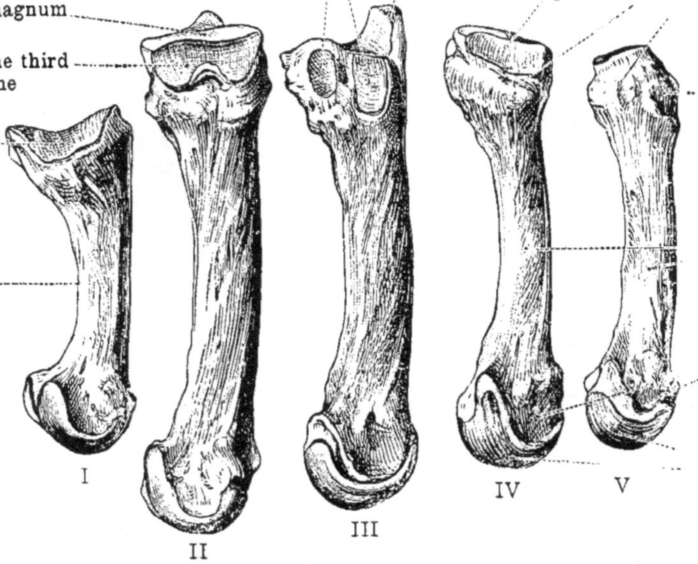

FIG. 297.—ULNAR ASPECT OF THE FIVE METACARPAL BONES OF THE RIGHT HAND.

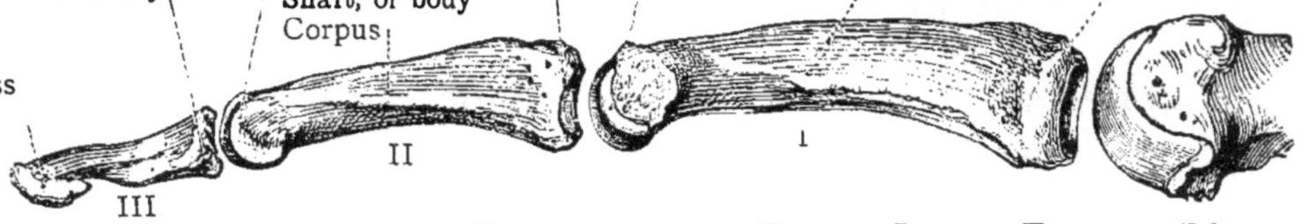

FIG. 298.—RADIAL ASPECT OF THE BONES OF THE RIGHT INDEX FINGER (MARGO RADIALIS DIGITI SECUNDI).

The Metacarpal Bones of the Hand and the Phalanges of the Fingers.

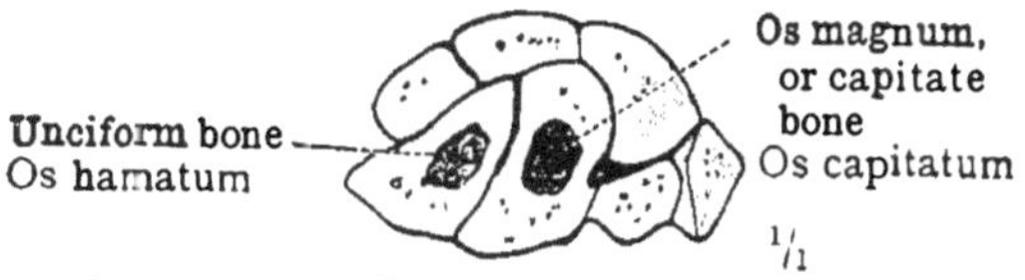

FIG. 299.—IN THE SECOND YEAR OF LIFE.

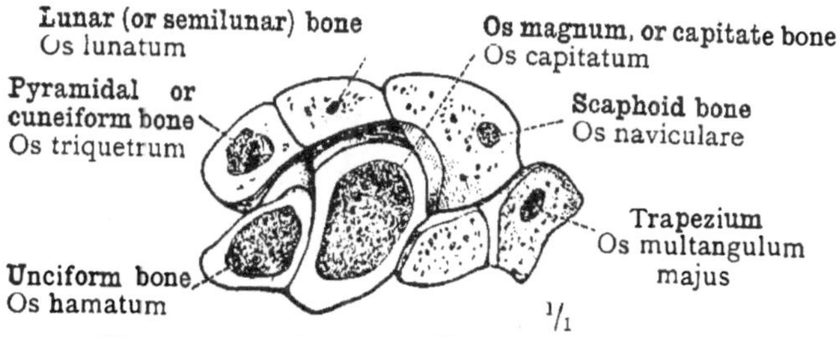

FIG. 300.—IN THE SEVENTH YEAR OF LIFE.

CENTRES OF OSSIFICATION OF THE CARPUS (SECTIONS PARALLEL TO THE POSTERIOR SURFACE).

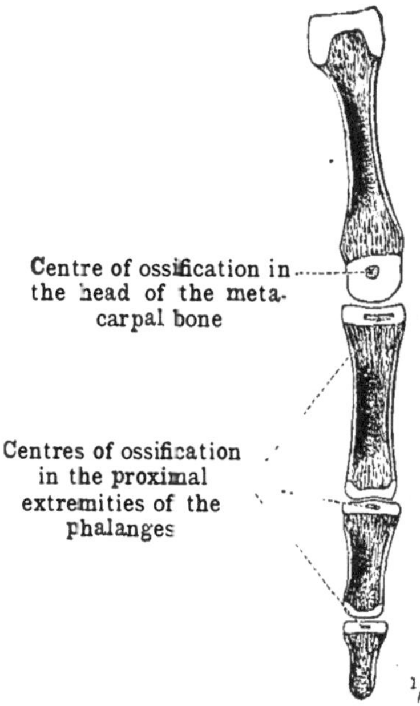

FIG. 301.—MIDDLE FINGER IN THE SECOND YEAR OF LIFE.

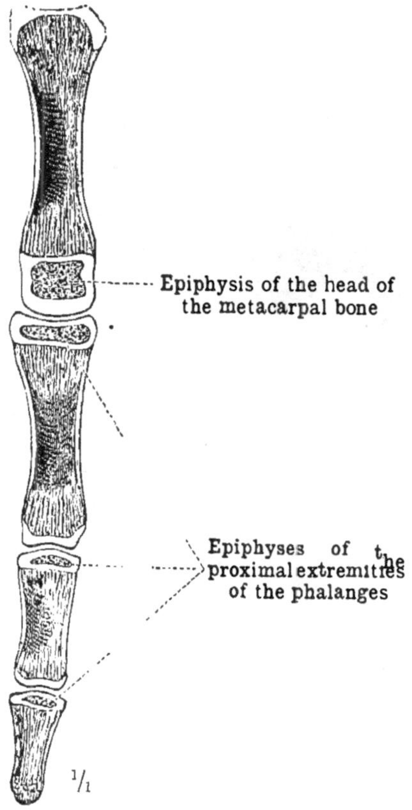

FIG. 302.—MIDDLE FINGER IN THE SEVENTH YEAR OF LIFE.

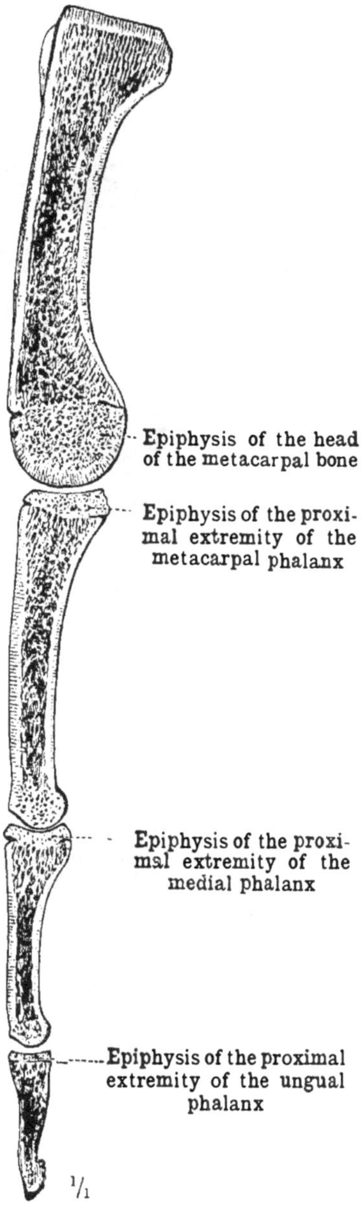

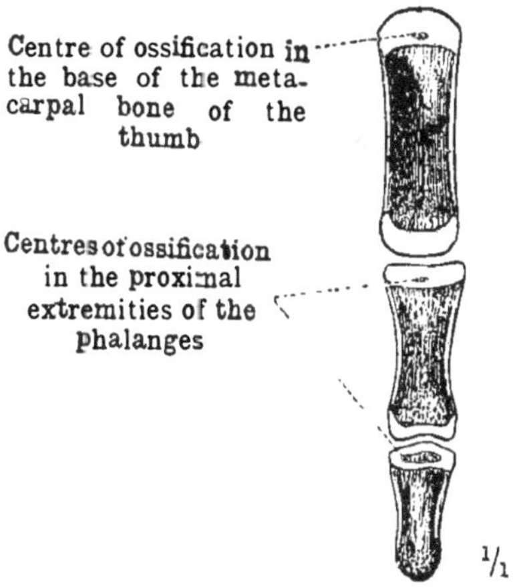

FIG. 304.—BONES OF THE THUMB IN THE FOURTH YEAR OF LIFE.

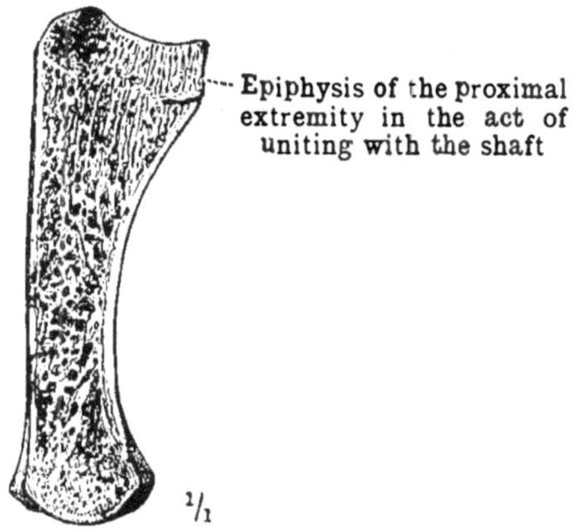

FIG. 305.—METACARPAL BONE OF THE THUMB IN THE EIGHTEENTH YEAR OF LIFE.

FIG. 303.—EPIPHYSES OF THE BONES OF THE MIDDLE FINGER IN THE ACT OF UNITING WITH THE SHAFTS: SEVENTEENTH YEAR OF LIFE.

Development of the Bones of the Hand.

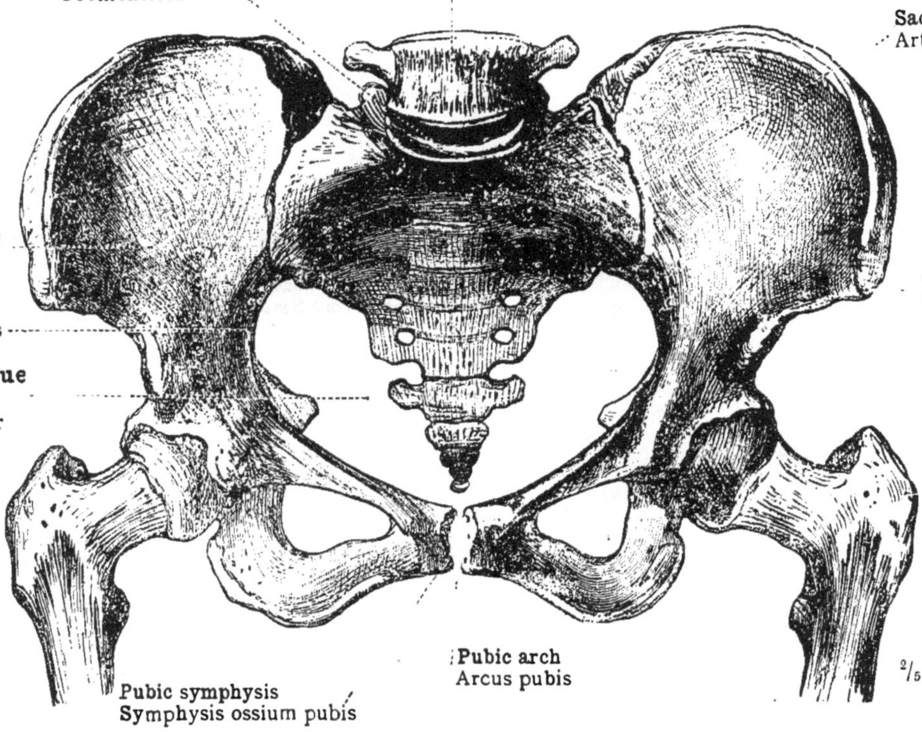

FIG. 306.—PELVIS MULIEBRIS—THE FEMALE PELVIS. ANTERIOR ASPECT.

The formation of the pelvis out of the sacrum and coccyx and the two innominate bones. The iliac portions of the innominate bones with the base of the sacrum constitute the upper or false pelvis; the pubic and ischiatic portions of the innominate bones with the sacrum and the coccyx constitute the lower or true pelvis; the boundary between the false and the true pelvis corresponds with the upper aperture or entrance of the true pelvis, the line separating the two being known as the brim or inlet of the true pelvis. Regarded as the means of attachment of the lower limb to the trunk, the pelvis is the cingulum extremitatis inferioris, or pelvic girdle.

Cingulum extremitatis inferioris—Pelvic girdle.

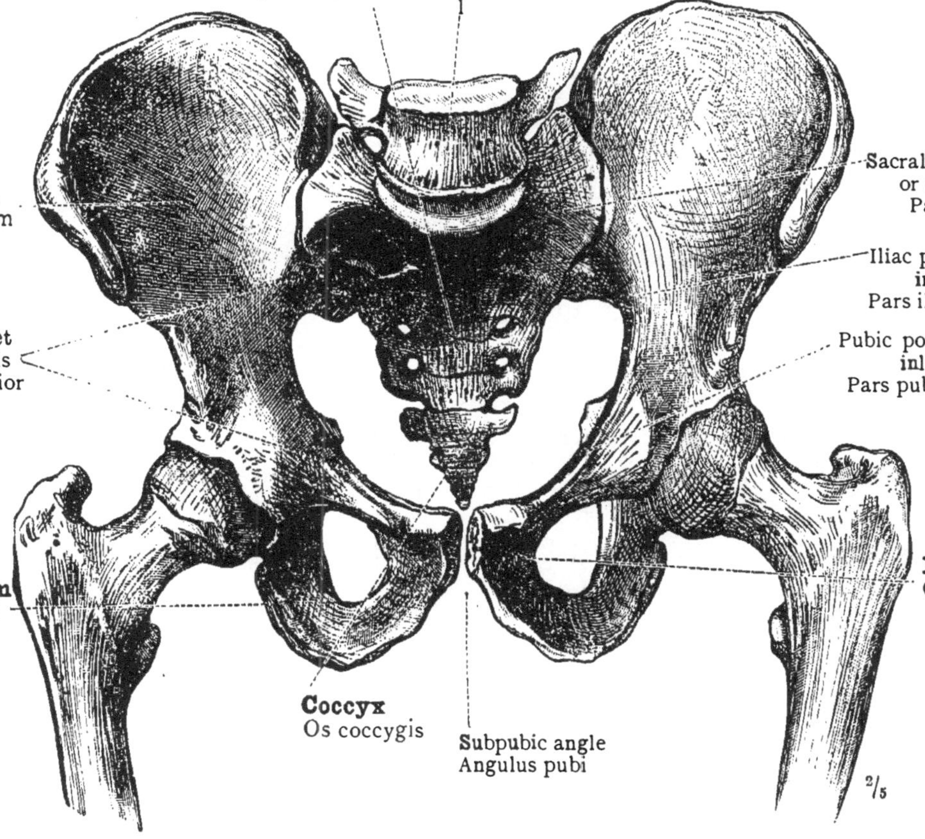

FIG. 307.—PELVIS VIRILIS—THE MALE PELVIS. ANTERIOR ASPECT.

The upper or false and the lower or true pelvis, pelvis major and pelvis minor. The brim of the true pelvis is divided into a sacral, an iliac, and a pubic portion.

Cingulum extremitatis inferioris—Pelvic girdle.

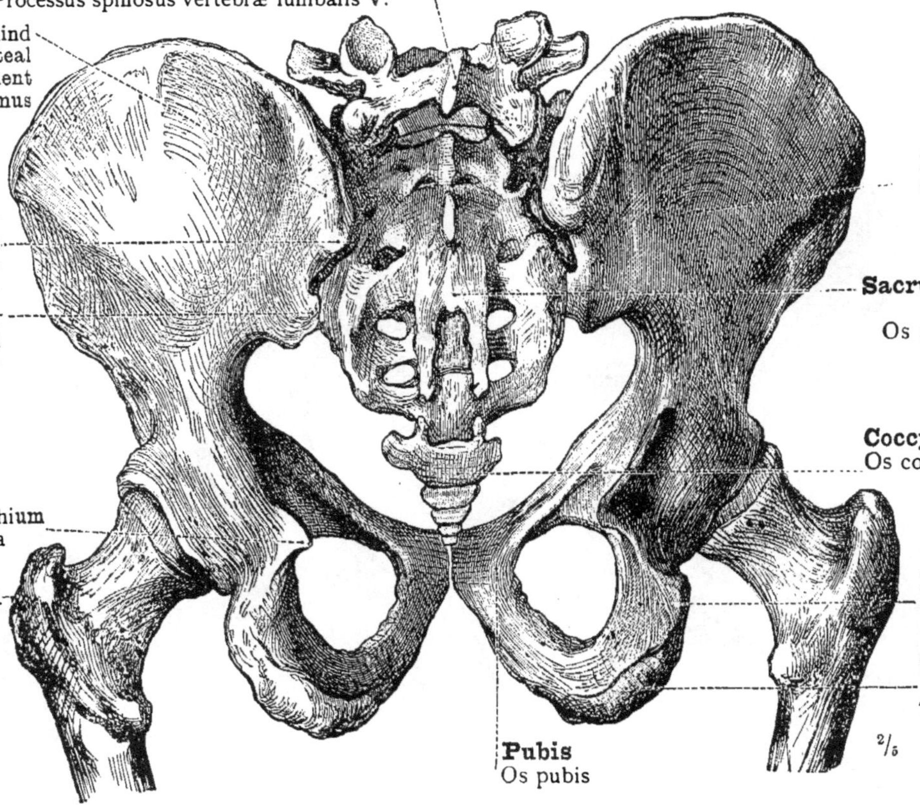

FIG. 308.—PELVIS VIRILIS—THE MALE PELVIS. POSTERIOR ASPECT.

The pelvic outlet, apertura pelvis (minoris) inferior, in the bony pelvis appears to be bounded on either side by the lower borders of the pubis and the ischium and the greater and lesser sciatic notches, incisuræ ischiadicæ major et minor, and behind by the projecting part of the sacrum and by the coccyx. But inasmuch as on either side there are two strong ligaments arising from the sacrum and coccyx, the great and the small sacrosciatic ligaments, ligamenta sacrotuberosum et sacrospinosum, which stretch across the two sciatic notches, and thus enlarge the posterior and lateral walls of the true pelvis, by this means the sciatic notches are filled in, and the outlet of the pelvis is notably diminished in size.

Cingulum extremitatis inferioris—Pelvic girdle.

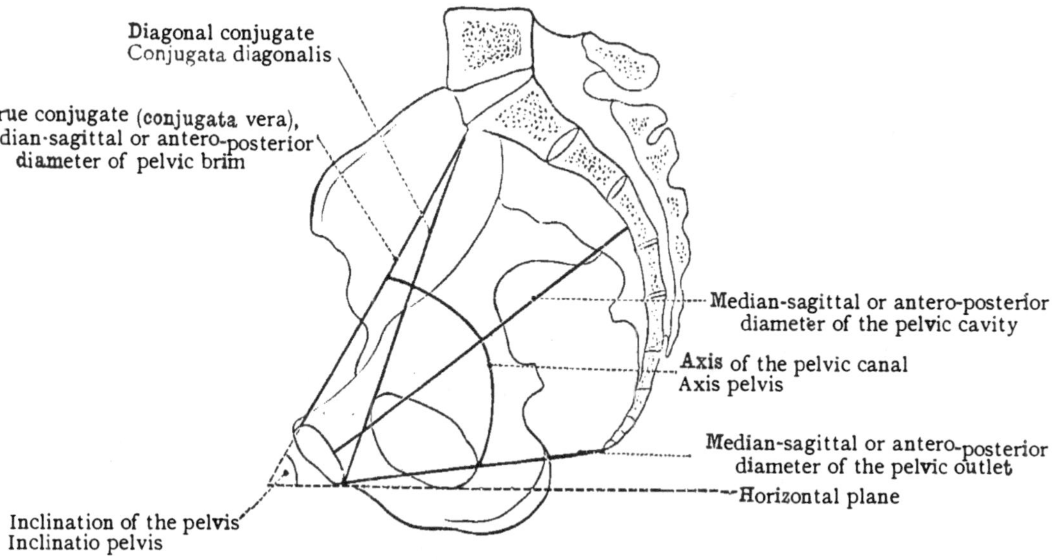

FIG. 309.—THE MEDIAN-SAGITTAL OR ANTERO-POSTERIOR DIAMETERS OF THE TRUE PELVIS.

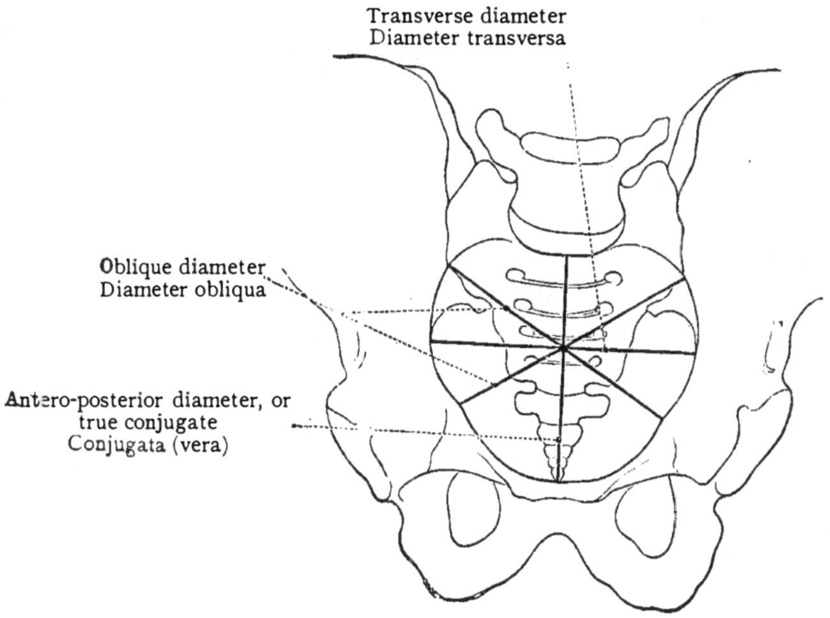

FIG. 310.—THE DIAMETERS OF THE PELVIC INLET (APERTURA PELVIS SUPERIOR).

The Principal Diameters of the True Pelvis.

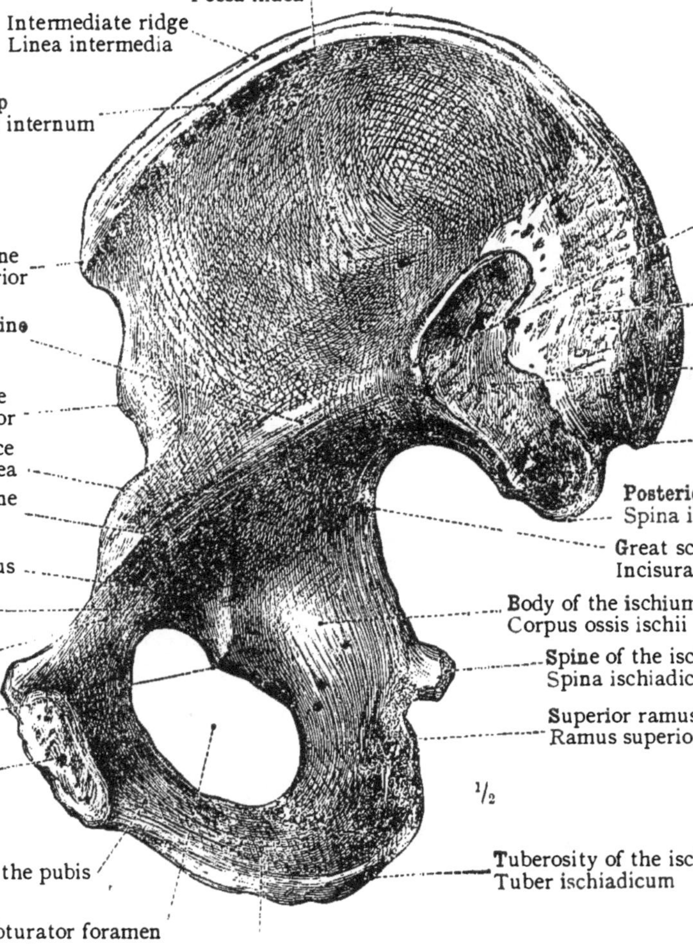

[1] This term, which is seldom used by English anatomists, denotes the posterior fifth of the crest of the ilium and the rough surface of bone immediately below the crest on either side.—Tr.

Fig. 311.—The Right Hip-Bone. Inner Aspect.

The ilium forms the upper part of the os innominatum. The slightly concave inner surface of the upper and anterior part of the ilium, known as the iliac fossa, is directed towards the observer; behind the fossa is the auricular surface for articulation with the sacrum; and behind the auricular surface is the internal rough surface of the *tuberosity of the ilium[1]. The upper border of the ilium is the iliac crest, the anterior extremity of which forms the anterior superior iliac spine, the posterior extremity, the posterior superior iliac spine. From the anterior border of the ilium projects the anterior inferior iliac spine, from the posterior border, the posterior inferior iliac spine. The superior or ascending and the inferior or descending ramus of the pubis and the superior and inferior ramus of the ischium, surrounding the obturator foramen, are all seen from the internal or pelvic aspect. The surface of the pubic symphysis, by means of which the two pubic bones articulate, forms the internal limiting surface of the os pubis.

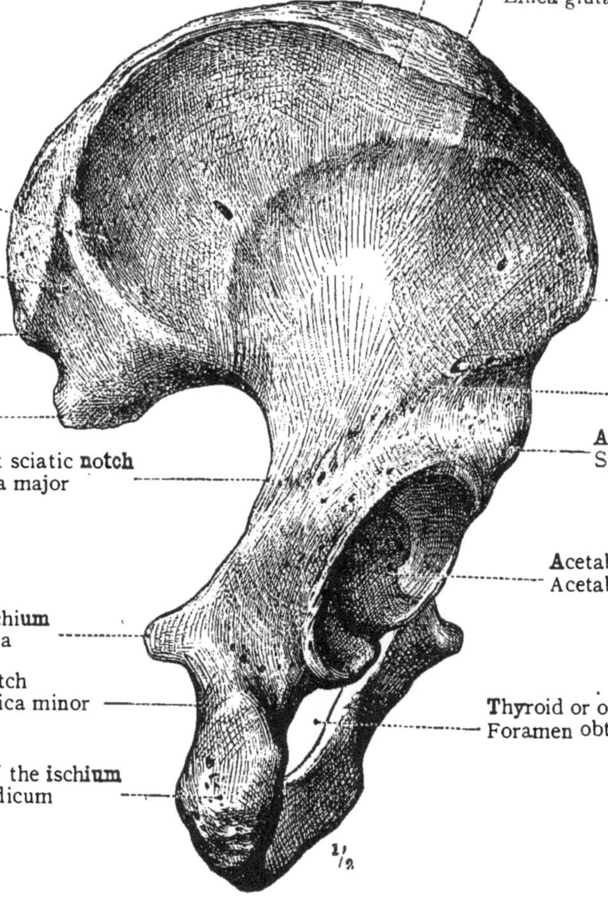

FIG. 312.—THE RIGHT HIP-BONE, OUTER SIDE. POSTERIOR ASPECT.

The outer surface of the ilium is seen, divided by the three gluteal lines into areas from which the three gluteal muscles respectively arise. The spine of the ischium projects backwards from the posterior border of the hip-bone ; above this spine is the iliosciatic or great sciatic notch, below it is the small sciatic notch. The lowest portion of the bone is formed by the backwardly projecting tuberosity of the ischium. The acetabulum is viewed obliquely from behind.

Os coxæ—Hip-bone.

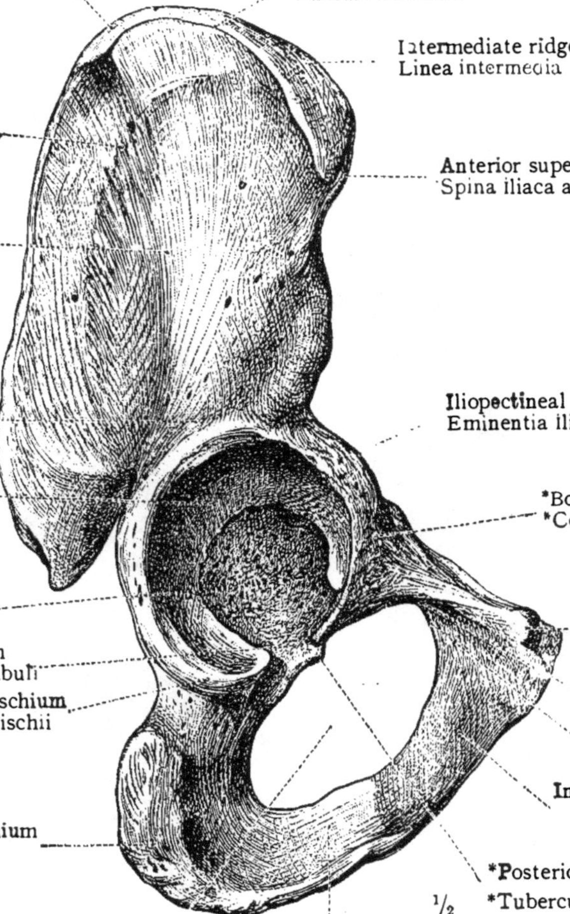

Body of the pubis: The use of this term by English anatomists is a variable one. Macalister, whose terminology here, as usual, is in conformity with that of Continental anatomists, writes: "The pubis consists of a body which forms a little less than one-fifth of the acetabulum . . ."; Quain, on the other hand, writes: "The flat portion between the rami [of the pubis] is the body"; and Young, in his "Synopsis of Human Anatomy" (U.S.), follows Quain's usage. The Continental application of the term has, however, the advantage in the point of consistency, the *body* being then, in the case of each of the three elements of the hip-bone, the thickened portion taking part in the formation of the acetabulum, of which the *body of the pubis* constitutes about one-fifth, the *body of the ilium* nearly two-fifths, and the *body of the ischium* the remainder.—TR.

FIG. 313.—THE RIGHT HIP-BONE, OUTER SIDE. SEEN FROM THE RIGHT.

For this illustration the hip-bone has been so placed that a direct view of the interior of the acetabulum is obtained; this consists of two portions, the rough, nearly circular fossa of the acetabulum, and the horse-shoe shaped articular surface (facies lunata—covered in the recent state with cartilage); opposite the fossa of the acetabulum, the rim bounding the depression is interrupted by the cotyloid notch (incisura acetabuli). The three bones which, separate at first, subsequently unite to form the hip-bone, all take part in the formation of the acetabulum (*see note [1] above*).

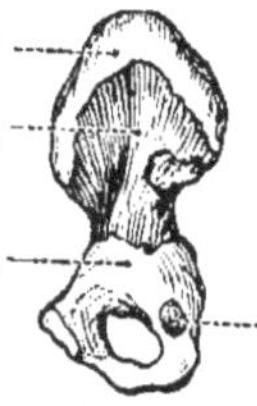

FIG. 314.—IN THE FIFTH MONTH OF FŒTAL LIFE (MONTHS OF FOUR WEEKS EACH).

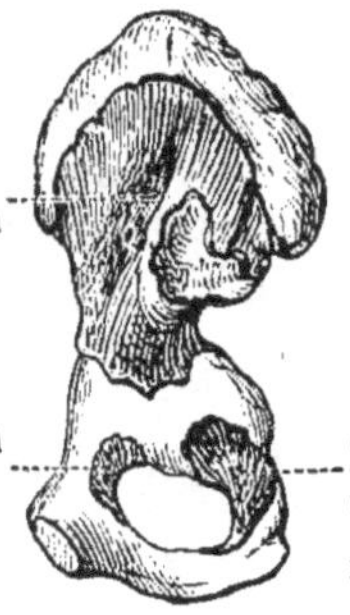

FIG. 315.—IN THE SIXTH MONTH OF FŒTAL LIFE (MONTHS OF FOUR WEEKS EACH).

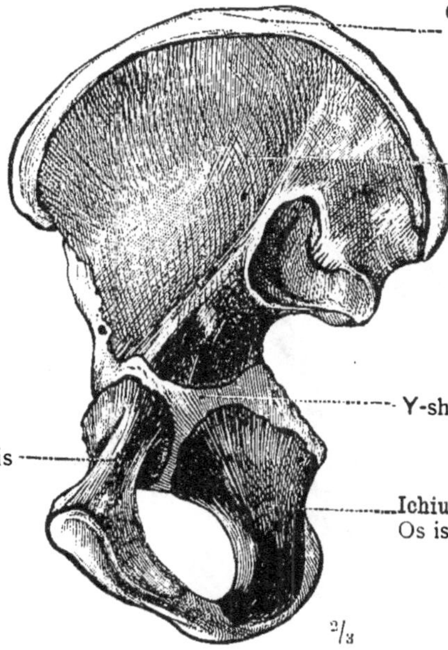

FIG. 316.—IN THE FOURTH YEAR OF LIFE.

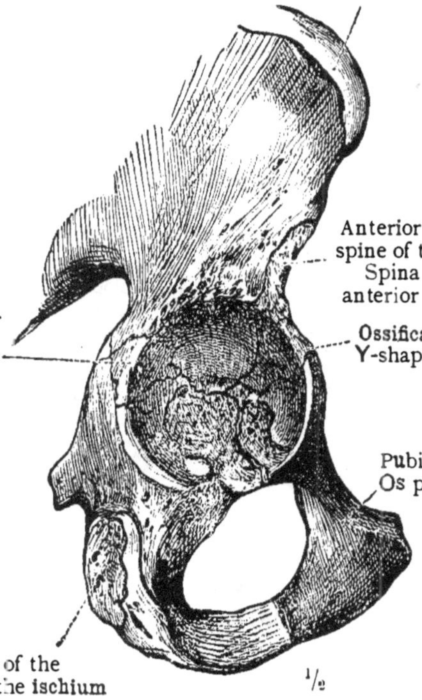

FIG. 317.—IN THE FOURTEENTH YEAR OF LIFE.

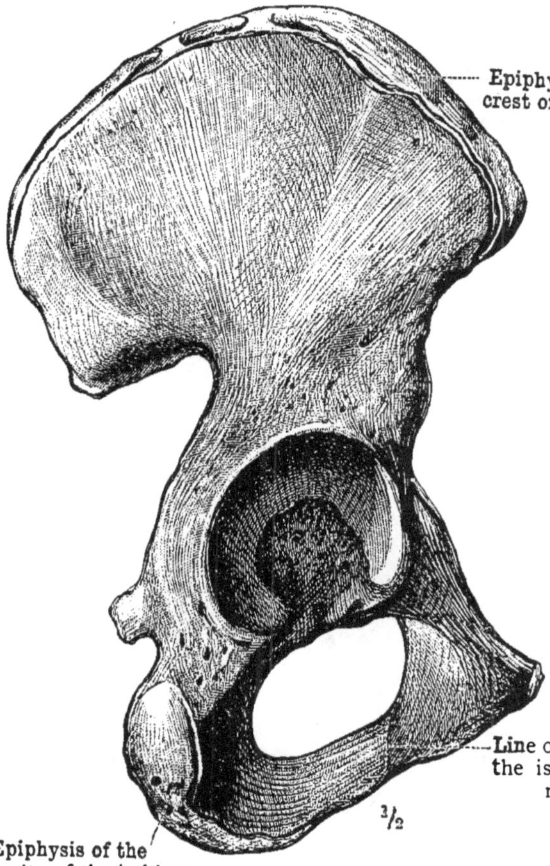

FIG. 318.—IN THE SEVENTEENTH YEAR OF LIFE.

Development of the Hip-Bone.

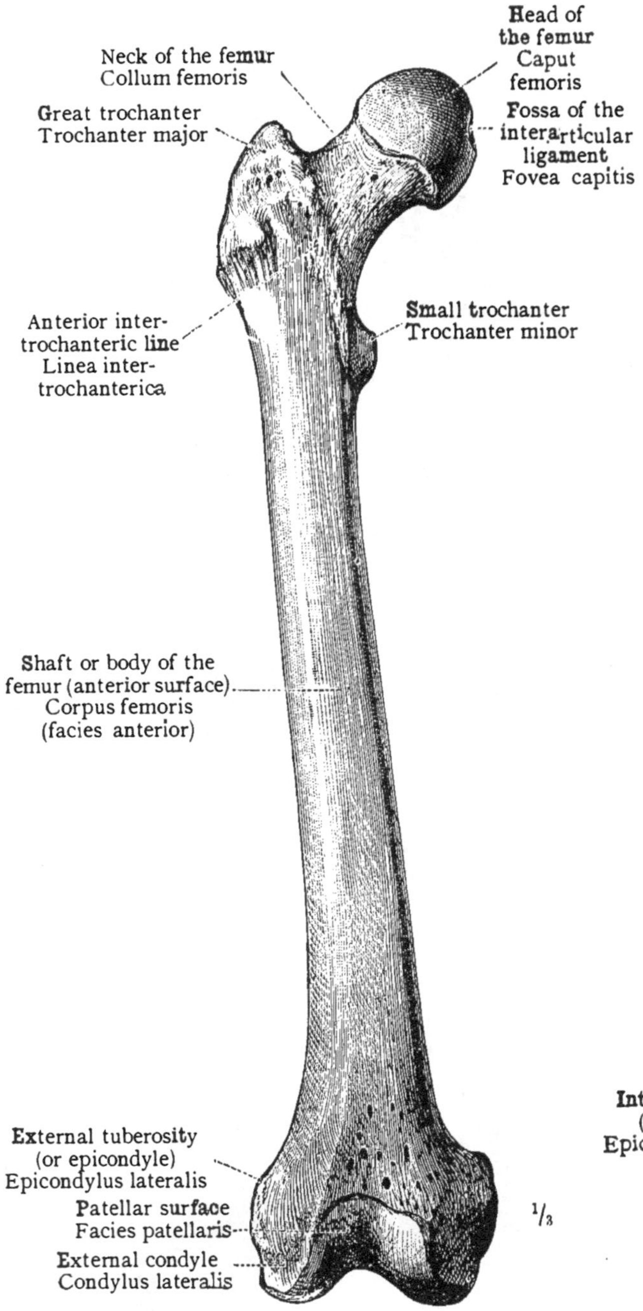

FIG. 319.—THE RIGHT FEMUR, ANTERIOR ASPECT.

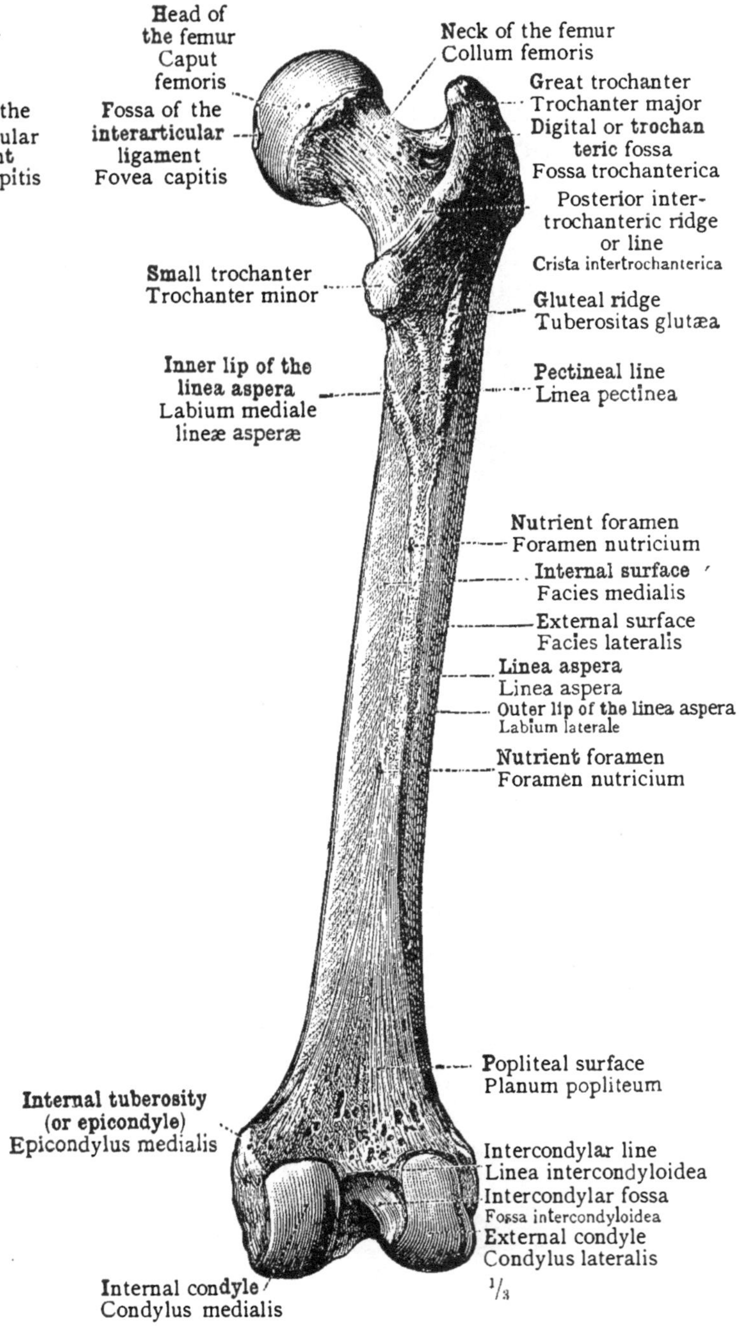

FIG. 320.—THE RIGHT FEMUR, POSTERIOR ASPECT.

Femur—The femur, or thigh-bone.

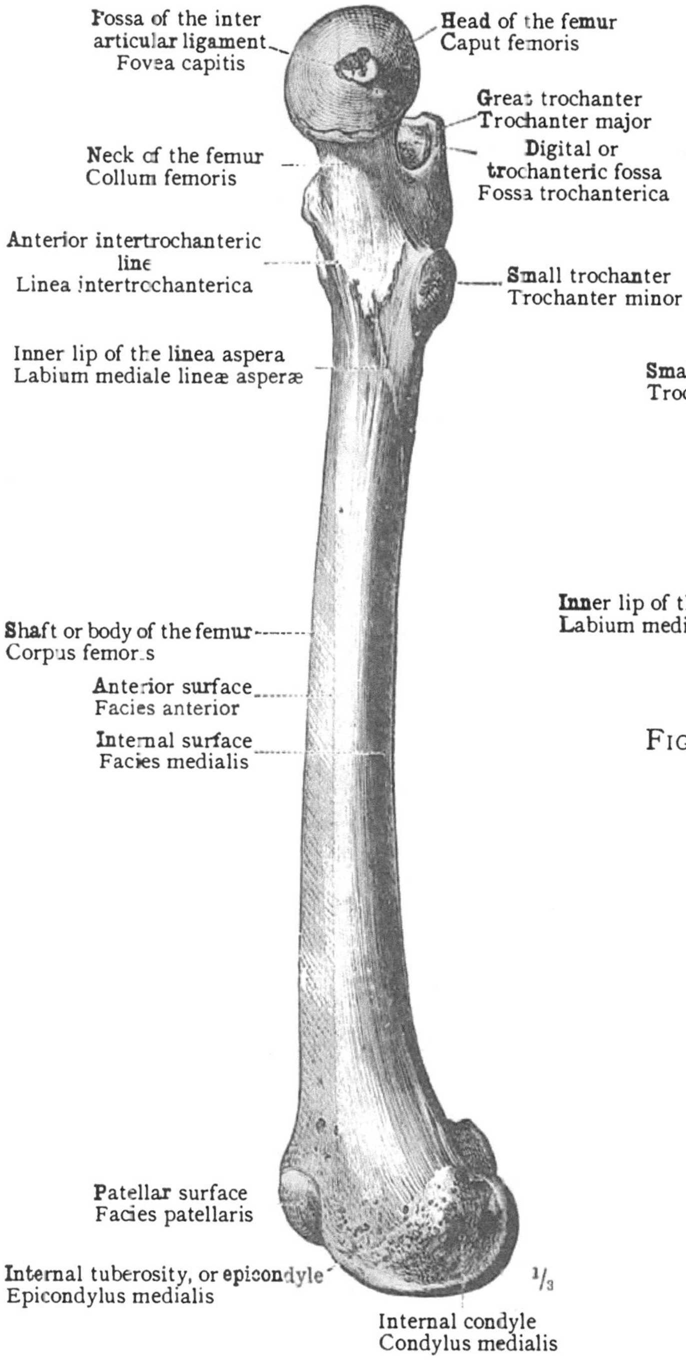

FIG. 321.—THE RIGHT FEMUR, INTERNAL ASPECT.

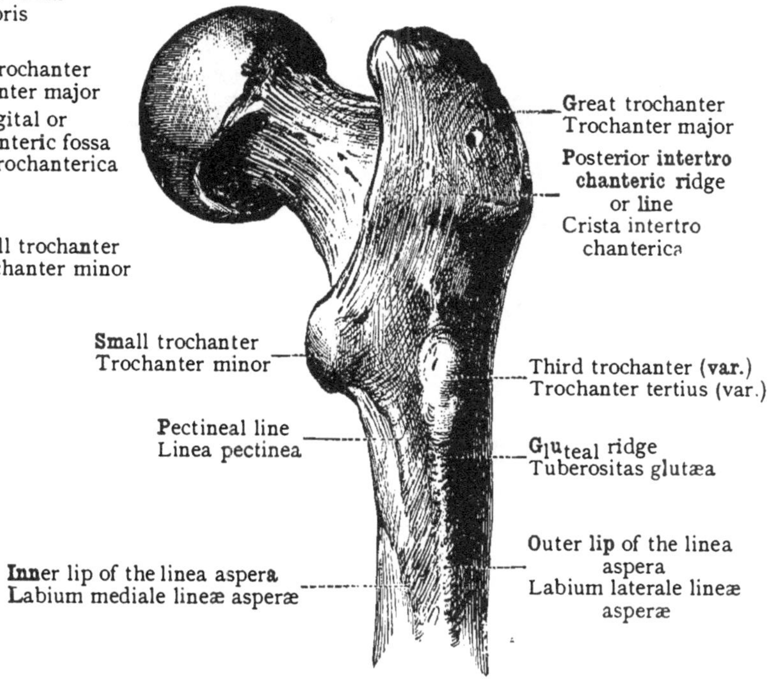

FIG. 322.—THE UPPER PORTION OF THE RIGHT FEMUR: THIRD TROCHANTER (VAR.). SEEN FROM BEHIND.

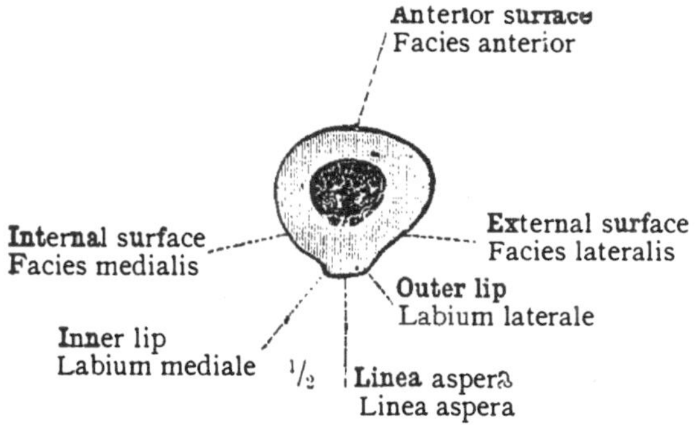

FIG. 323.—TRANSVERSE SECTION THROUGH THE MIDDLE OF THE SHAFT OF THE RIGHT FEMUR.

Femur—The femur.

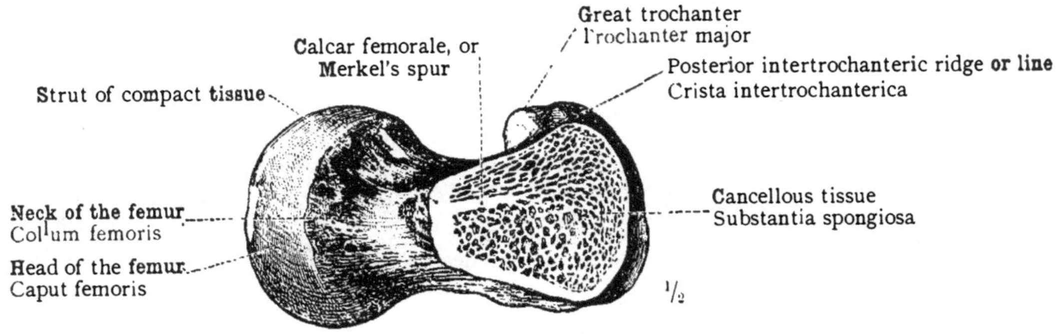

FIG. 324.—HORIZONTAL SECTION THROUGH THE PROXIMAL EXTREMITY OF THE RIGHT FEMUR, ABOVE THE SMALL TROCHANTER, TO SHOW THE CALCAR FEMORALE.

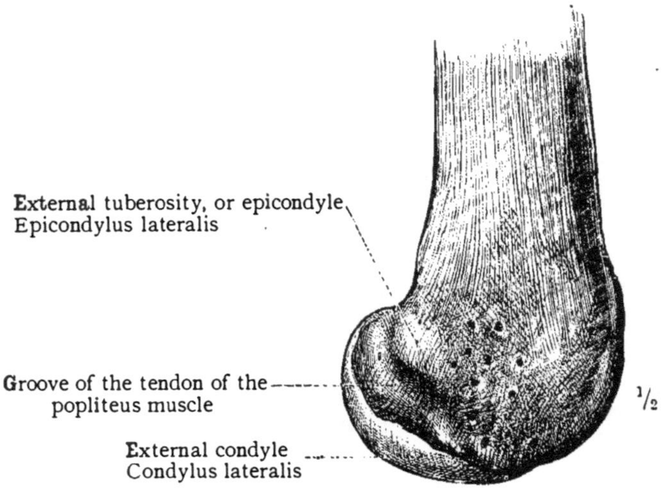

FIG. 325.—DISTAL EXTREMITY OF THE RIGHT FEMUR. SEEN FROM THE OUTER SIDE.

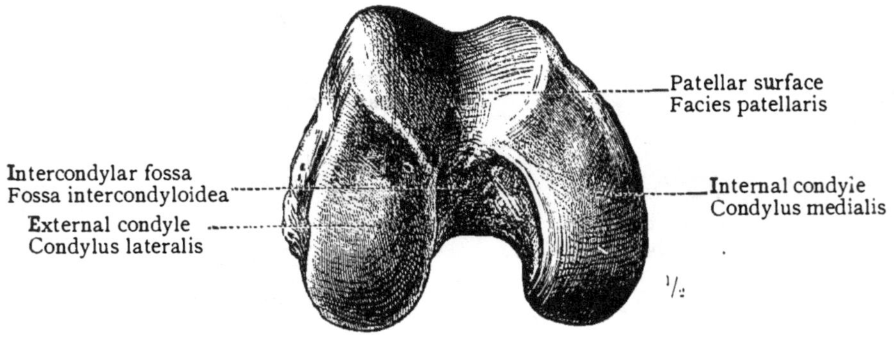

FIG. 326.—DISTAL ARTICULAR EXTREMITY OF THE RIGHT FEMUR. SEEN FROM BELOW.

Femur—The femur.

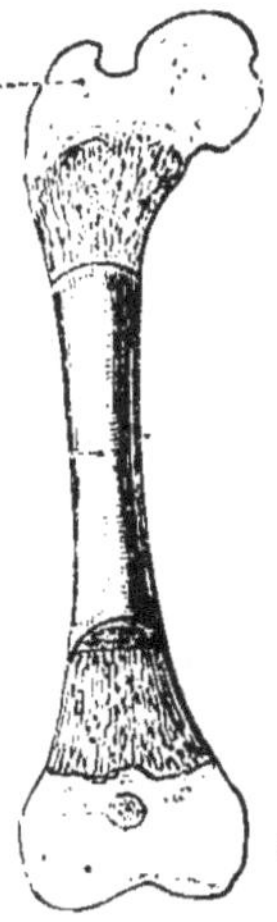

FIG. 327.—FROM A BOY STILL-BORN AT FULL TERM.
Body-length, 21 inches.

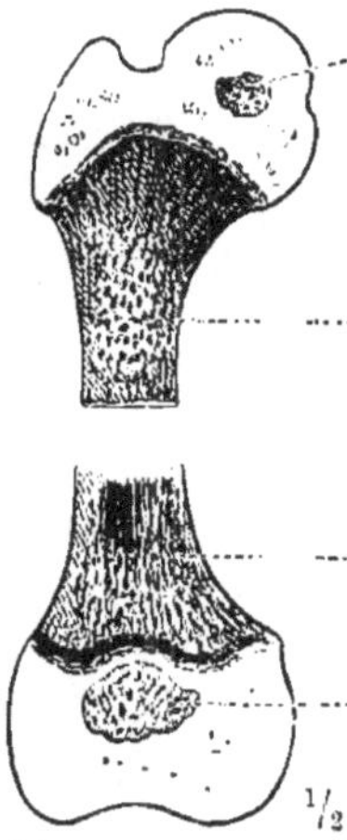

FIG. 328.—FROM A BOY AGED NINE AND A HALF MONTHS.

THE CENTRES OF OSSIFICATION OF THE PROXIMAL AND DISTAL EPIPHYSES.

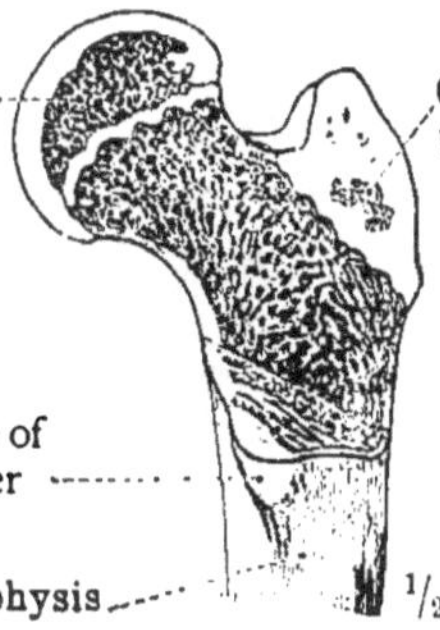

FIG. 329.—FROM A GIRL AGED SEVEN YEARS.

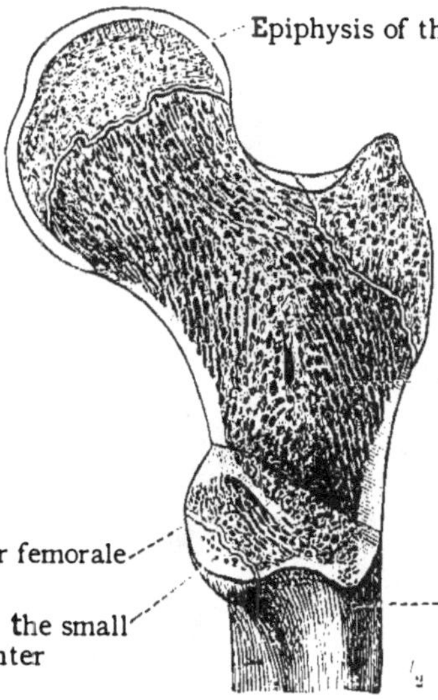

FIG. 330.—FROM A GIRL AGED FIFTEEN YEARS.

THE EPIPHYSES OF THE PROXIMAL EXTREMITY.

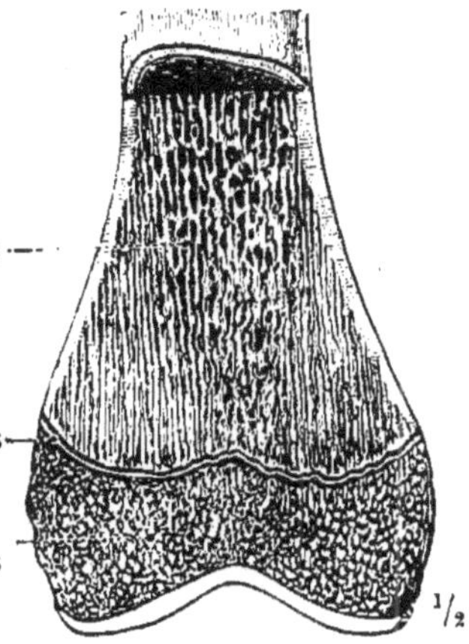

FIG. 331.—IN FRONTAL SECTION.

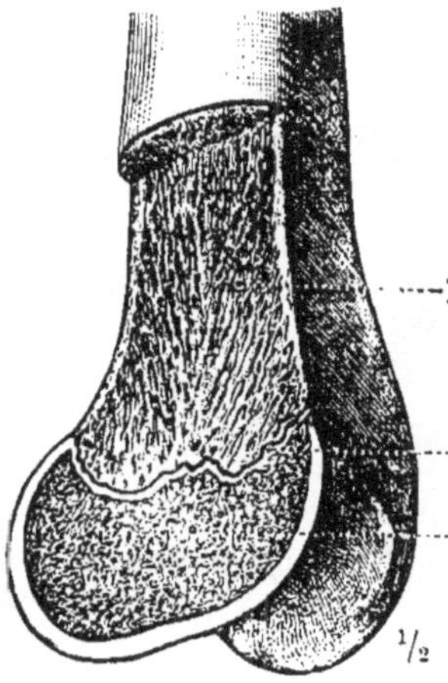

FIG. 332.—IN SAGITTAL SECTION.

THE EPIPHYSIS OF THE DISTAL EXTREMITY FROM A GIRL AGED FIFTEEN YEARS.

Development of the Femur.

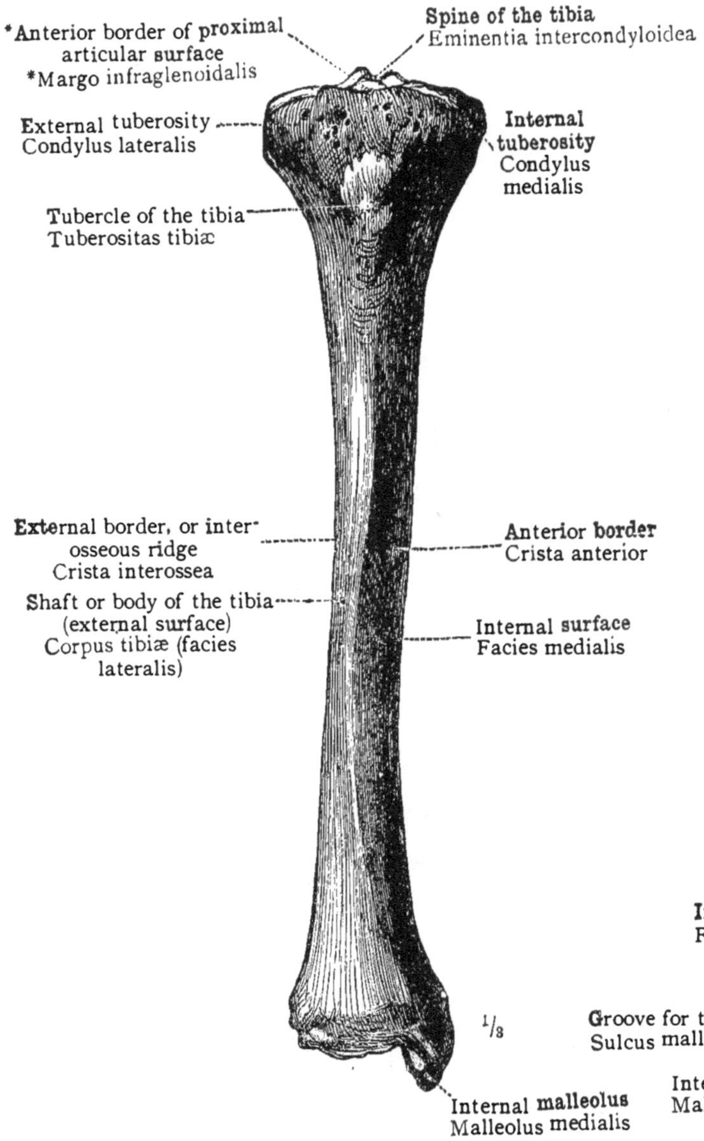

FIG. 333.—ANTERIOR ASPECT.

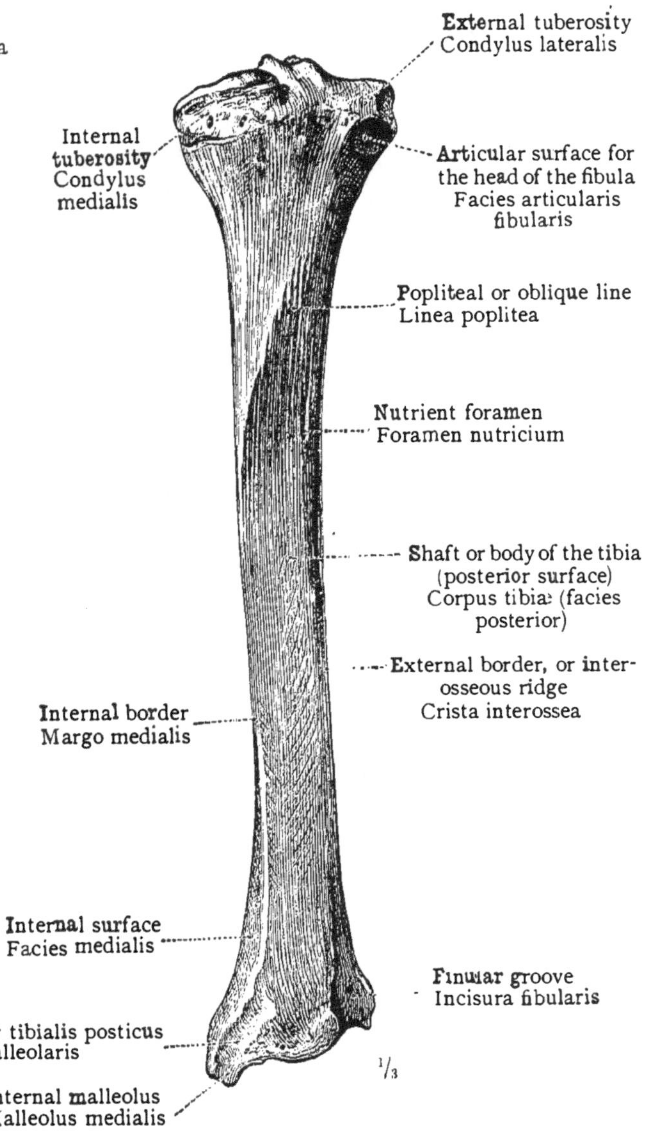

FIG. 334.—POSTERIOR ASPECT.

THE RIGHT TIBIA.

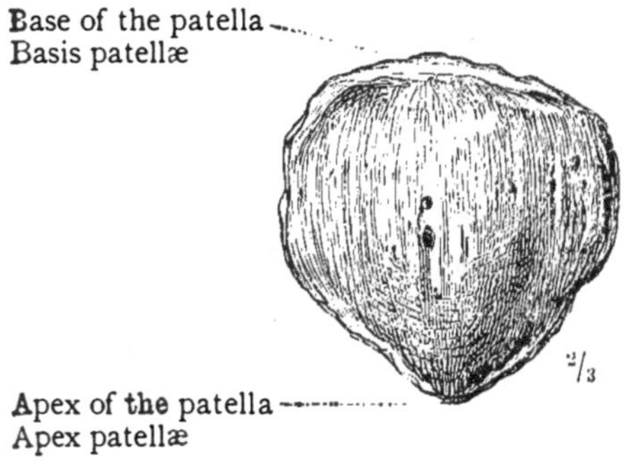

FIG. 335.—ANTERIOR SURFACE.

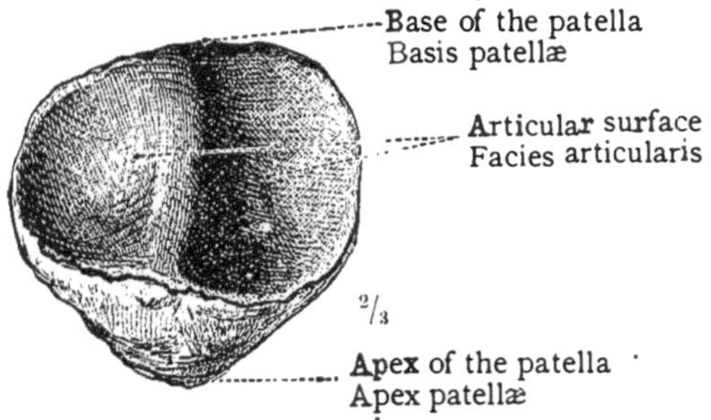

FIG. 336.—POSTERIOR SURFACE.

THE RIGHT PATELLA.

Ossa cruris—The bones of the leg: the patella, rotula, or knee-pan.

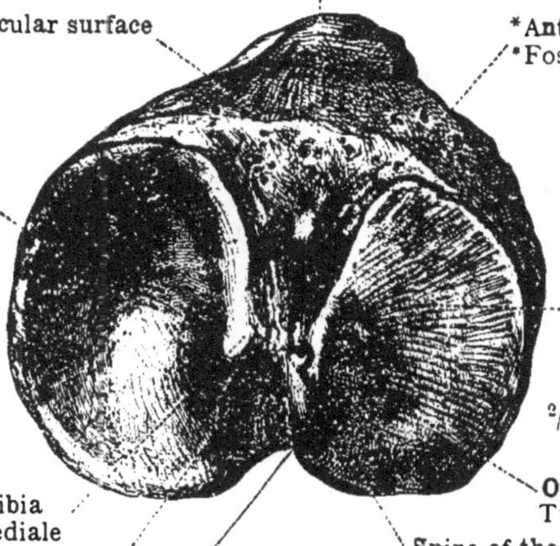

FIG. 338.—FACIES ARTICULARIS SUPERIOR TIBIÆ—THE PROXIMAL ARTICULAR SURFACE OF THE RIGHT TIBIA.

Note to Fig. 338.—*Anterior* and *Posterior Intercondylar Fossa.*—These terms are used neither by Quain nor by Macalister. The latter speaks of the hollows in question as *depressions for the crucial ligaments.*—TR.

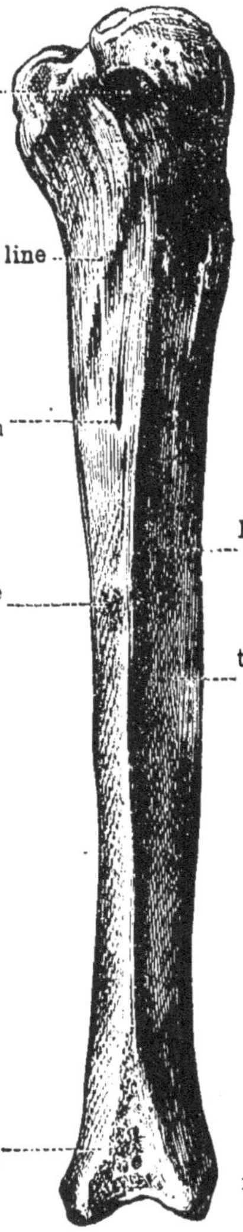

FIG. 337.—RIGHT TIBIA SEEN FROM THE OUTER SIDE.

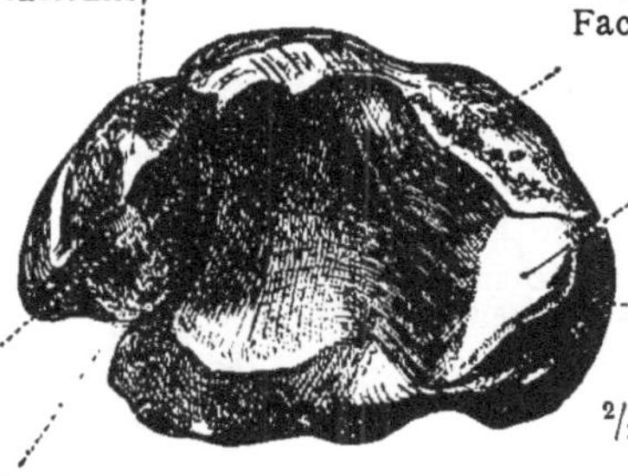

FIG. 339.—THE DISTAL ARTICULAR SURFACES OF THE BONES OF THE RIGHT LEG.

Ossa cruris—Bones of the leg.

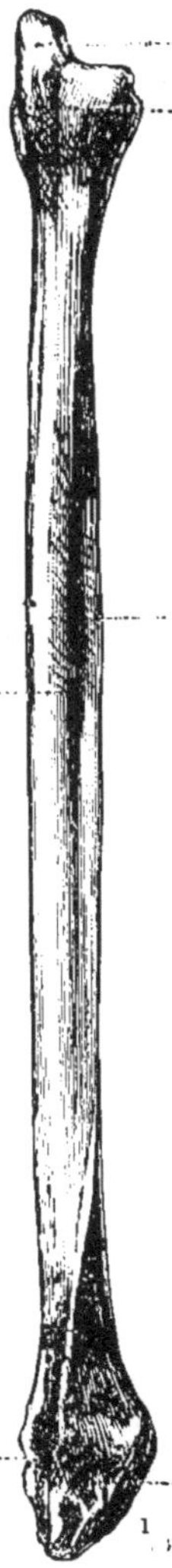

FIG. 340.—EXTERNAL ASPECT.

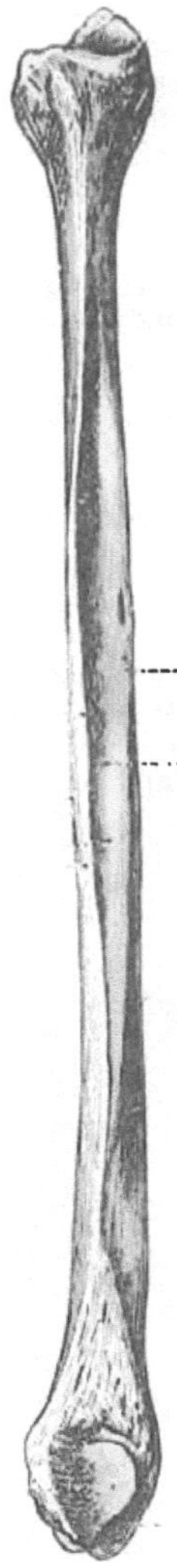

FIG. 341.—INTERNAL ASPECT.

THE RIGHT FIBULA OR PERONEAL BONE.

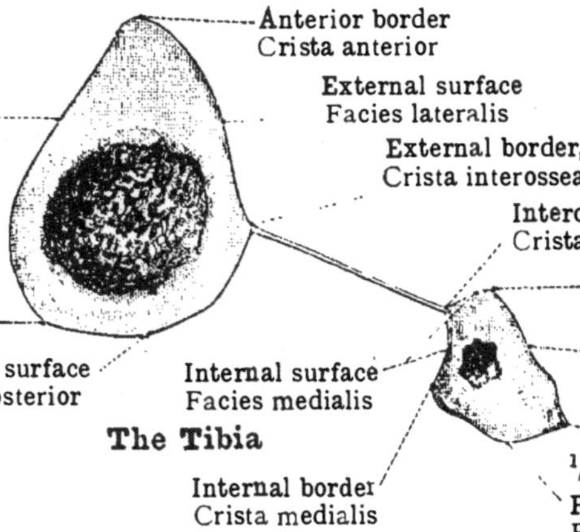

FIG. 342.—TRANSVERSE SECTION THROUGH THE MIDDLE OF THE BONES OF THE RIGHT LEG, WITH THE INTEROSSEOUS MEMBRANE.

Ossa cruris—Bones of the leg.

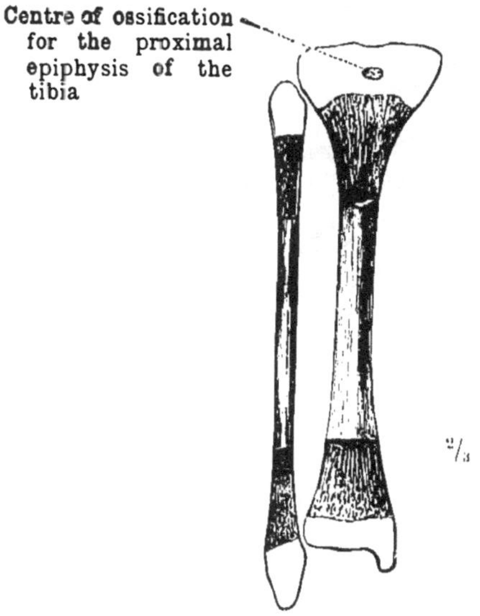

FIG. 343.—FROM A BOY STILL-BORN AT FULL TERM.
Body length, 21 inches.

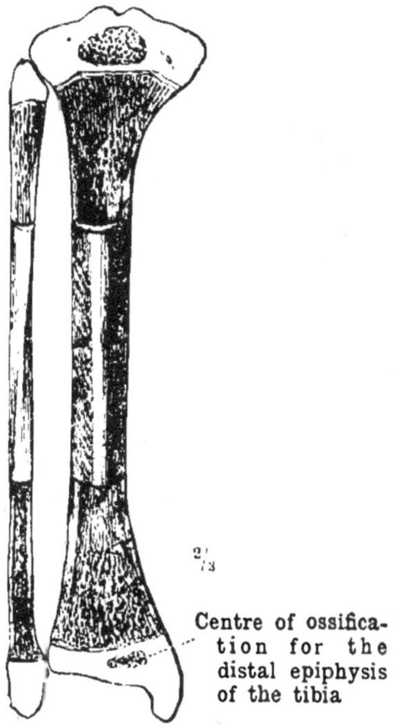

FIG. 344.—FROM A BOY AGED NINE AND HALF MONTHS.

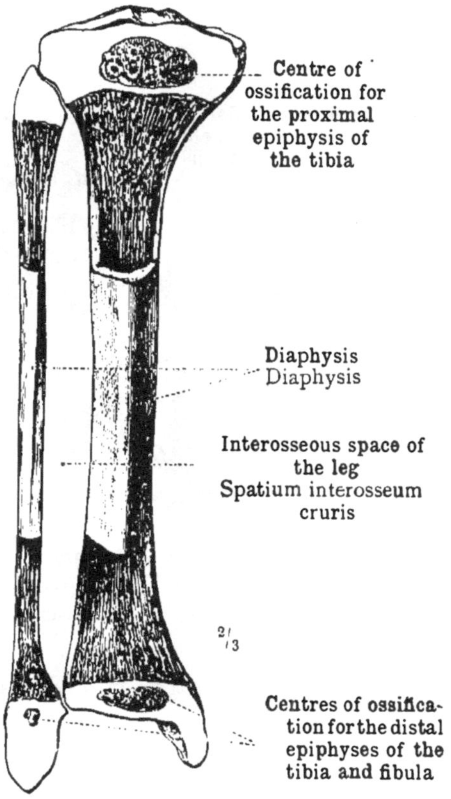

FIG. 345.—FROM A BOY AGED ONE AND A HALF YEARS.

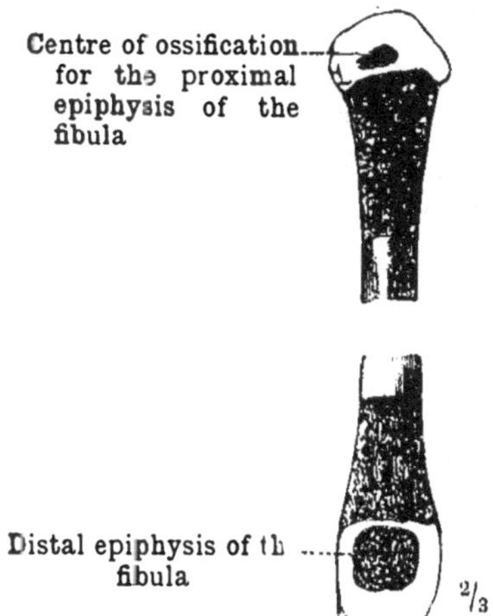

FIG. 346.—PROXIMAL AND DISTAL PORTIONS OF THE FIBULA OF A GIRL AGED FOUR AND A HALF YEARS.

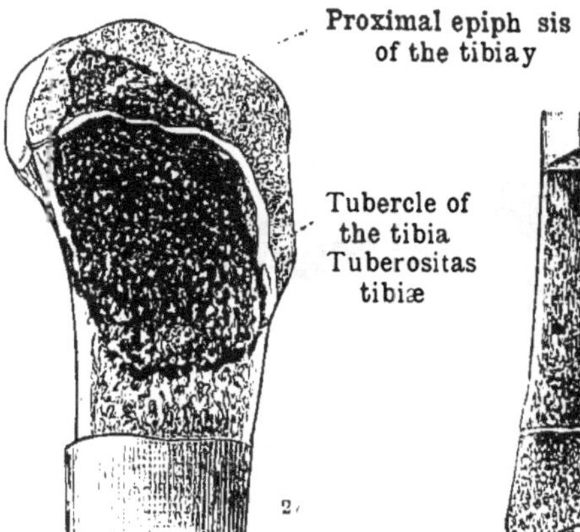

FIG. 347.—PROXIMAL PORTION OF THE TIBIA OF A GIRL AGED FIFTEEN YEARS. SAGITTAL SECTION

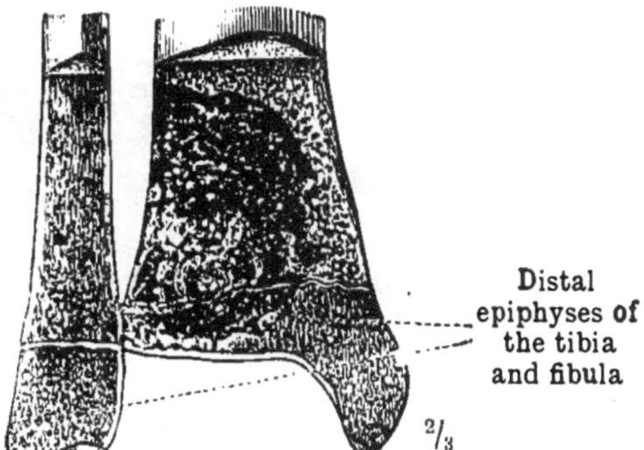

FIG. 348.—THE DISTAL PORTIONS OF THE BONES OF THE LEG OF A GIRL AGED FIFTEEN YEARS. FRONTAL SECTION.

Development of the Bones of the Leg.

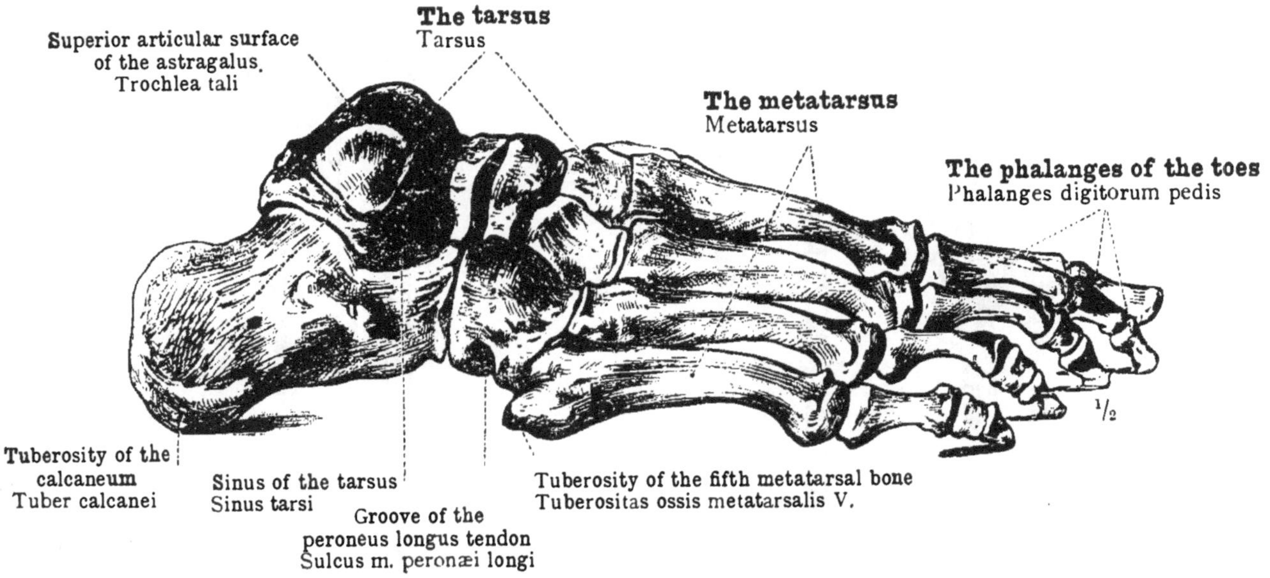

FIG. 349.—BONES OF THE RIGHT FOOT SEEN FROM THE OUTER SIDE FACIES DORSALIS PEDIS ET MARGO LATERALIS PEDIS.

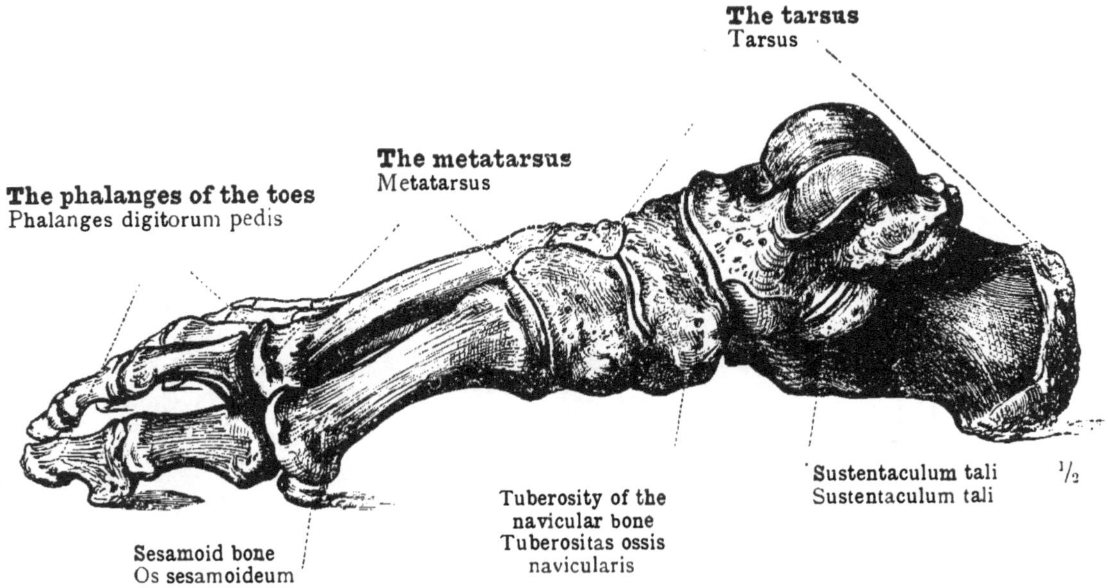

FIG. 350.—THE BONES OF THE RIGHT FOOT SEEN FROM THE INNER SIDE MARGO MEDIALIS PEDIS.

Skeleton pedis—Bones of the foot.

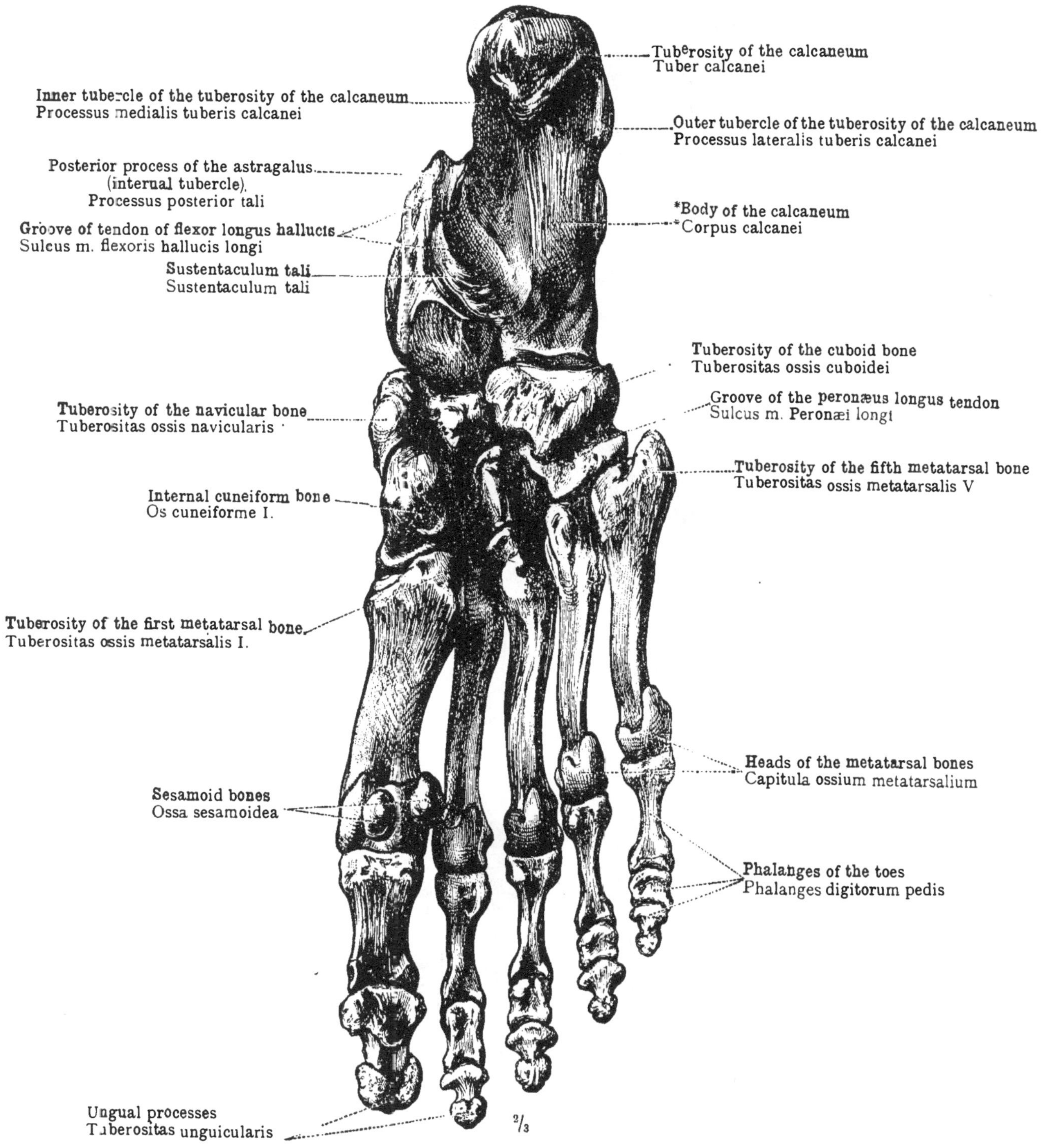

FIG. 351.—THE BONES OF THE RIGHT FOOT SEEN FROM THE PLANTAR SIDE: FACIES PLANTARIS PEDIS.

Skeleton pedis—Bones of the foot.

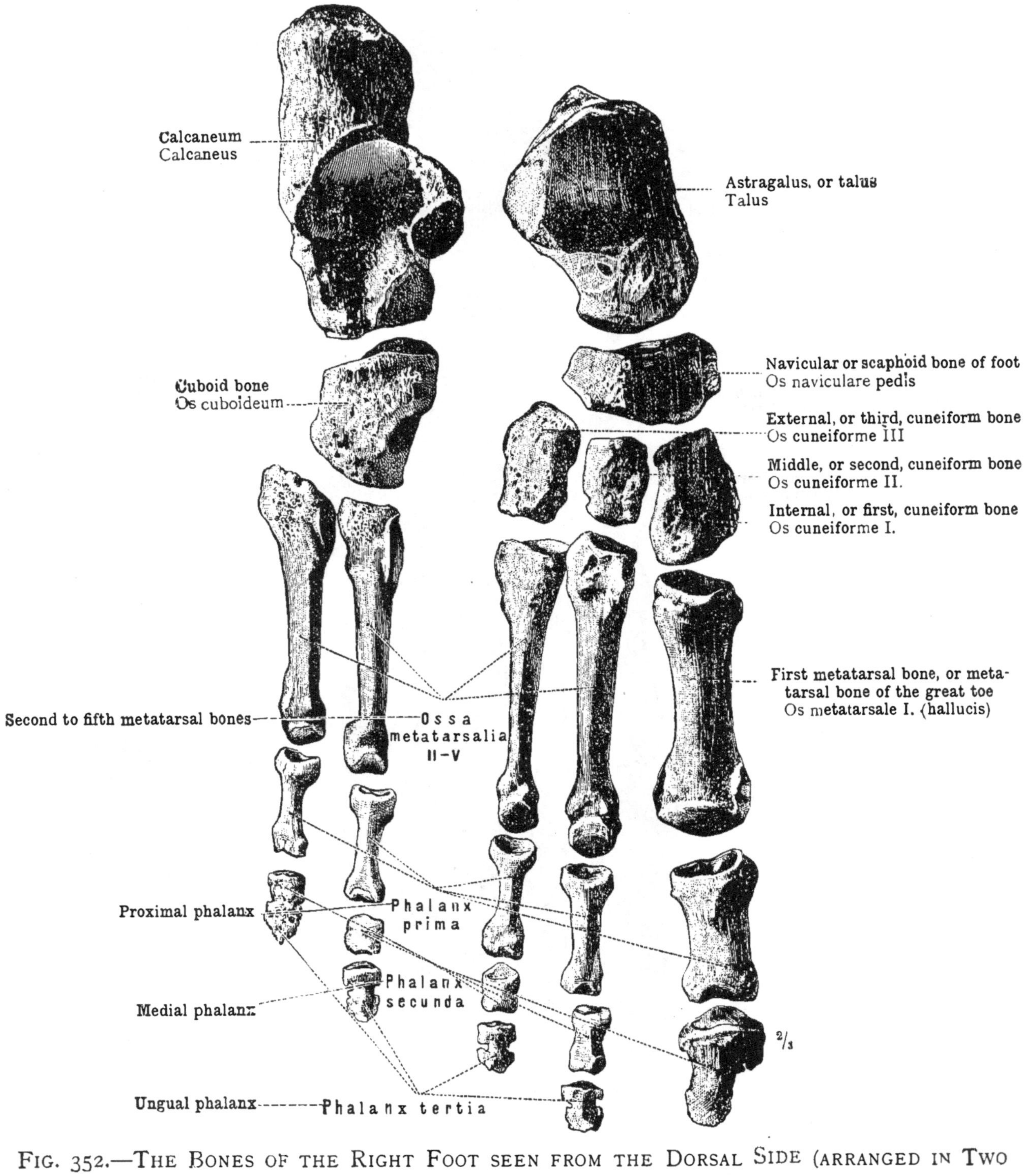

FIG. 352.—THE BONES OF THE RIGHT FOOT SEEN FROM THE DORSAL SIDE (ARRANGED IN TWO LONGITUDINAL ROWS).

Skeleton pedis—Bones of the foot.

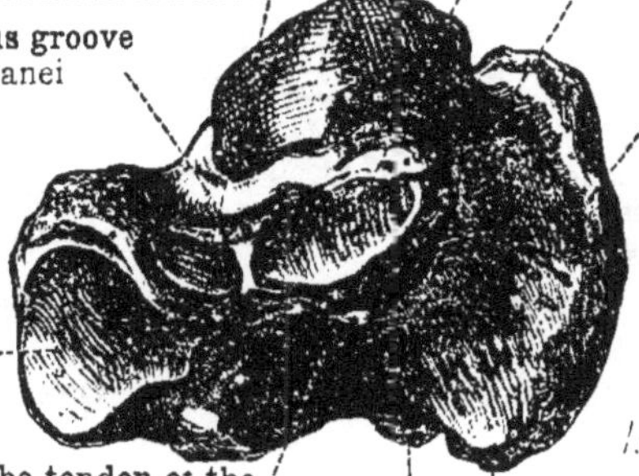

FIG. 353.—SEEN OBLIQUELY FROM WITHIN AND BEFORE.

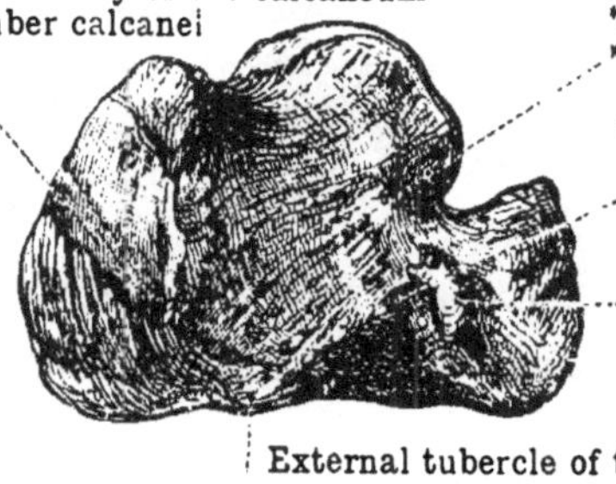

FIG. 354.—SEEN OBLIQUELY FROM WITHOUT AND BEHIND.

THE RIGHT CALCANEUM OR OS CALCIS.

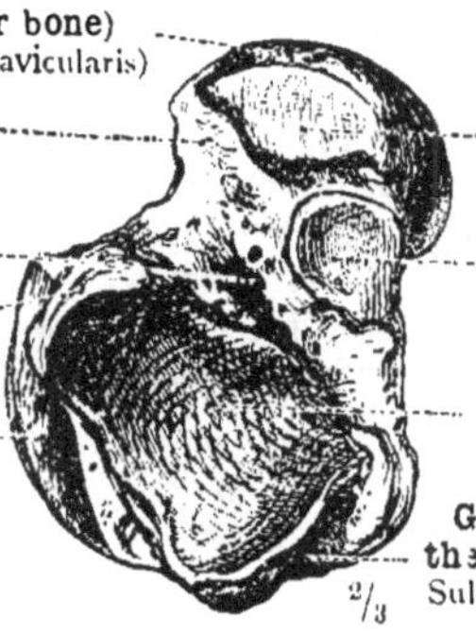

FIG. 355.—SEEN FROM BELOW.

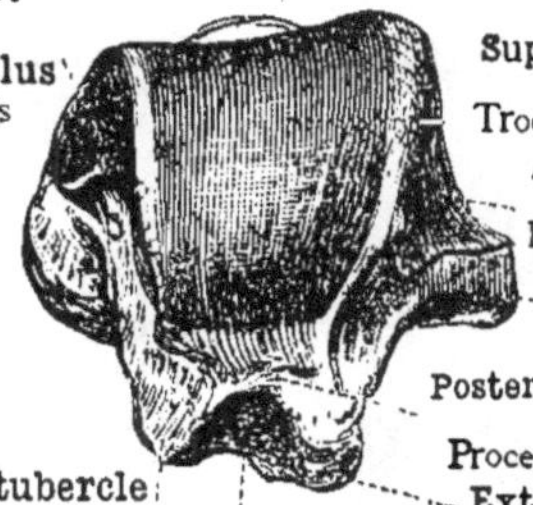

FIG. 356.—SEEN FROM BEHIND.

THE RIGHT ASTRAGALUS.

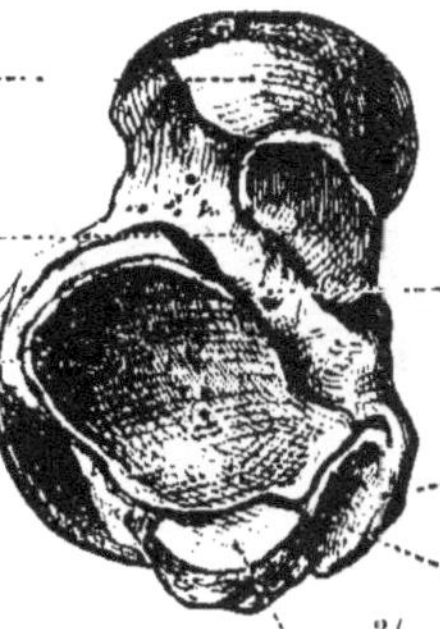

FIG. 357.—THE RIGHT ASTRAGALUS, WITH AN OS TRIGONUM (VAR.). SEEN FROM BELOW.

Ossa tarsi—Bones of the tarsus.

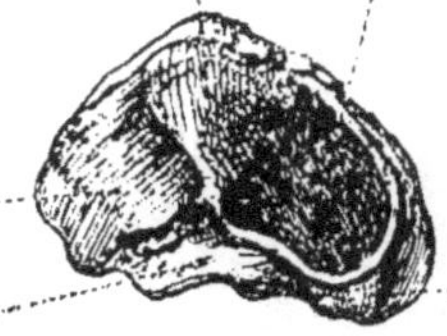

FIG. 358.—ANTERIOR ASPECT.

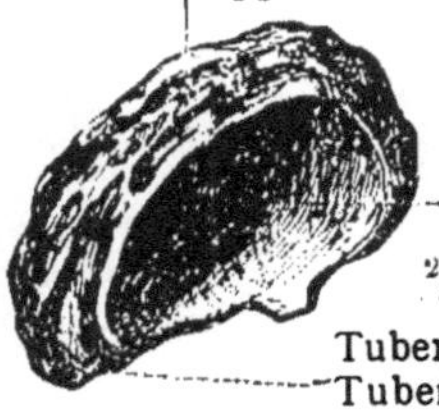

FIG. 359.—POSTERIOR ASPECT

OS NAVICULARE PEDIS—THE RIGHT NAVICULAR OR SCAPHOID BONE OF THE FOOT.

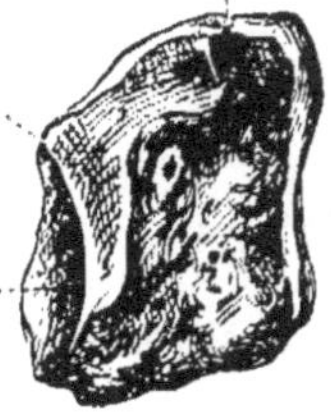

FIG. 360.—EXTERNAL ASPECT.

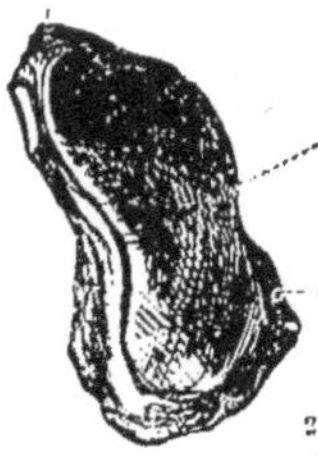

FIG. 361.—ANTERIOR ASPECT.

OS CUNEIFORME I.—THE RIGHT INTERNAL CUNEIFORM BONE.

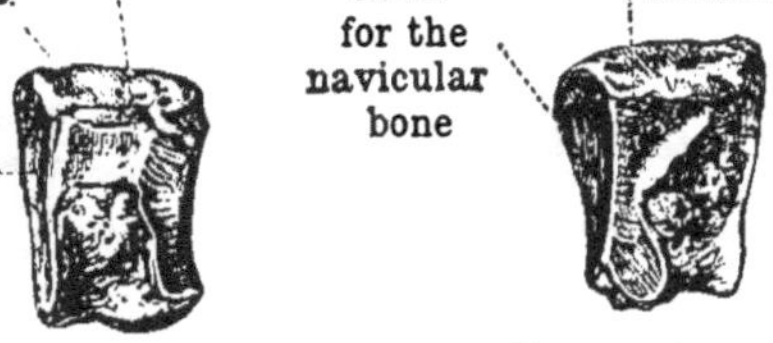

FIG. 362.—OS CUNEIFORME II.—THE RIGHT MIDDLE CUNEIFORM BONE.

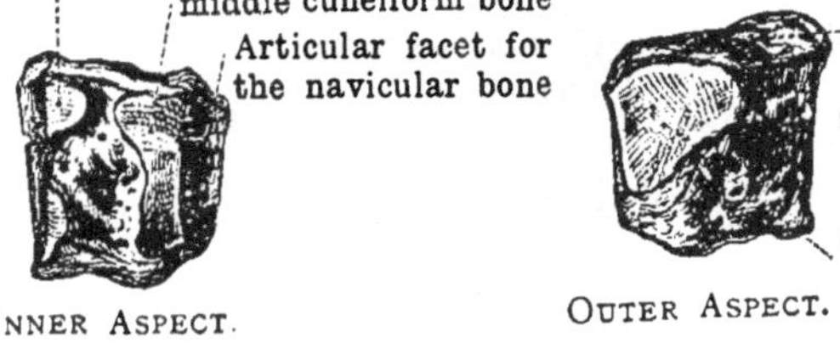

FIG. 363.—OS CUNEIFORME III.—THE RIGHT EXTERNAL CUNEIFORM BONE.

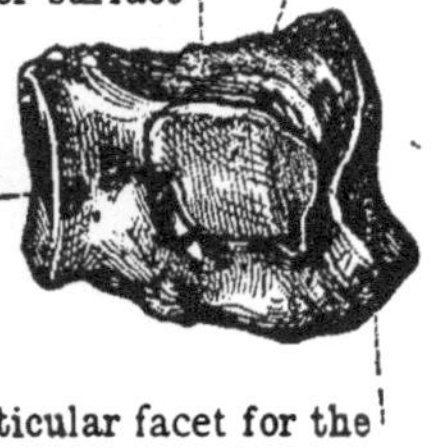

FIG. 364.—INNER ASPECT.

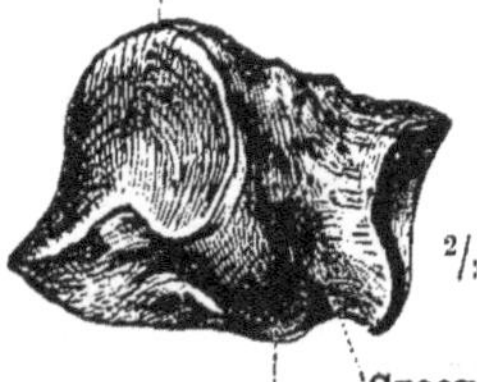

FIG. 365.—SEEN OBLIQUELY FROM WITHOUT AND BEHIND.

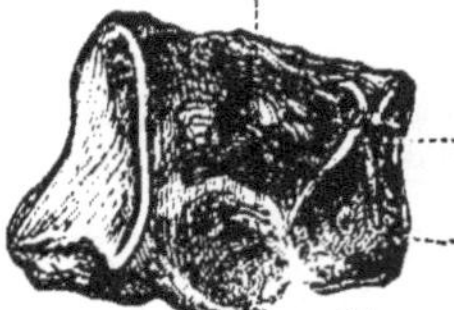

FIG. 366.—OUTER ASPECT.

OS CUBOIDEUM—THE RIGHT CUBOID BONE.

Ossa tarsi—Bones of the tarsus.

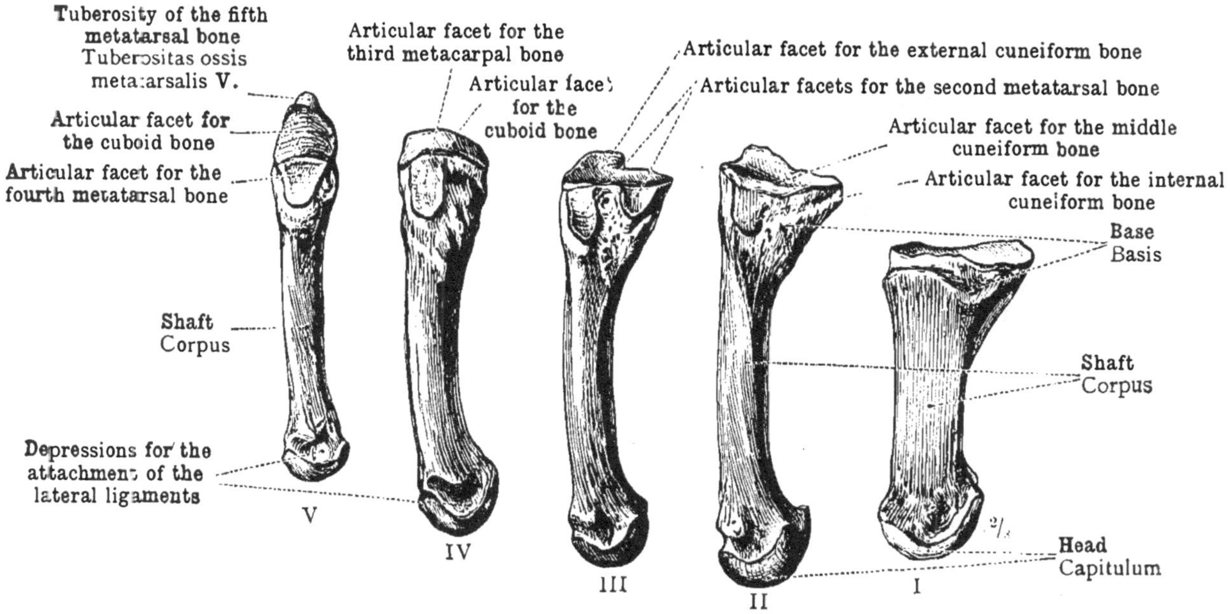

FIG. 367.—THE METATARSAL BONES OF THE RIGHT FOOT SEEN FROM THE INNER SIDE.

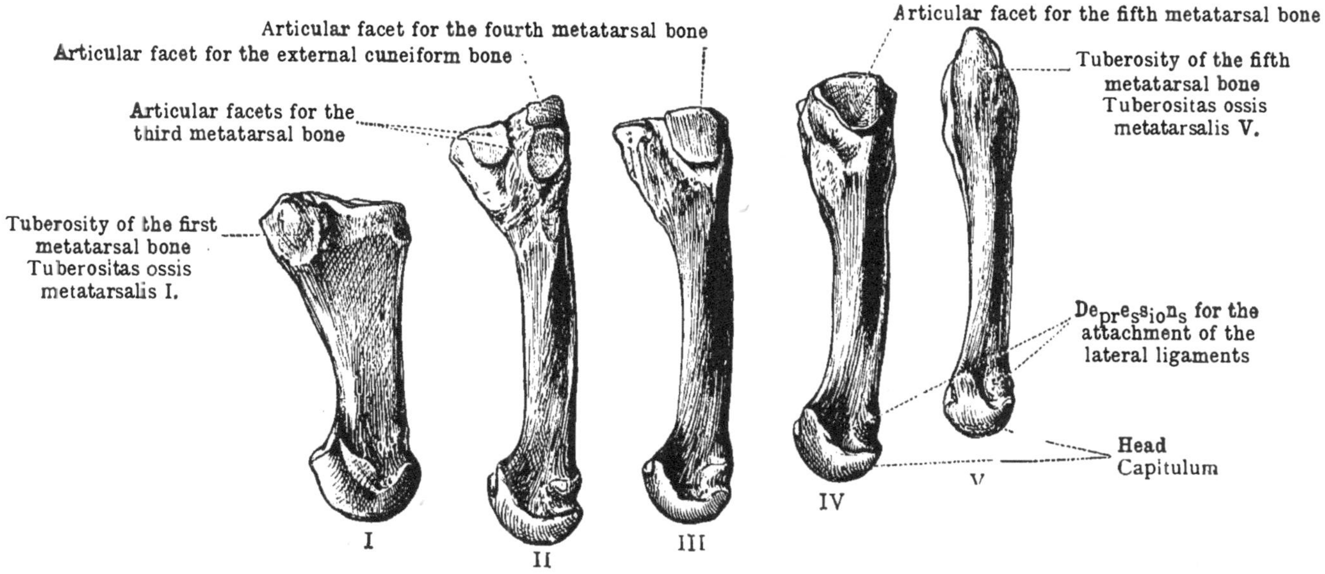

FIG. 368.—THE METATARSAL BONES OF THE RIGHT FOOT SEEN FROM THE OUTER SIDE.

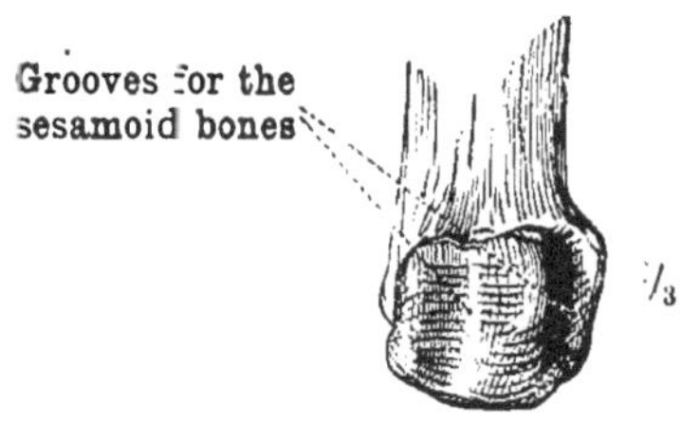

FIG. 369.—PLANTAR ASPECT OF THE HEAD OF THE METATARSAL BONE OF THE GREAT TOE (CAPITULUM OSSIS METATARSALIS HALLUCIS).

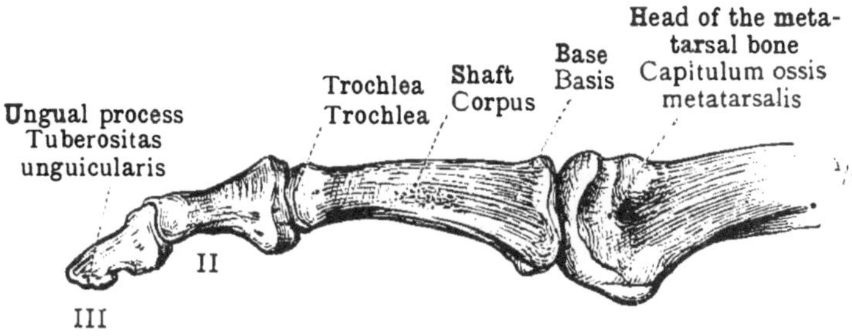

FIG. 370.—THE PHALANGES OF THE SECOND TOE SEEN FROM THE INNER SIDE (MARGO MEDIALIS DIGITI SECUNDI PEDIS).

Metatarsal Bones and Phalanges of the Toes.

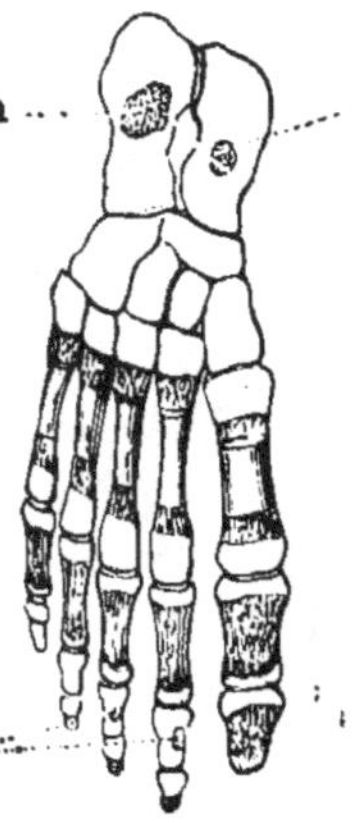

FIG. 371.—FROM A HUMAN FŒTUS IN THE MIDDLE OF THE NINTH MONTH (MONTHS OF FOUR WEEKS EACH).
Body-length, 17½ inches.

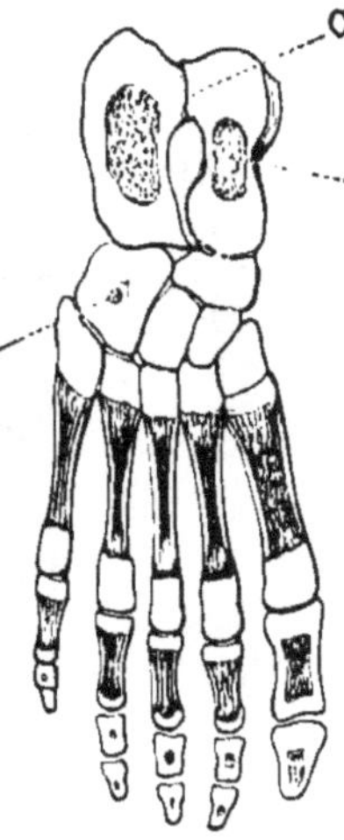

FIG. 372.—FROM A BOY STILL-BORN AT FULL TERM
Body-length, 22 inches.

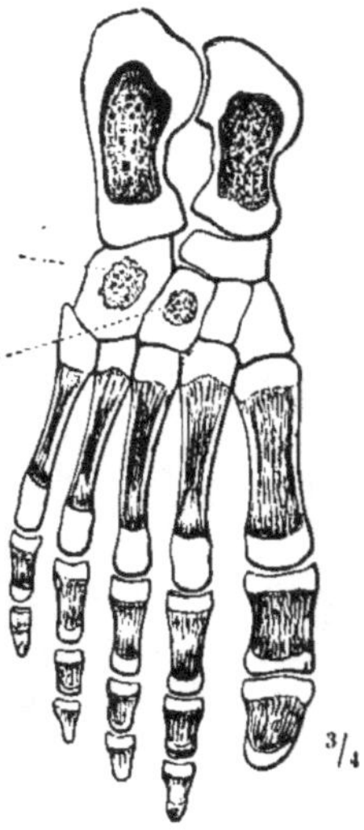

FIG. 373.—FROM A BOY AGED TWELVE WEEKS.

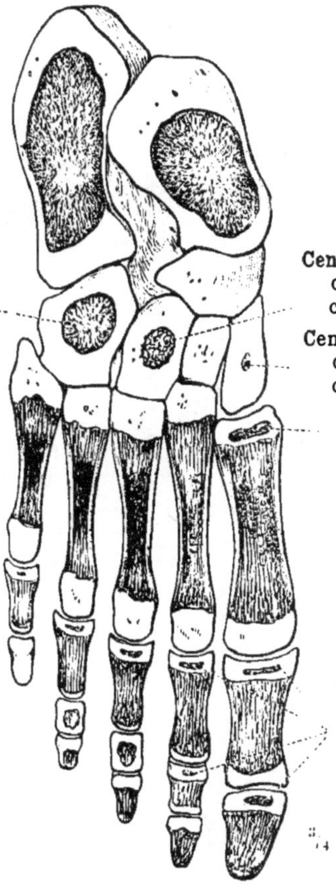

FIG. 374.—FROM A BOY AGED THREE YEARS.

Development of the Bones of the Foot.

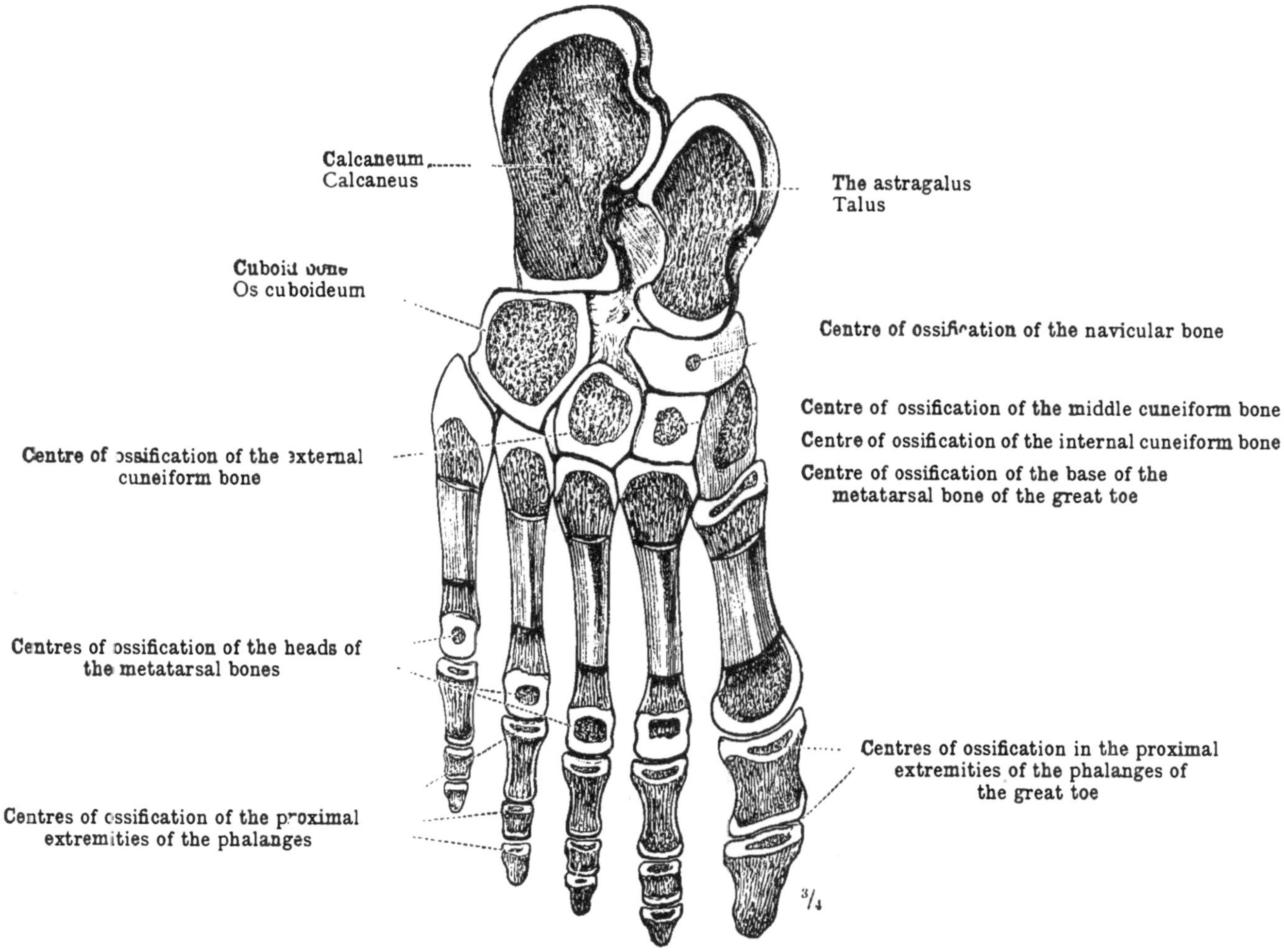

FIG. 375.—OSSIFICATION OF THE BONES OF THE FOOT IN A GIRL AGED SIX YEARS.

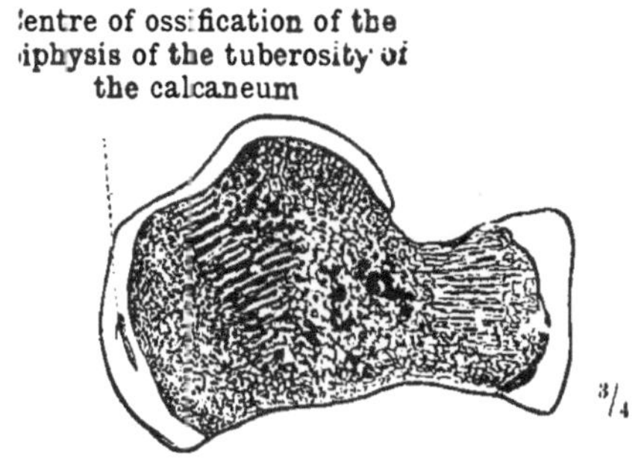

IG. 376.—FROM A GIRL AGED EIGHT YEARS.

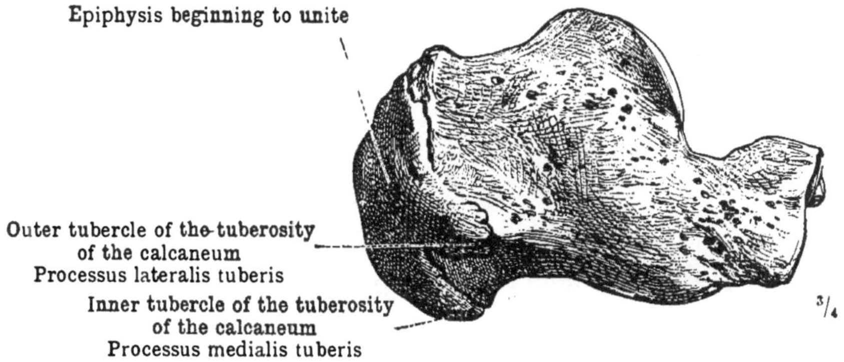

FIG. 377.—FROM A YOUNG MAN AGED EIGHTEEN YEARS (EPIPHYSIS BEGINNING TO UNITE).

EPIPHYSIS OF THE TUBEROSITY OF THE CALCANEUM.

Development of the Bones of the Foot.

INDEX

TO THE

REGIONS OF THE HUMAN BODY

AND TO THE

OSTEOLOGY

INDEX

TO THE REGIONS OF THE HUMAN BODY

R

S.

T.

U.

Z.

INDEX

TO THE OSTEOLOGY

Certain names in this Index have an asterisk (*) prefixed; these, as more fully explained in the Translator's Preface, being terms that form part of the English nomenclature used in this work, but which are not commonly employed by English anatomists. To other names a dagger (†) is prefixed; these are Latin names used by the author in the original work, but not included in the official nomenclature of the "Anatomische Gesellschaft."

A.

INDEX

TO THE OSTEOLO

Certain names in this Index have an asterisk (*) prefixed; these, as more fully explained he Translator's Preface, being terms that form part of the English nomenclature used in this work, but which are not commonly employed by English a n ists. To other names a dagger (†) is prefixed; these are Latin names used by the author in the original work, but not included in the official nomenclatur the "Anatomische Gesellschaft."

A.

R.

S.

U.

V.

W.

X.

Z.

SYNDESMOLOGIA

ARTHROLOGY

THE ARTICULATIONS IN GENERAL

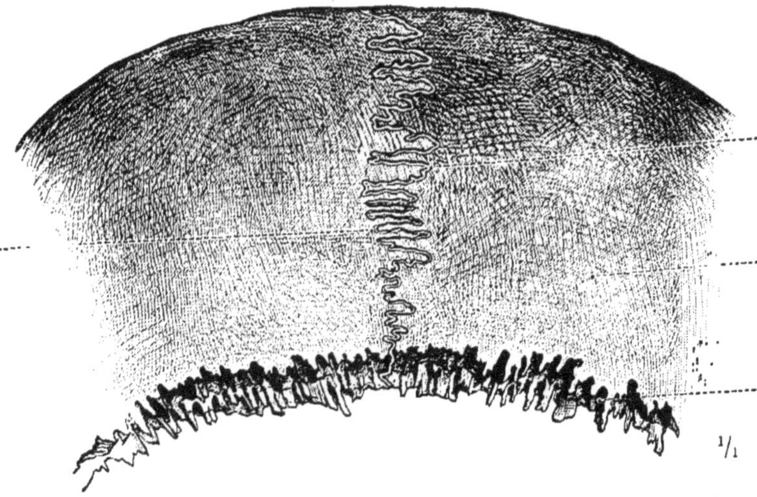

FIG. 378.—SUTURA SERRATA—SERRATED OR DENTATED SUTURE.

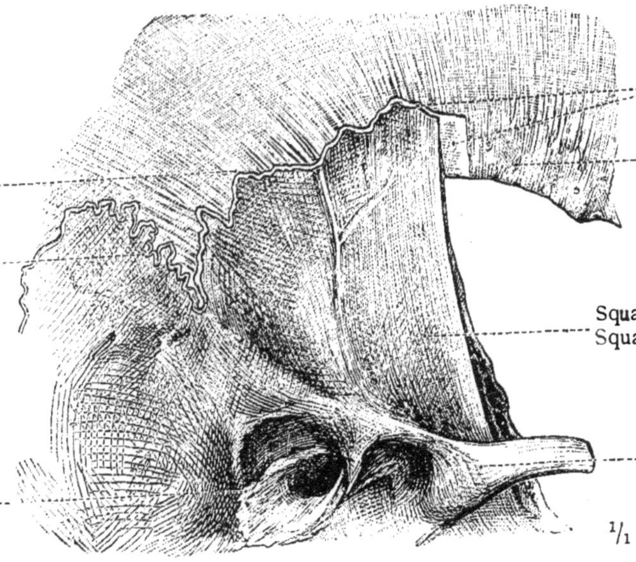

FIG. 379.—SUTURA SQUAMOSA—SQUAMOUS OR SCALY SUTURE.

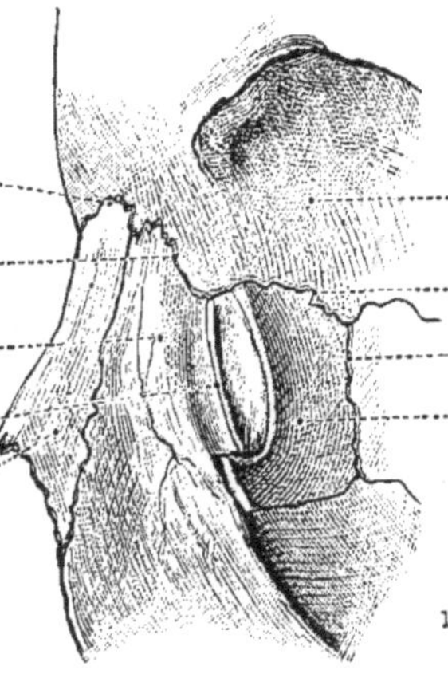

FIG. 380.—HARMONIA—HARMONIC SUTURE.

Synarthrosis, or Continuous Articulation.

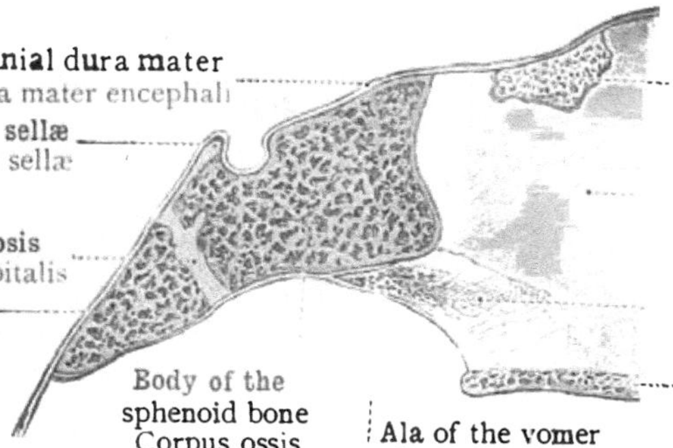

FIG. 381.—SYNCHONDROSIS. (THE SPHENO-OCCIPITAL SYNCHONDROSIS OF A GIRL AT THE AGE OF TWO YEARS; MEDIAN SAGITTAL SECTION.)

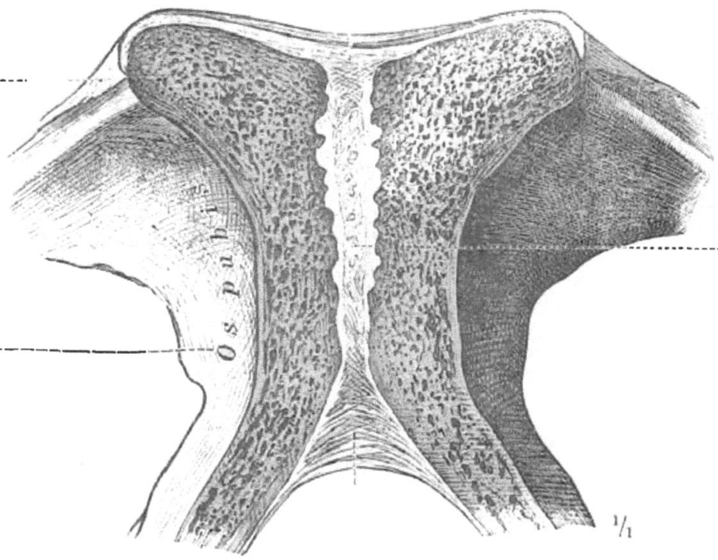

FIG. 382.—SYMPHYSIS. (THE PUBIC SYMPHYSIS; FRONTAL SECTION, POSTERIOR PORTION.)

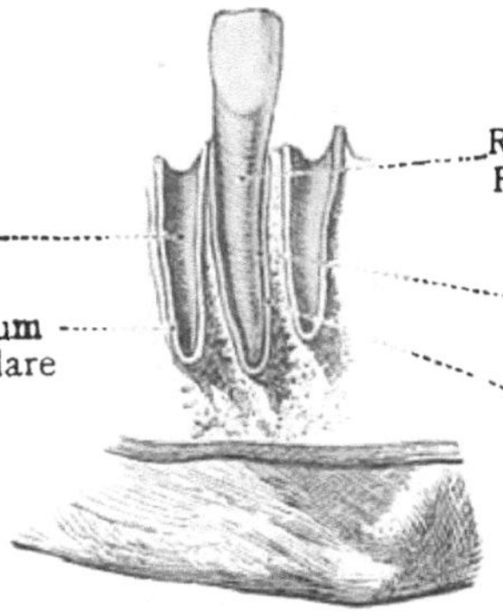

FIG. 383.—GOMPHOSIS.

Synarthrosis, or Continuous Articulation.

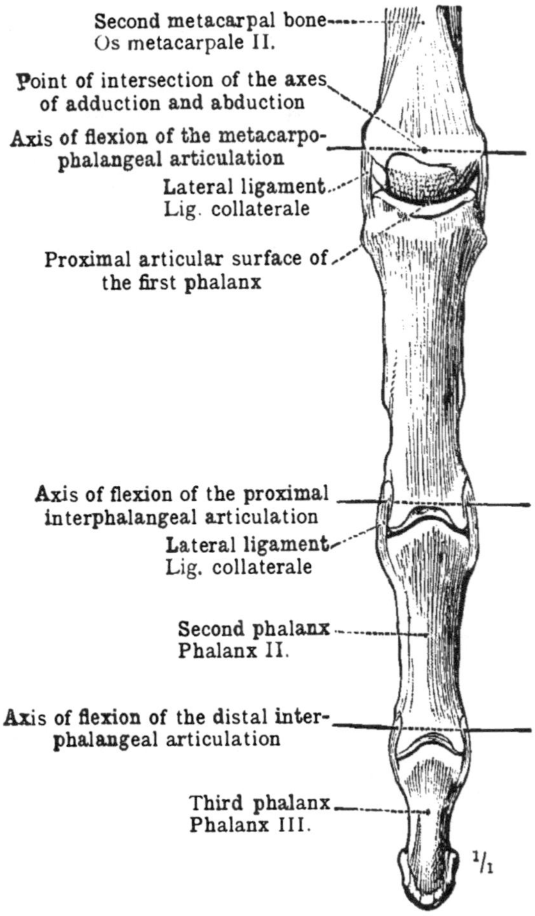

FIG. 384.—EXTENSION. POSTERIOR ASPECT

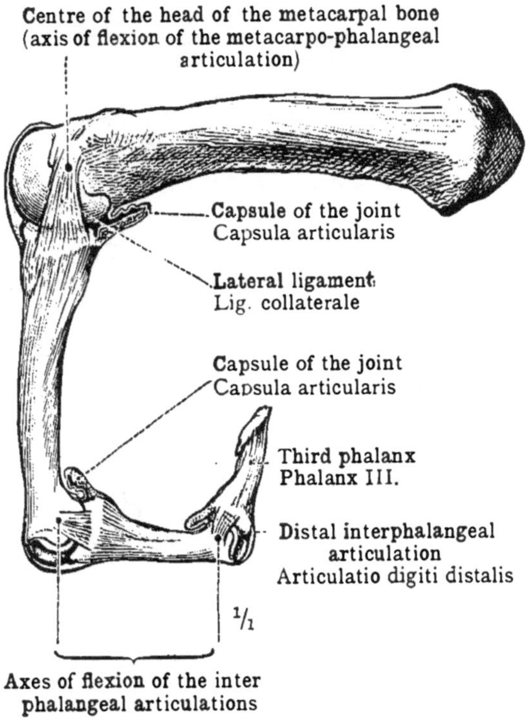

FIG. 385.—FLEXION. LATERAL ASPECT.

DIARTHROSIS (METACARPO-PHALANGEAL ARTICULATION).—GINGLYMUS, OR HINGE JOINT (ARTICULATIONS OF THE FINGERS).

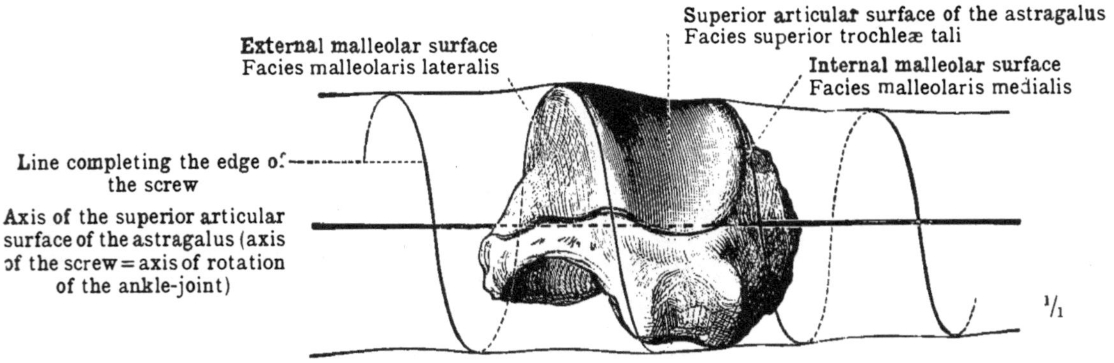

FIG. 386.—ARTICULATIO COCHLEARIS, COCHLEOID OR SCRE GINGLYMUS. (SUPERIOR ARTICULAR SURFACE OF THE LEFT ASTRAGALUS, SEEN FROM BEHIND, SHOWING THE SCREW FORM OF THE ANKLE-JOINT.

Diarthrosis, or Discontinuous Articulation—Articulatio simplex, simple joint.

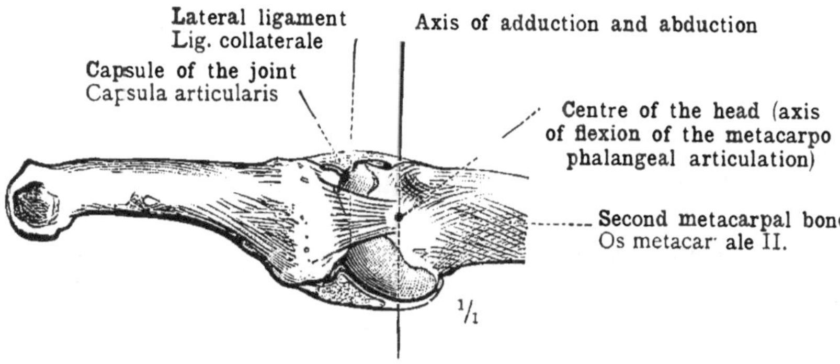

FIG. 387.—CONDYLARTHROSIS, OR CONDYLOID JOINT. (THE METACARPO-PHALANGEAL ARTICULATION OF THE INDEX-FINGER; LATERAL VIEW.)

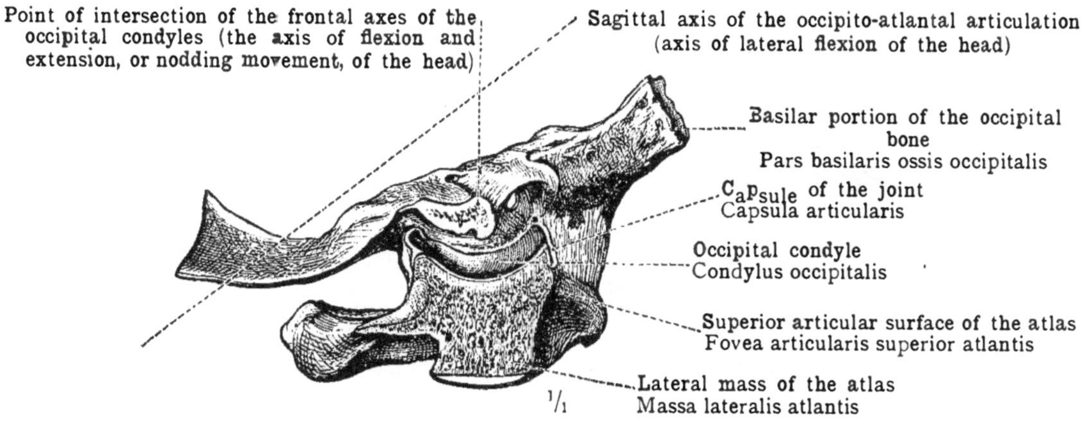

FIG. 388.—CONDYLARTHROSIS, OR CONDYLOID JOINT. (RIGHT OCCIPITO-ATLANTAL ARTICULATION; SEEN FROM THE OUTER SIDE.)

The outer half of the lateral mass of the atlas has been removed by a sagittal section passing through the joint.

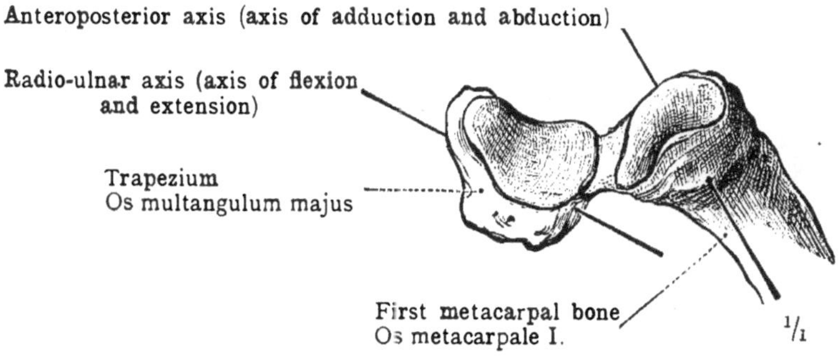

FIG. 389.—ARTICULATIO SELLARIS—SADDLE JOINT. (ARTICULATIO CARPOMETACARPEA POLLICIS—CARPOMETACARPAL JOINT OF THE THUMB.)

Diarthrosis, or Discontinuous Articulation—Articulatio simplex, simple joint.

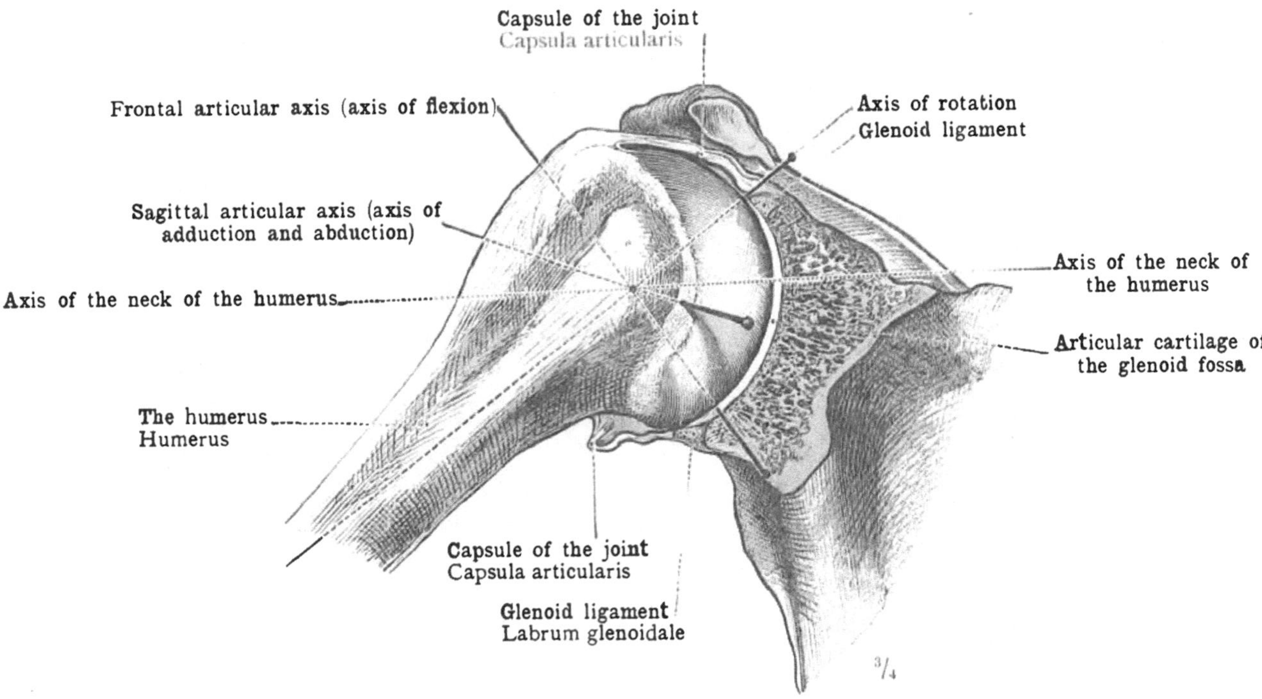

FIG. 390.—ENARTHROSIS,[1] OR ARTHRODIA; BALL-AND-SOCKET JOINT. (THE RIGHT SHOULDER-JOINT SEEN FROM BEFORE, THE ANTERIOR HALF OF THE GLENOID FOSSA AND OF THE CAPSULE OF THE JOINT HAVING BEEN REMOVED.)

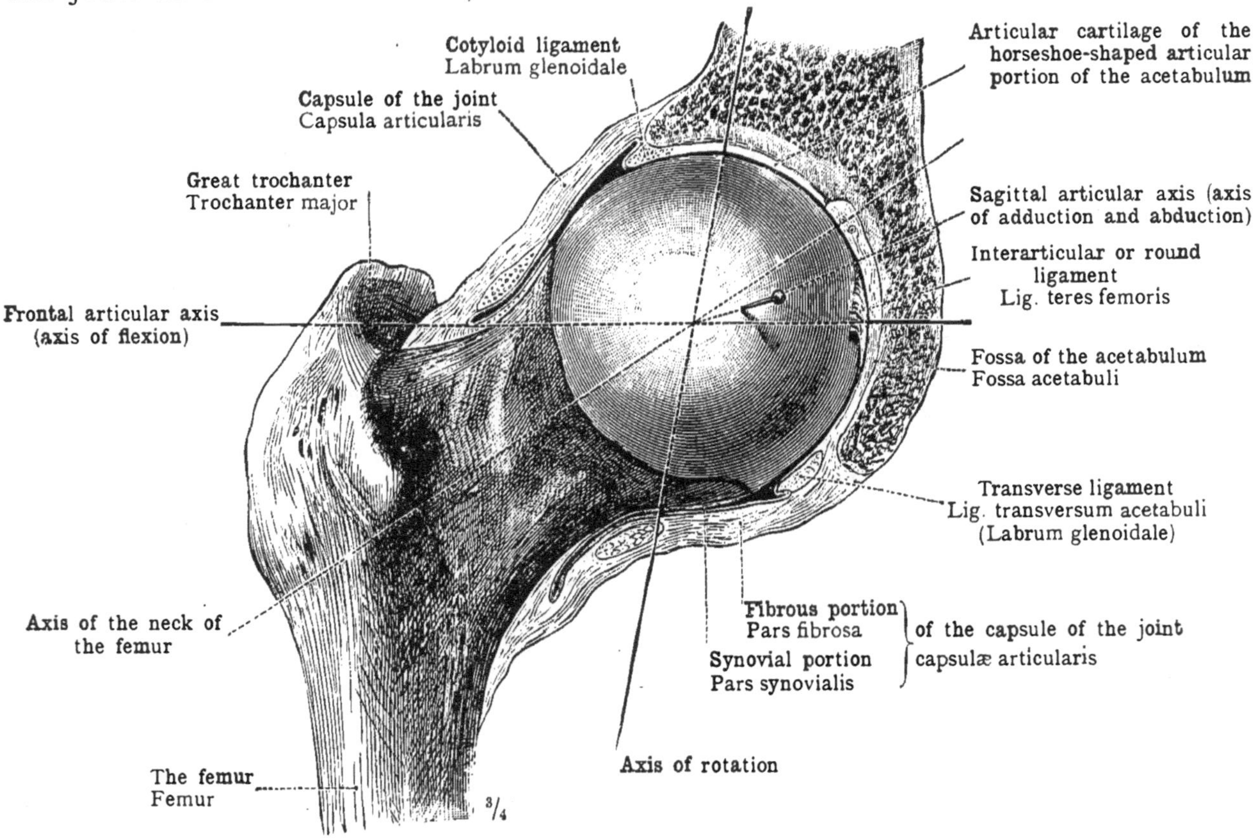

FIG. 391.—ENARTHROSIS,[1] OR ARTHRODIA; BALL-AND-SOCKET JOINT. (THE RIGHT HIP-JOINT SEEN FROM BEFORE, THE ANTERIOR HALF OF THE ACETABULUM AND OF THE CAPSULE OF THE JOINT HAVING BEEN REMOVED.)

[1] I have departed a little on this page from the author's terminology, which differs slightly from that in use in England. Both the hip and the shoulder joint are classed by him as examples of ARTICULATIO SPHÆROIDEA, *Kugelgelenk*—lit., "ball joint"; one of these, the shoulder-joint, in which the concave articular surface is considerably less than a hemisphere in extent, is called by him ARTHRODIA, *freies Gelenk*—lit., "free joint"; while the other, the hip-joint, in which the concave articular surface is considerably more than a hemisphere in extent, is called ENARTHROSIS, *Nussgelenk*—lit., "nut joint." English anatomists do not, as a rule, draw this distinction. The movements of the hip and the shoulder joint are identical in character, and the greater extent of the rigid portion of the enveloping surface in the one case than in the other has not been considered a difference sufficiently important to warrant a separation into two classes. Hence, in England the terms ENARTHROSIS and ARTHRODIA are applied indifferently to all ball-and-socket joints.—TR.

Diarthrosis, or Discontinuous Articulation—Articulatio simplex, simple joint; articulatio

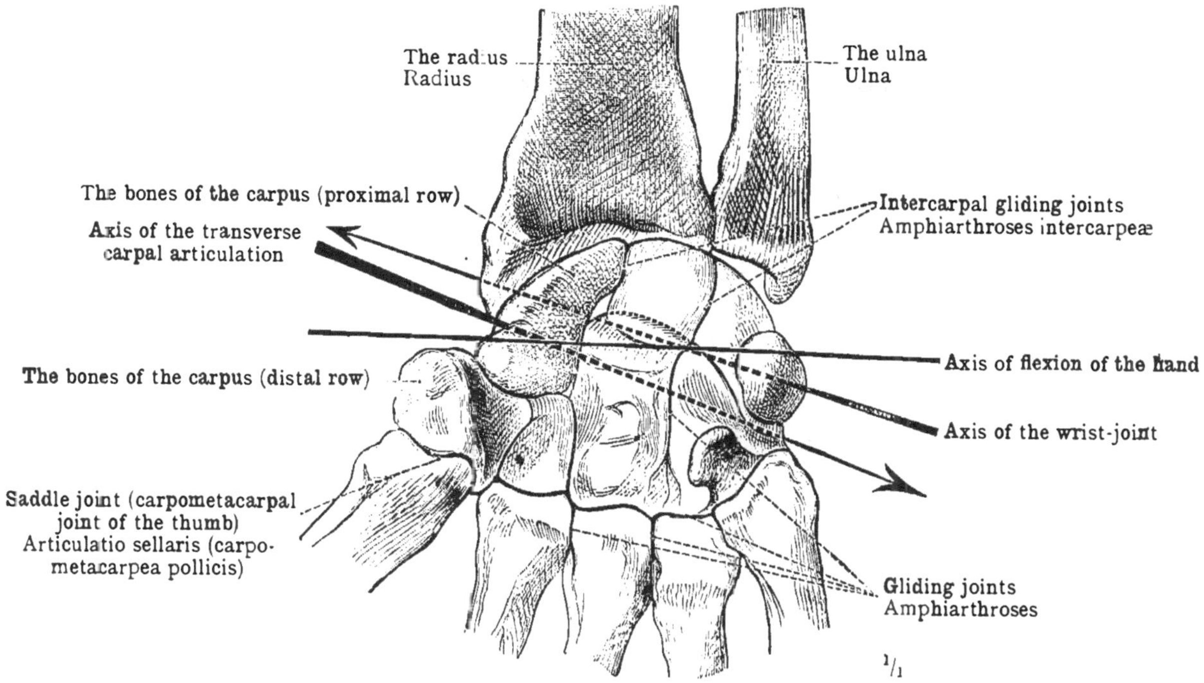

FIG. 392.—ARTICULATIO COMPOSITA, COMPOUND JOINTS (ARTICULATIONS OF THE HAND).—AMPHIARTHROSIS = ARTHRODIA OR GLIDING JOINT, AS SEEN IN THE INTERCARPAL, CARPO-METACARPAL, AND INTERMETACARPAL JOINT.

The arrows show the dorsal emergence of the axes of the wrist-joint and of the transverse carpal articulation respectively.

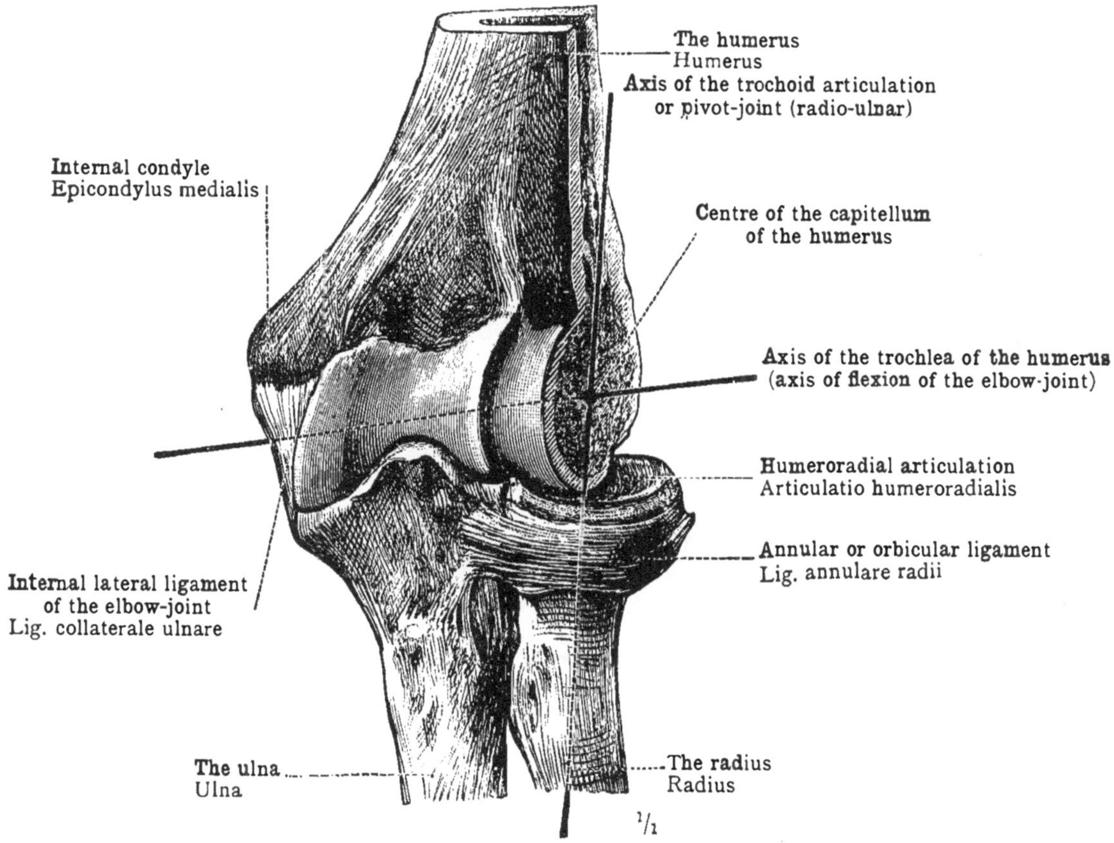

FIG. 393.—ARTICULATIO TROCHOIDEA, TROCHOID OR PIVOT JOINT.—GINGLYMUS, HINGE JOINT. (PALMAR ASPECT OF THE ELBOW-JOINT.)

The radial half of the capitellum of the humerus has been removed by a sagittal section passing through its centre of curvature.

Diarthrosis, or Discontinuous Articulation.
Amphiarthrosis, arthrodia or gliding joint—Articulatio composita, compound joint.

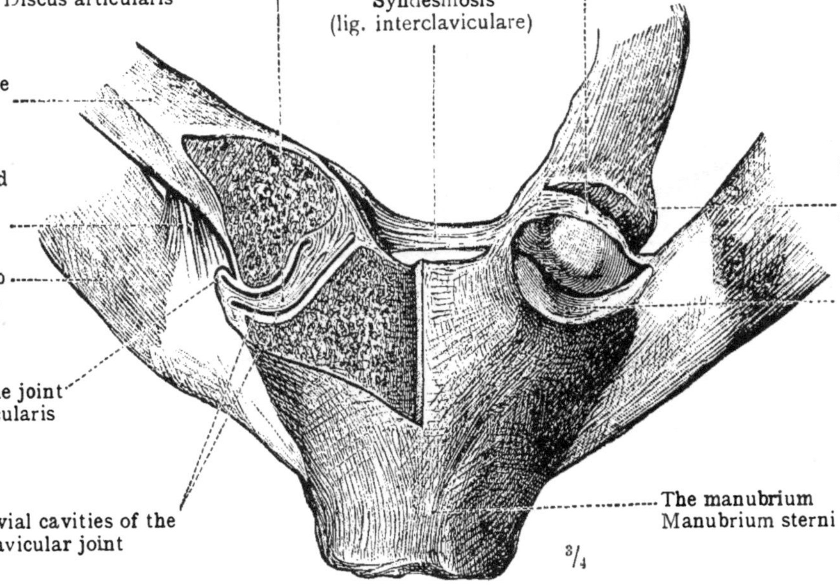

FIG. 394.—SYNDESMOSIS.—INTERARTICULAR FIBROCARTILAGE. (THE STERNOCLAVICULAR ARTICULATION, ANTERIOR ASPECT.)

The right articulation is divided through the middle by a frontal secti n ; in the left, the front portion of the capsule has been removed, and the clavicle has been drawn backwards.

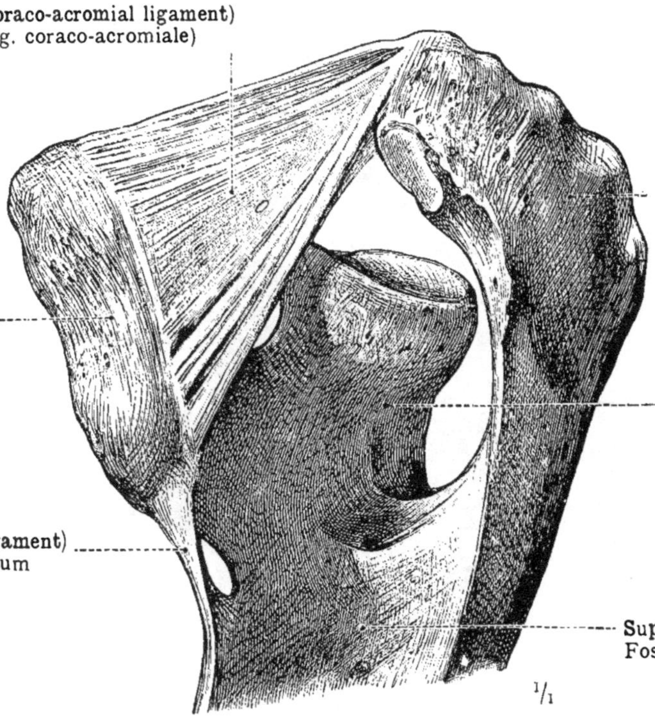

FIG. 395.—SYNDESMOSES SCAPULÆ, PROPER LIGAMENTS OF THE SCAPULA ; SEEN FROM ABOVE.

Syndesmosis, fibrous or gamentous union—Discus articularis, interarticular fibrocartilage.

JUNCTURÆ OSSIUM TRUNCI

THE ARTICULATIONS OF THE TRUNK

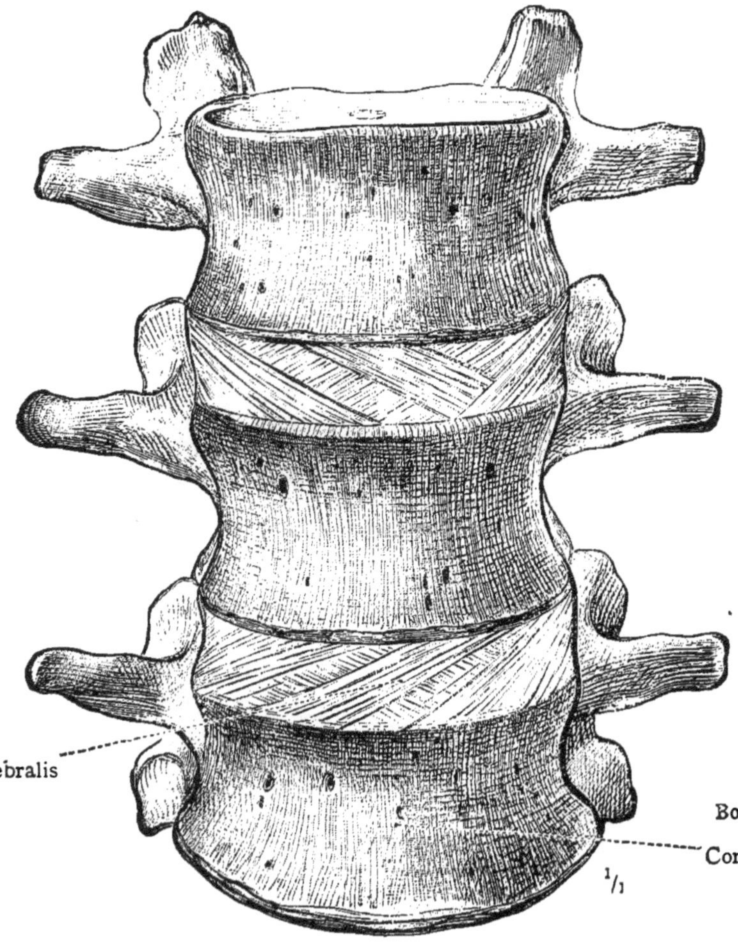

FIG. 396.—FIBROCARTILAGINES INTERVERTEBRALES, INTERVERTEBRAL DISCS. (SECOND, THIRD, AND FOURTH LUMBAR VERTEBRÆ; SEEN FROM BEFORE.)

Ligamenta columnæ vertebralis—The ligaments of the vertebral column.

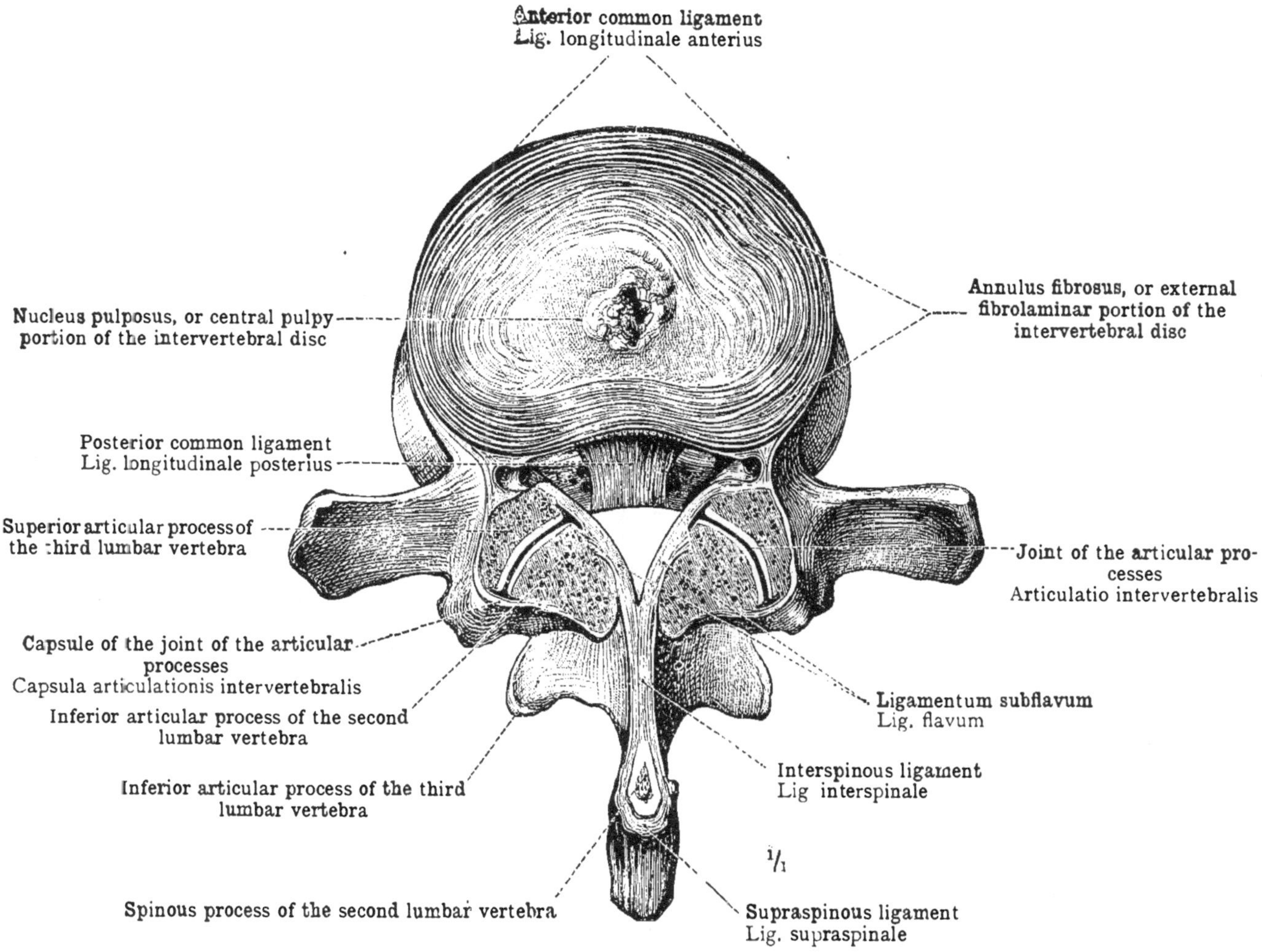

FIG. 397.—INTERVERTEBRAL DISC BETWEEN THE SECOND LUMBAR VERTEBRA AND THE THIRD. (LOWER HALF OF A HORIZONTAL SECTION.)

columnæ vertebralis—The ligaments of the vertebral column.

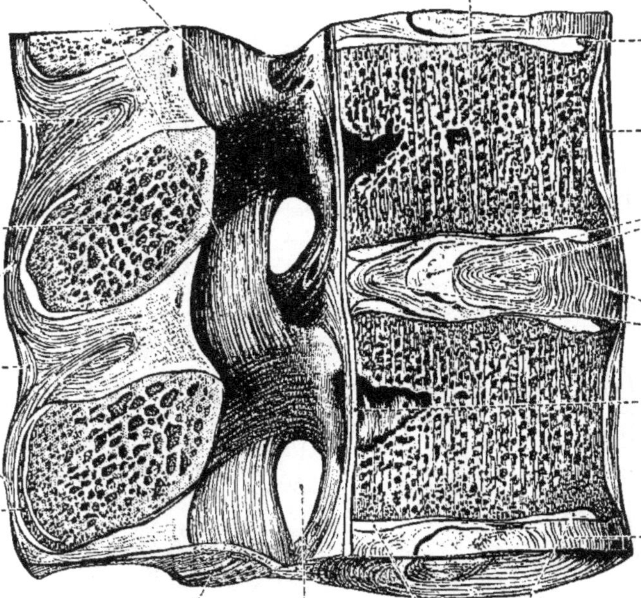

FIG. 398.—FIBROCARTILAGINES INTERVERTEBRALES, INTERVERTEBRAL DISCS. LIGAMENTA FLAVA, OR SUBFLAVA. LIGAMENTA INTERSPINALIA, INTERSPINOUS LIGAMENTS. LIGAMENTUM SUPRASPINALE, SUPRASPINOUS LIGAMENT. (MEDIAN SECTION THROUGH THE TWELFTH DORSAL AND THE FIRST LUMBAR VERTEBRÆ, LEFT HALF.)

Ligamenta columnæ vertebralis—The ligaments of the vertebral column.

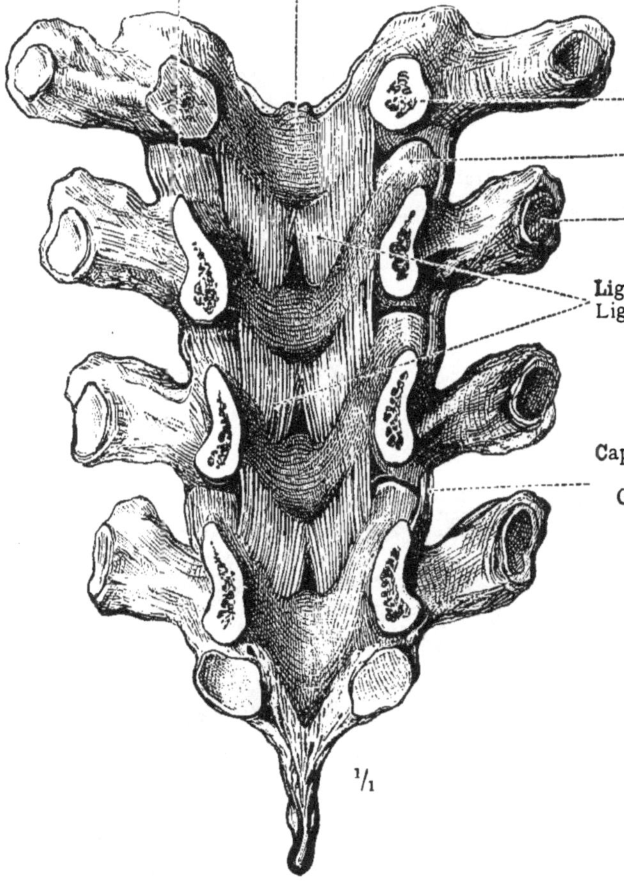

FIG. 399.—LIGAMENTA FLAVA, LIGAMENTA SUBFLAVA. ARTICULATIONES INTERVERTEBRALES, INTERVERTEBRAL ARTICULATIONS. OF THESE LATTER THE RIGHT ARE UNOPENED, THE LEFT OPENED. (THE ARCHES OF THE FIRST FOUR DORSAL VERTEBRÆ, SEPARATED FROM THE BODIES BY A FRONTAL SECTION. SEEN FROM BEFORE.)

Ligamenta columnæ vertebralis—The ligaments of the vertebral column.

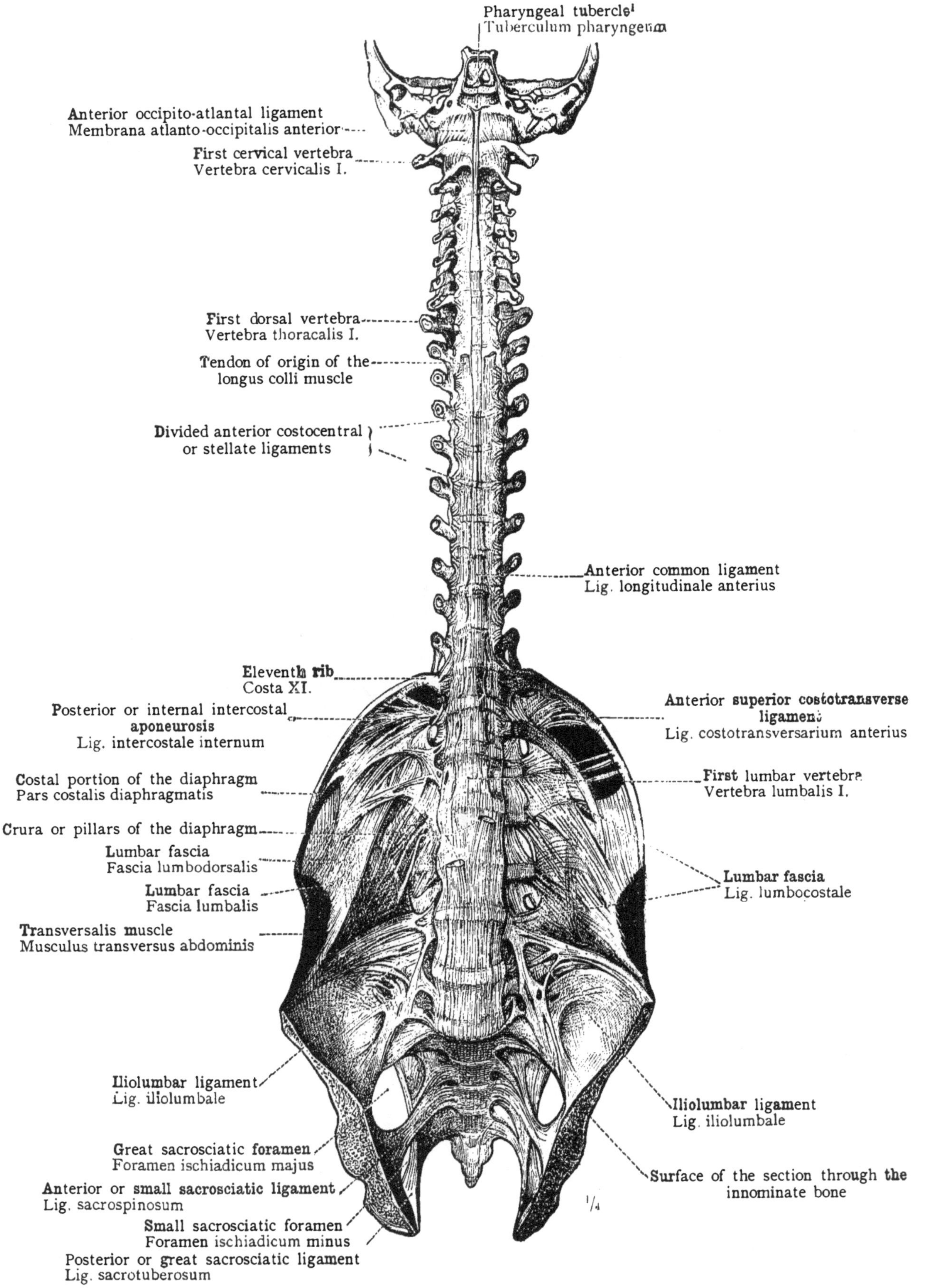

[1] U.S.: Pharyngeal spine.

FIG. 400.—LIGAMENTUM LONGITUDINALE ANTERIUS, THE ANTERIOR COMMON LIGAMENT. LIGAMENTUM LUMBOCOSTALE, LUMBOCOSTAL LIGAMENT. (THE VENTRAL ASPECT OF THE VERTEBRAL COLUMN, THE ANTERIOR HALF OF THE BASE OF THE SKULL AND THE ANTERIOR HALF OF THE PELVIS HAVING BEEN REMOVED.)

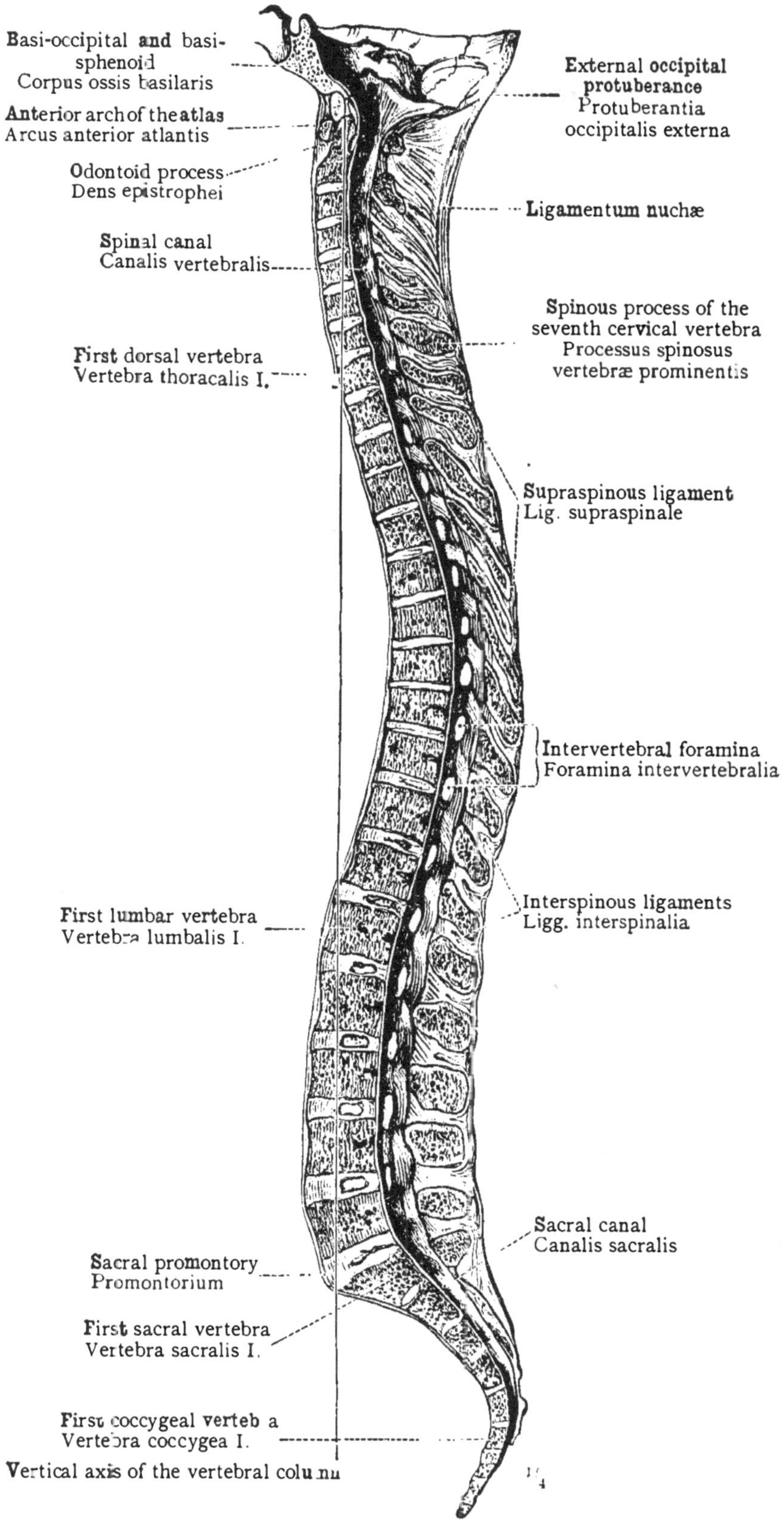

FIG. 401.—INTERVERTEBRAL DISCS, INTERSPINOUS LIGAMENTS, SUPRASPINOUS LIGAMENT, LIGAMENTUM NUCHÆ. SPINAL CANAL; INTERVERTEBRAL FORAMINA. VERTICAL AXIS OF THE VERTEBRAL COLUMN. (MEDIAN SECTION THROUGH THE VERTEBRAL COLUMN.)

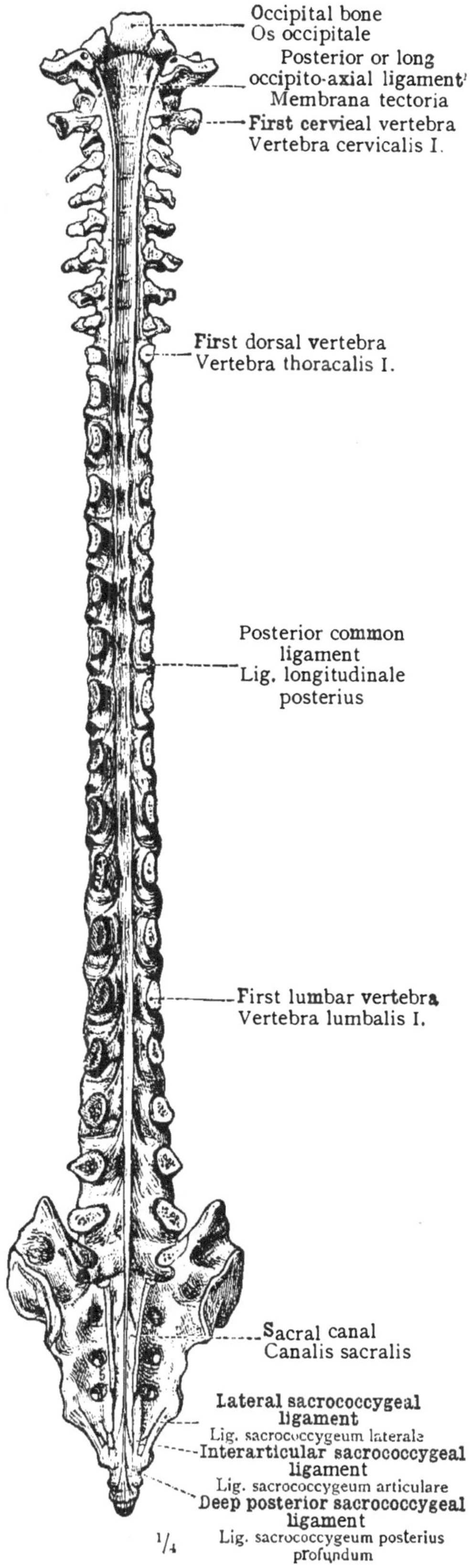

FIG. 402.—POSTERIOR COMMON LIGAMENT AND ITS RELATION WITH THE POSTERIOR OCCIPITO-AXIAL AND THE DEEP POSTERIOR SACROCOCCYGEAL LIGAMENTS. (THE VERTEBRAL COLUMN WITH THE SPINAL CANAL OPENED BY THE REMOVAL OF THE NEURAL ARCHES; SEEN FROM BEHIND.)

[1] Macalister calls this ligament *ligamentum latum axiale*, the broad axial ligament.—TR.

Ligamenta columnæ vertebralis—The ligaments of the vertebral column.

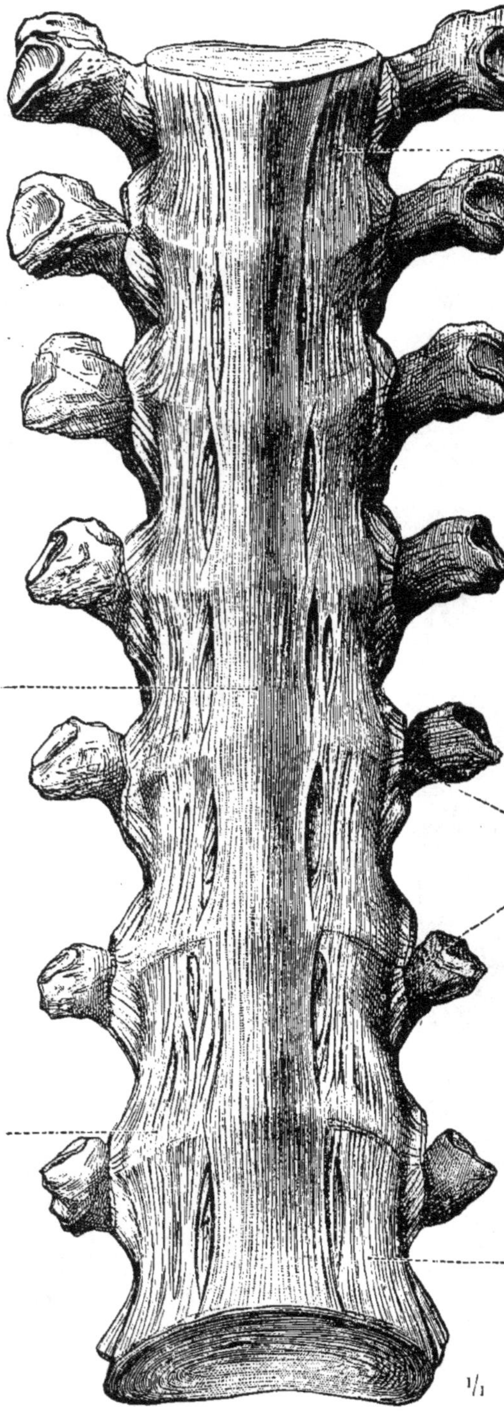

FIG. 403.—LIGAMENTUM LONGITUDINALE ANTERIUS, THE ANTERIOR COMMON LIGAMENT OF THE VERTEBRAL COLUMN. (THE FOURTH TO THE TENTH DORSAL VERTEBRÆ; SEEN FROM BEFORE.)

Ligamenta columnæ vertebralis—The ligaments of the vertebral column.

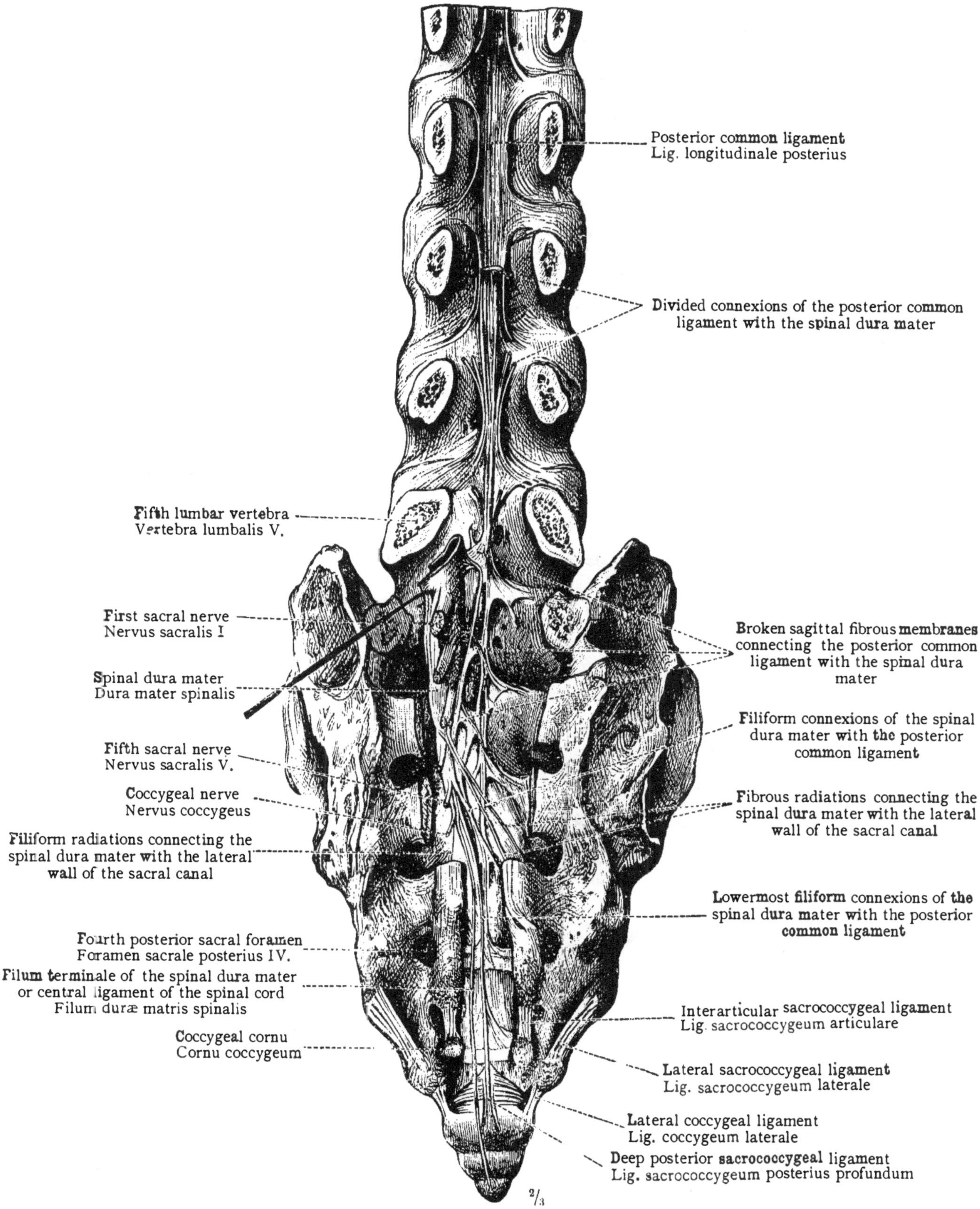

FIG. 404.—LUMBAR AND SACRAL PORTIONS OF THE POSTERIOR COMMON LIGAMENT, AND THE CONNEXIONS OF THIS LIGAMENT WITH THE SPINAL DURA MATER AND WITH THE DEEP POSTERIOR SACROCOCCYGEAL LIGAMENT. (THE SACRUM AND THE LUMBAR PORTION OF THE VERTEBRAL COLUMN WITH THE SPINAL CANAL LAID OPEN FROM BEHIND.)

The sacral portion of the dura mater has been drawn to the left side.

Ligamenta columnæ vertebralis—The ligaments of the vertebral column.

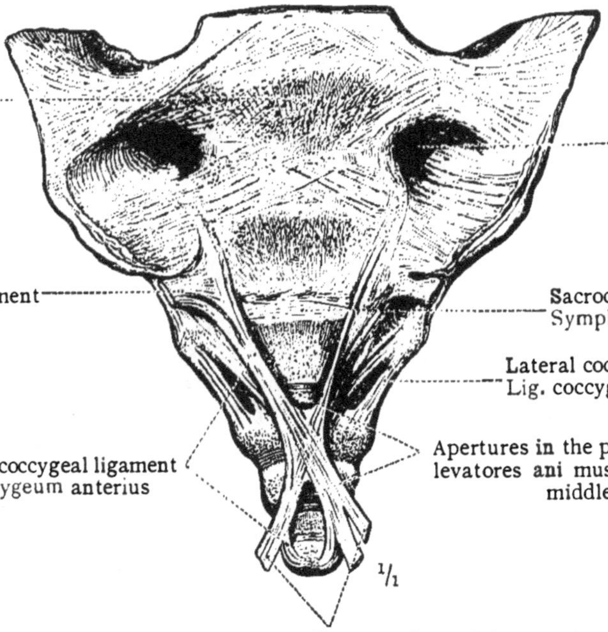

FIG. 405.—THE LIGAMENTS CONNECTING THE ANTERIOR SURFACES OF THE SACRUM AND COCCYX: THE ANTERIOR AND THE LATERAL SACROCOCCYGEAL LIGAMENTS.

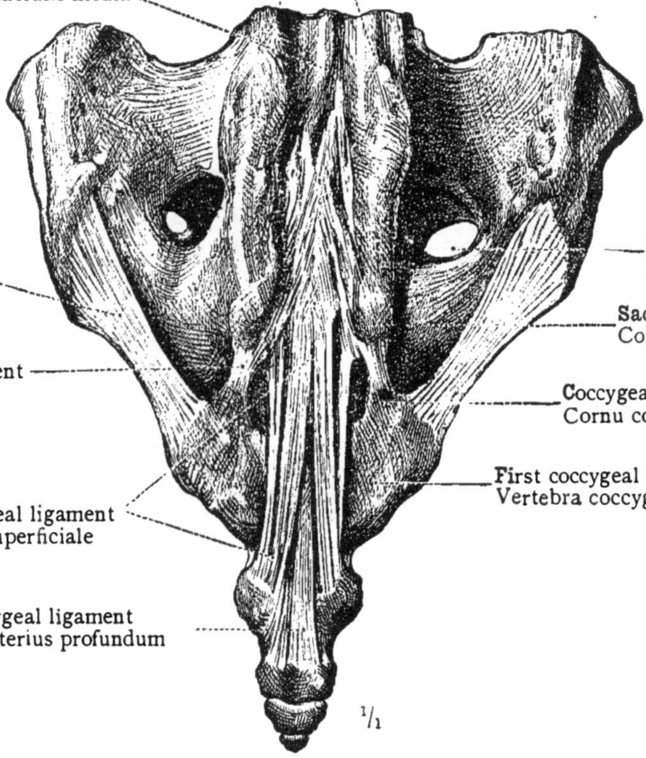

FIG. 406.—THE LIGAMENTS CONNECTING THE POSTERIOR SURFACES OF THE SACRUM AND COCCYX: THE SUPERFICIAL AND DEEP POSTERIOR SACROCOCCYGEAL LIGAMENTS, AND THE INTERARTICULAR AND LATERAL SACROCOCCYGEAL LIGAMENTS.

THE COCCYX WITH THE TWO LAST SACRAL VERTEBRÆ.

Ligamenta columnæ vertebralis—The ligaments of the vertebral column.

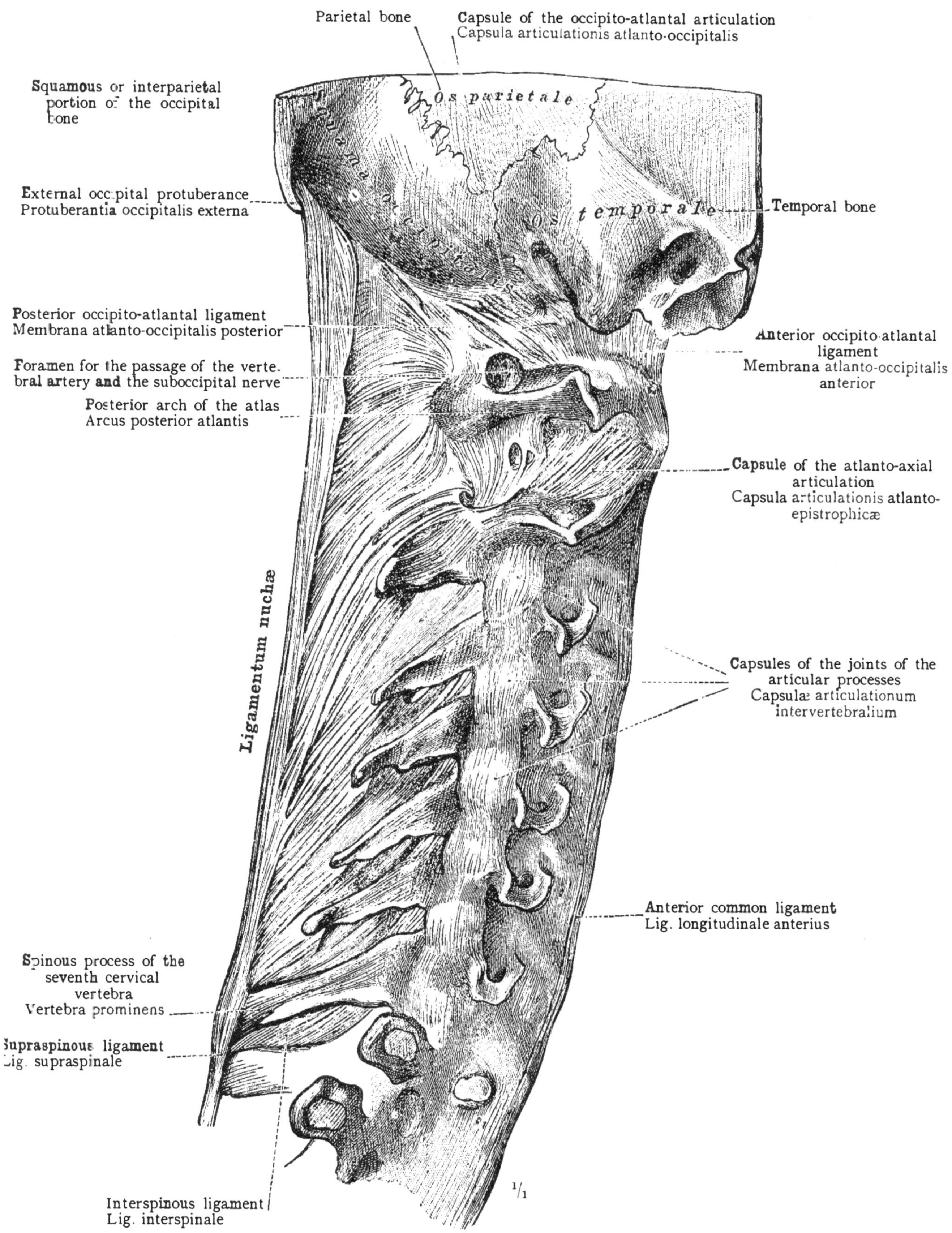

FIG. 407.—LIGAMENTUM NUCHÆ. (THE CERVICAL PORTION OF THE VERTEBRAL COLUMN AND THE POSTERIOR PORTION OF THE CRANIUM; SEEN FROM THE RIGHT SIDE.)

Ligamenta columnæ vertebralis—The ligaments of the vertebral column.

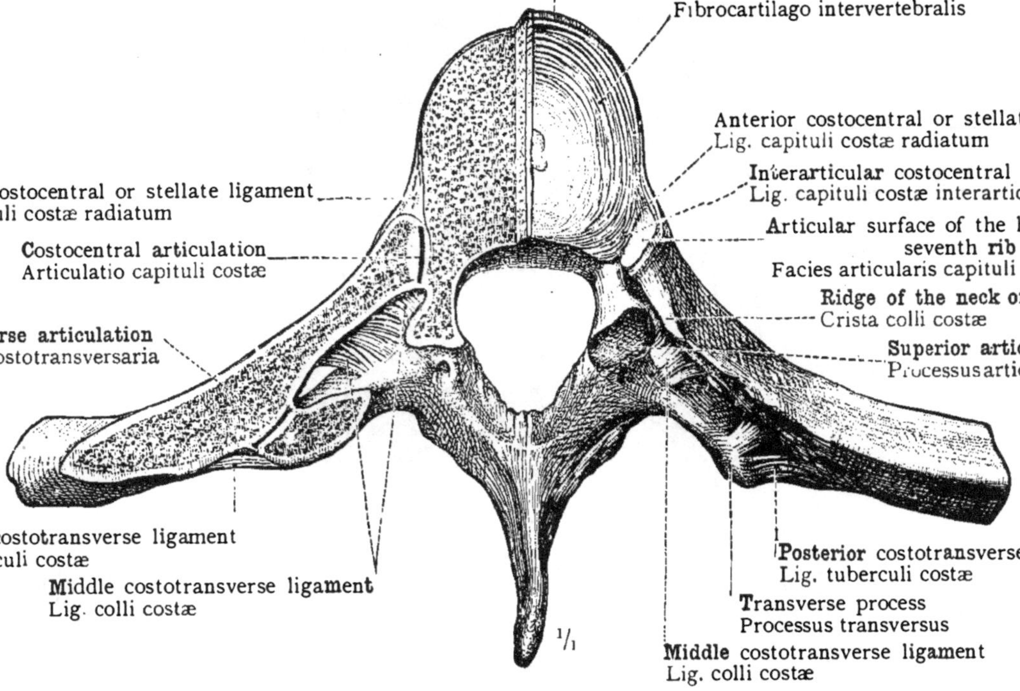

FIG. 408.—ARTICULATIONES CAPITULORUM ET COSTOTRANSVERSARIÆ, THE COSTOCENTRAL AND COSTOTRANSVERSE ARTICULATIONS: LIGAMENTUM CAPITULI COSTÆ INTERARTICULARE, THE INTERARTICULAR COSTOCENTRAL LIGAMENT; LIGAMENTUM COLLI COSTÆ ET LIGAMENTUM TUBERCULI COSTÆ, THE MIDDLE AND POSTERIOR COSTOTRANSVERSE LIGAMENTS. (THE SEVENTH DORSAL VERTEBRA WITH THE VERTEBRAL EXTREMITIES OF THE SEVENTH PAIR OF RIBS; SEEN FROM ABOVE.)

On the left side the costocentral and costotransverse articulations have been opened by a horizontal section through the rib and the vertebral body; on the right side the section passes through the intervertebral disc on a plane just above the attachment of the interarticular costocentral ligament to the ridge between the two articular facets on the vertebral extremity of the rib.

Articulationes costovertebrales—Costovertebral articulations.

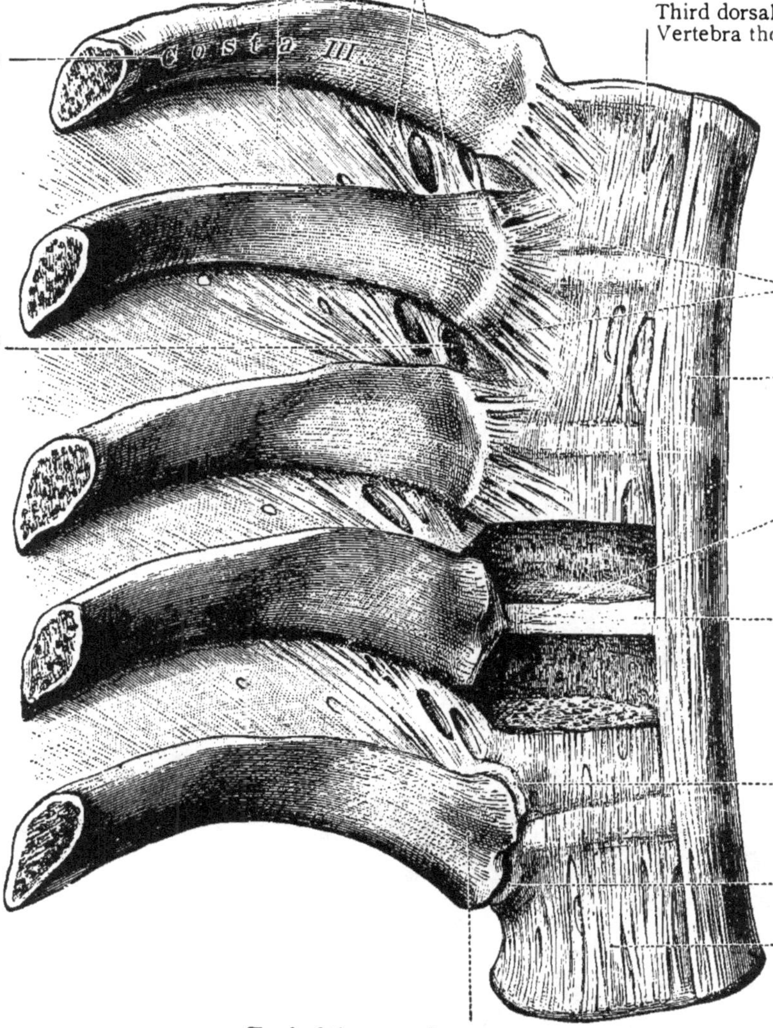

[1] This term, *costotransverse foramen*, is also used by English anatomists to denote the foramina in the transverse processes of the cervical vertebræ for the transmission of the vertebral artery.—TR.

[2] These are upper and lower costal facets respectively in relation to the articular surface of the head of the rib: but, strictly speaking, what is here called "upper costal facet" is the lower costal facet of the sixth dorsal vertebra; while what is here called "lower costal facet" is the upper costal facet of the seventh dorsal vertebra.—TR.

FIG. 409.—COSTOCENTRAL AND COSTOTRANSVERSE ARTICULATIONS: ANTERIOR COSTOCENTRAL OR STELLATE LIGAMENT; INTERARTICULAR COSTOCENTRAL LIGAMENT; ANTERIOR SUPERIOR COSTOTRANSVERSE LIGAMENT; AND COSTOTRANSVERSE FORAMINA. POSTERIOR OR INTERNAL INTERCOSTAL APONEUROSES. (THE THIRD TO THE SEVENTH DORSAL VERTEBRÆ WITH THE VERTEBRAL EXTREMITIES OF THE THIRD TO THE SEVENTH RIGHT RIBS; SEEN FROM THE RIGHT AND FROM BEFORE.)

The third, fourth, and fifth costocentral articulations are unopened; the sixth and the seventh have been opened from before. In the sixth articulation, by the partial removal of the bodies of the fifth and sixth dorsal vertebræ, the upper and lower surfaces of the intervertebral disc have been exposed, and the attachment of the disc to the ridge between the two articular facets on the head of the rib has been demonstrated.

Articulationes costovertebrales—Costovertebral articulations.

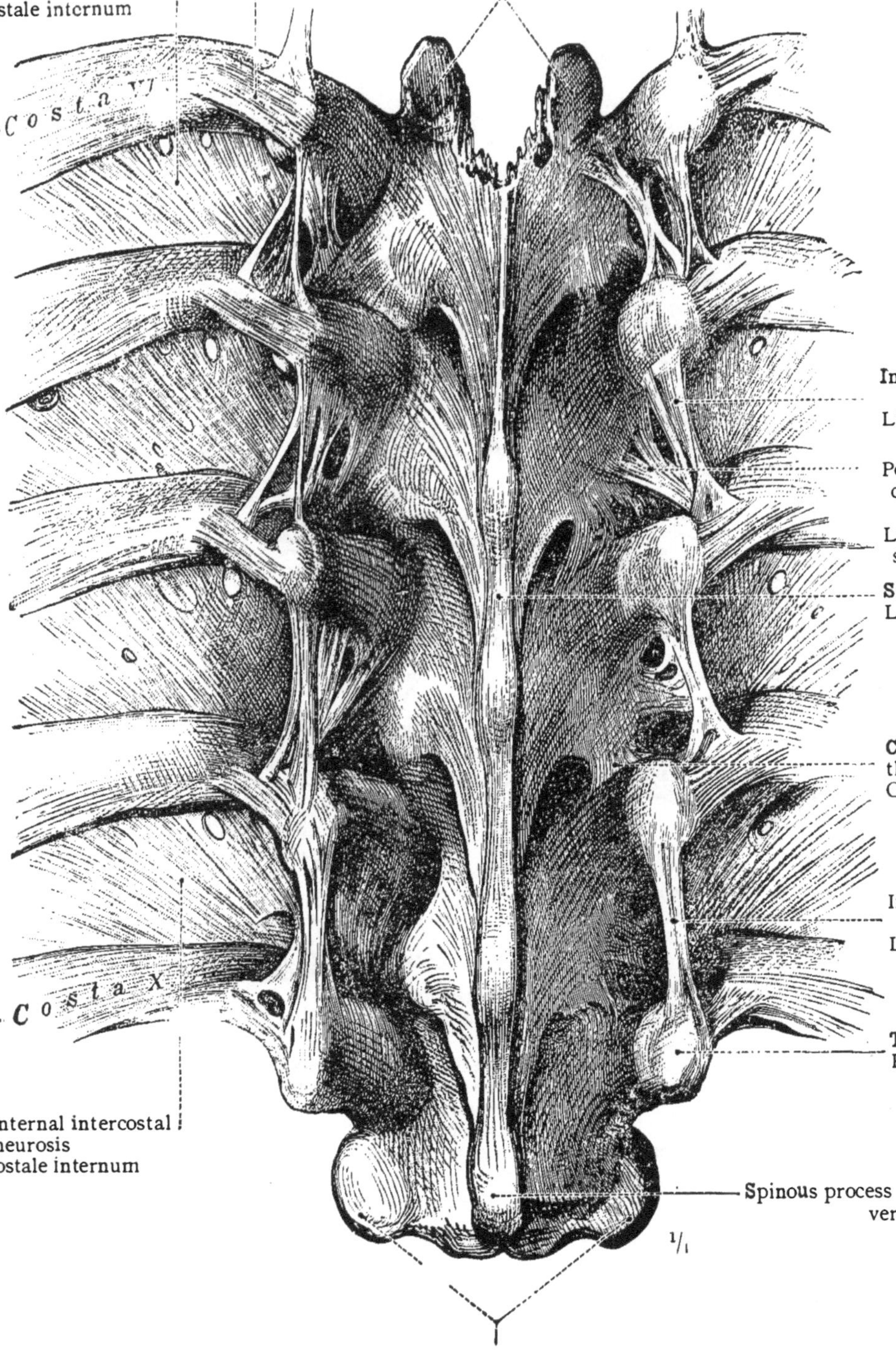

Fig. 410.—The Ligaments connecting the Dorsal Vertebræ with the Ribs posteriorly: Posterior and Posterior Superior Costotransverse Ligaments; Intertransverse Ligaments; Posterior or Internal Intercostal Aponeuroses; Supraspinous Ligament. (Sixth to Tenth Dorsal Vertebræ with the Vertebral Extremities of the Sixth to Tenth Ribs.)

Articulationes costovertebrales—Costovertebral articulations.

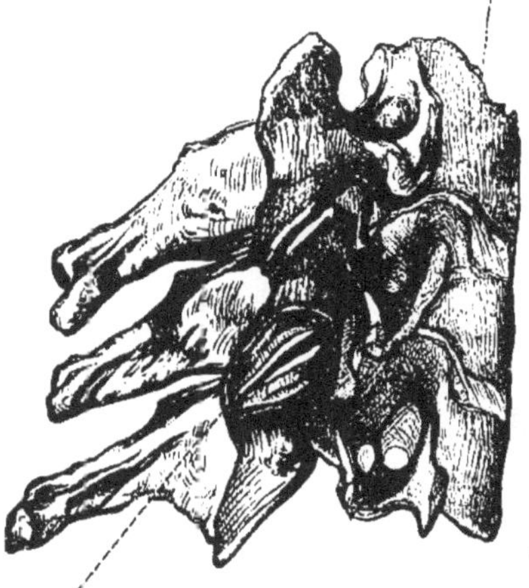

FIG. 411.—THIRD, FOURTH, AND FIFTH CERVICAL VERTEBRÆ SEEN FROM THE RIGHT SIDE.

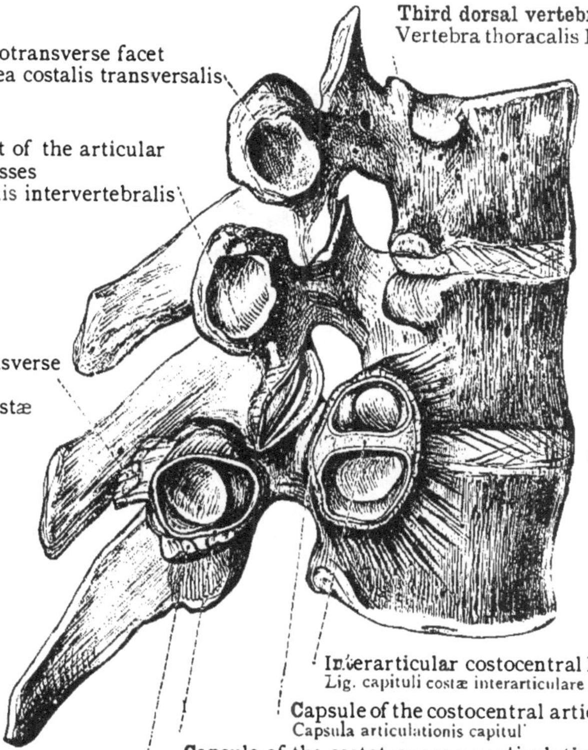

FIG. 412.—THIRD, FOURTH, AND FIFTH DORSAL VERTEBRÆ SEEN FROM THE RIGHT SIDE.

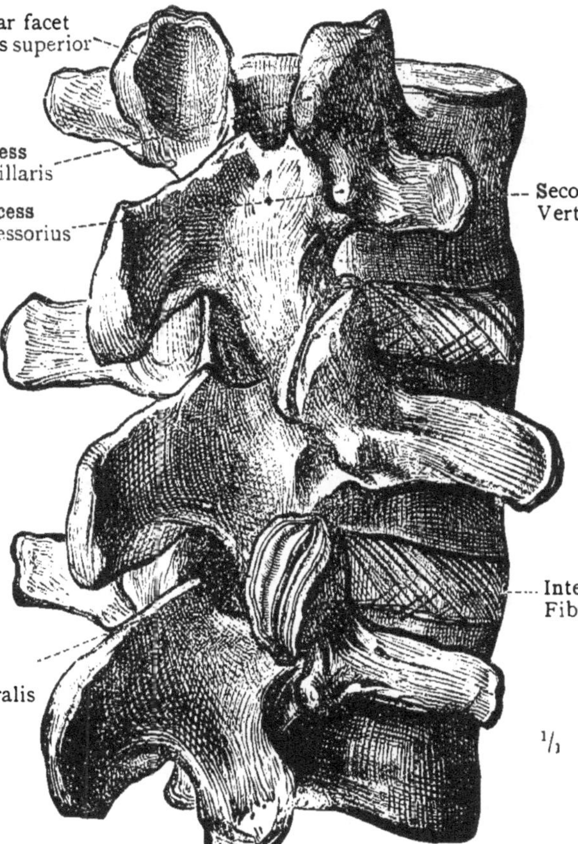

FIG. 413.—SECOND, THIRD, AND FOURTH LUMBAR VERTEBRÆ SEEN FROM THE RIGHT AND FROM BEHIND.

THE DIRECTION OF THE ARTICULAR SURFACES AND THE CONNEXIONS OF THE CAPSULES OF THE JOINTS OF THE ARTICULAR PROCESSES IN THE CERVICAL, DORSAL, AND LUMBAR VERTEBRÆ RESPECTIVELY.

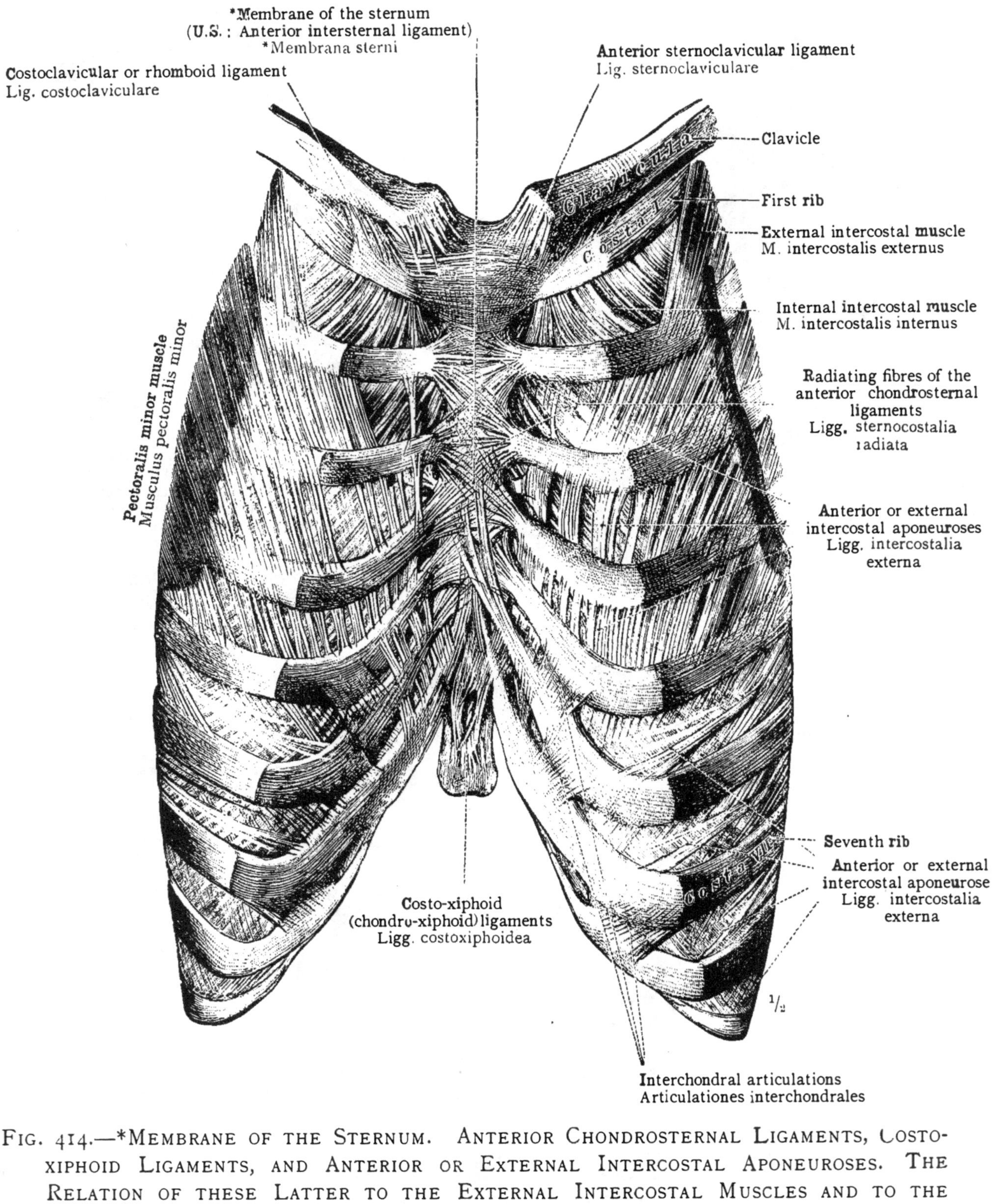

FIG. 414.—*MEMBRANE OF THE STERNUM. ANTERIOR CHONDROSTERNAL LIGAMENTS, COSTO-XIPHOID LIGAMENTS, AND ANTERIOR OR EXTERNAL INTERCOSTAL APONEUROSES. THE RELATION OF THESE LATTER TO THE EXTERNAL INTERCOSTAL MUSCLES AND TO THE PECTORALIS MINOR MUSCLE. (ANTERIOR WALL OF THE THORAX SEEN FROM BEFORE.)

Articulationes sternocostales—Chondrosternal articulations.

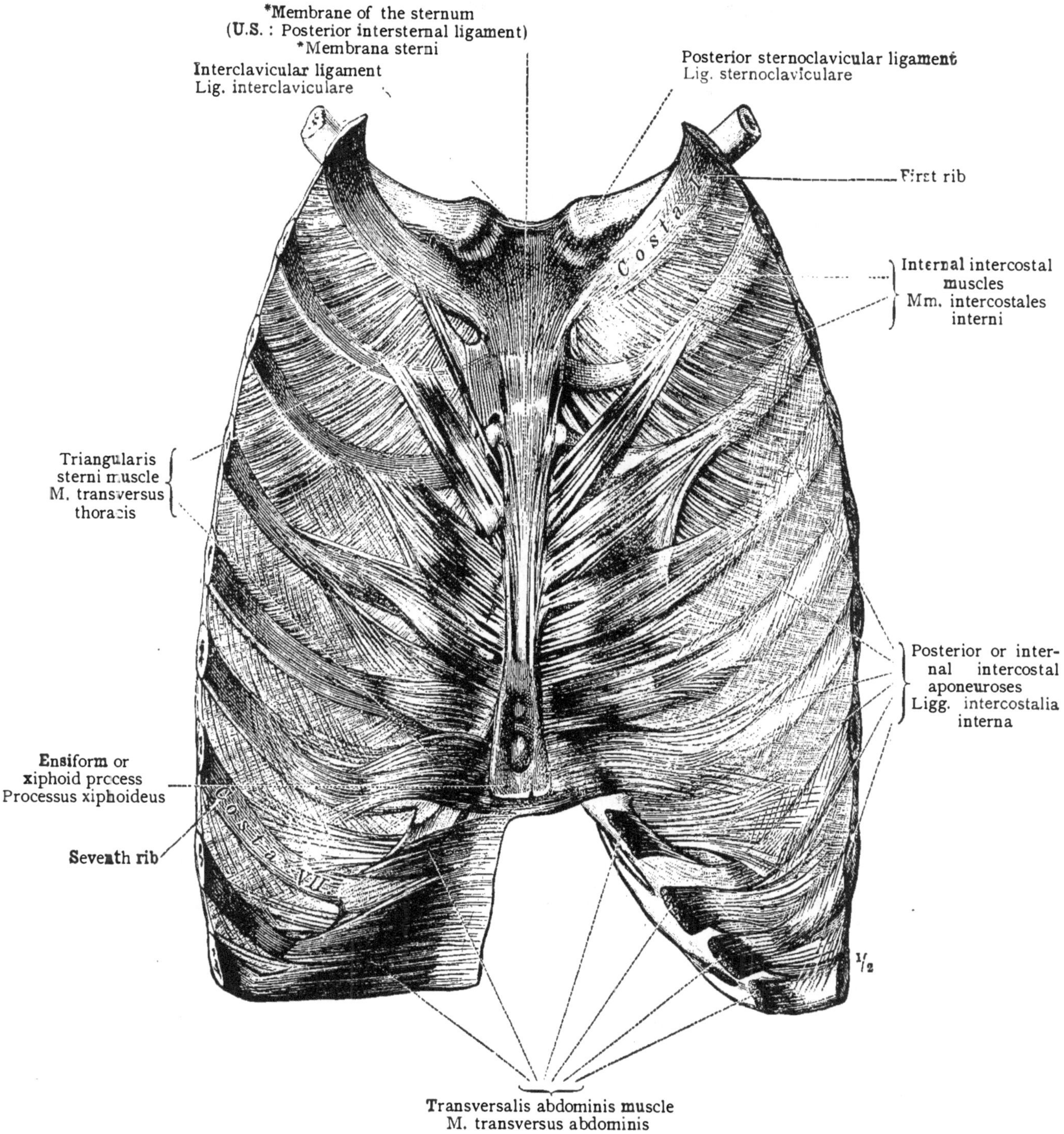

FIG. 415.—POSTERIOR OR INTERNAL INTERCOSTAL APONEUROSES, AND THEIR RELATION TO THE TRIANGULARIS STERNI AND TRANSVERSALIS ABDOMINIS MUSCLES. STERNOCLAVICULAR ARTICULATION. (ANTERIOR WALL OF THE THORAX SEEN FROM BEHIND.)

Articulationes sternocostales—Chondrosternal articulations.

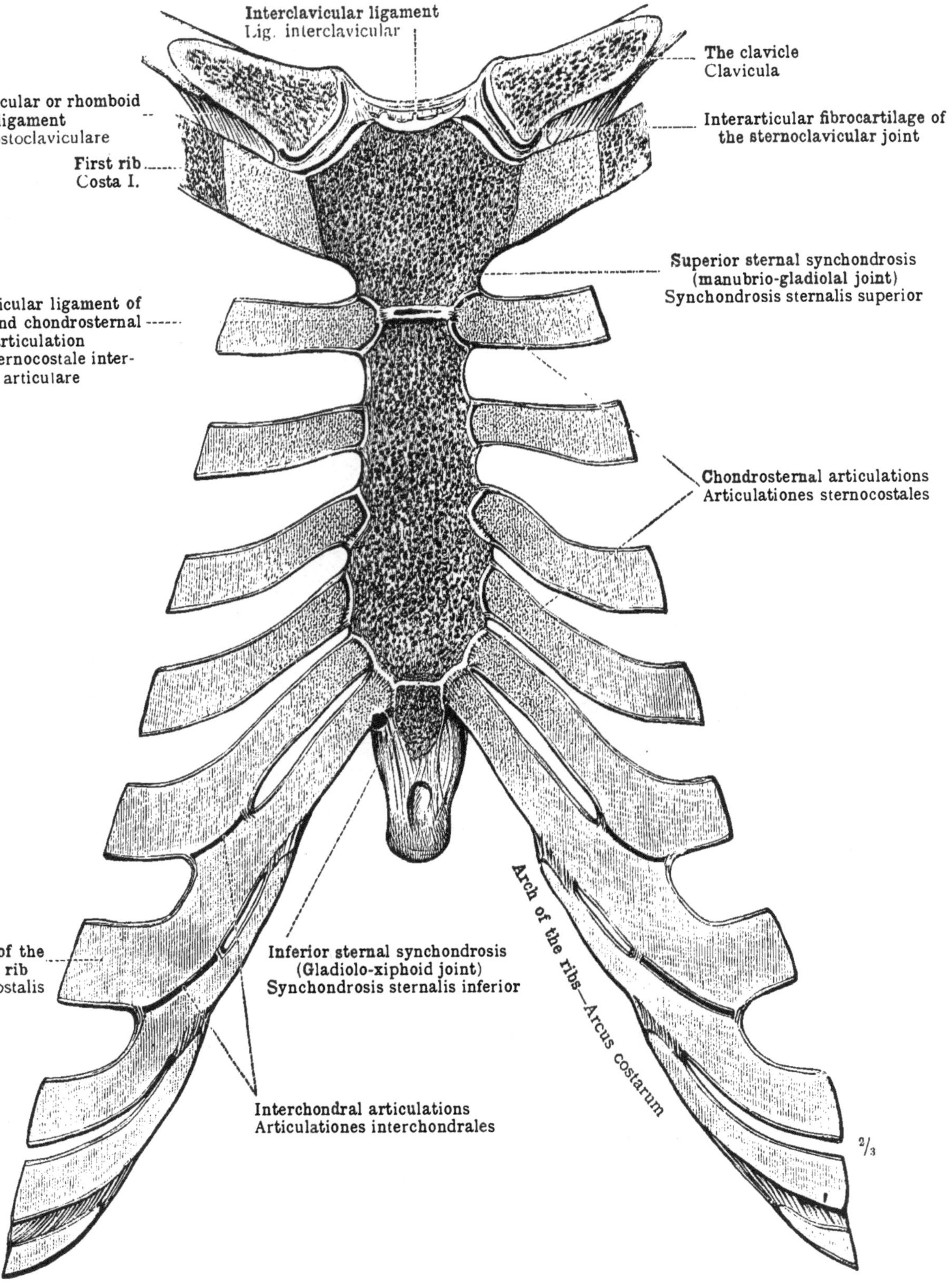

FIG. 416.—CHONDROSTERNAL ARTICULATIONS. INTERCHONDRAL ARTICULATIONS. INTERSTERNAL SYNCHONDROSES. STERNOCLAVICULAR ARTICULATION. (POSTERIOR HALF OF A FRONTAL SECTION THROUGH THE STERNUM, THE CARTILAGES OF THE RIBS, AND THE STERNAL EXTREMITIES OF THE CLAVICLES.)

Articulationes sternocostales—Chondrosternal articulations.

ARTICULATIONES
ET LIGAMENTA CAPITIS

THE ARTICULATIONS
AND LIGAMENTS OF THE HEAD

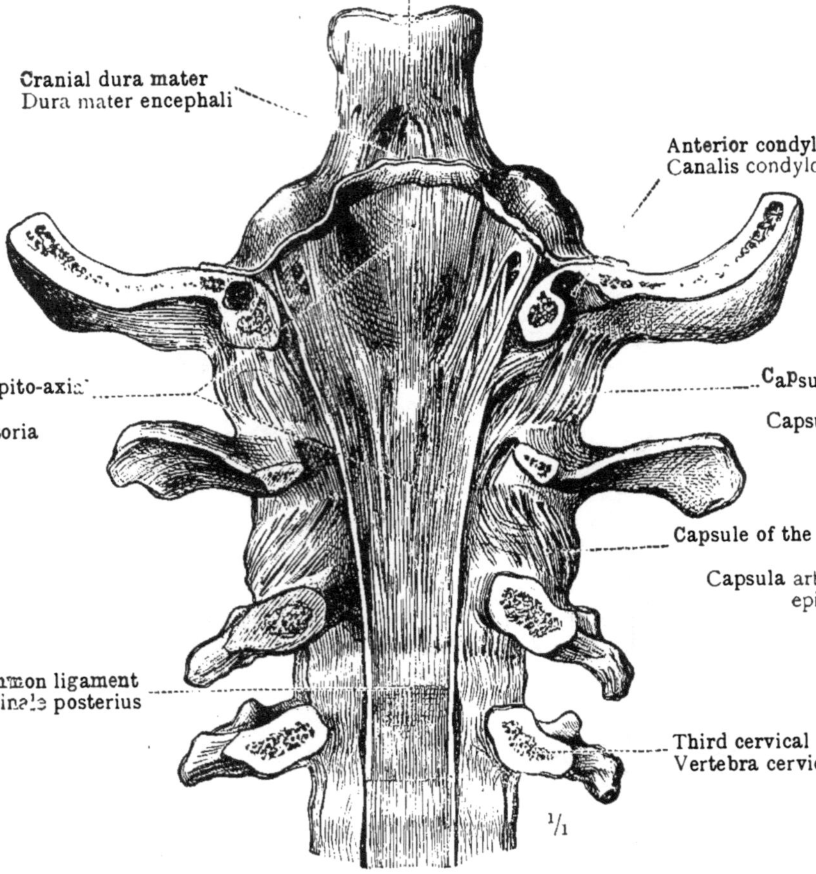

[1] See note to p. 177.

FIG. 417.—POSTERIOR OCCIPITO-AXIAL LIGAMENT. OCCIPITO-ATLANTAL AND ATLANTO-AXIAL SYNOVIAL JOINTS. (THE THREE UPPERMOST CERVICAL VERTEBRÆ AND THE OCCIPITAL BONE SEEN FROM BEHIND.)

By a frontal section behind the occipital condyles, the squamous portion of the occipital bone and the neural arches have been removed. The dura mater has been cut transversely in the basilar groove, and turned upwards

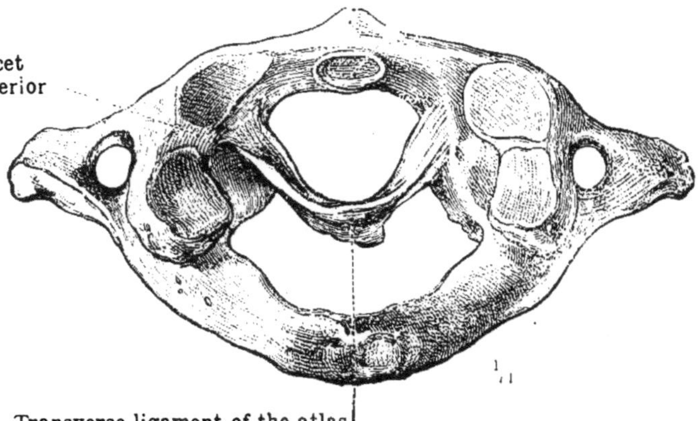

FIG. 418.—TRANSVERSE LIGAMENT OF THE ATLAS. (THE ATLAS SEEN FROM ABOVE.)

Articulationes atlanto-occipitalis et atlanto-epistrophica—Occipito-atlantal and atlanto-axial

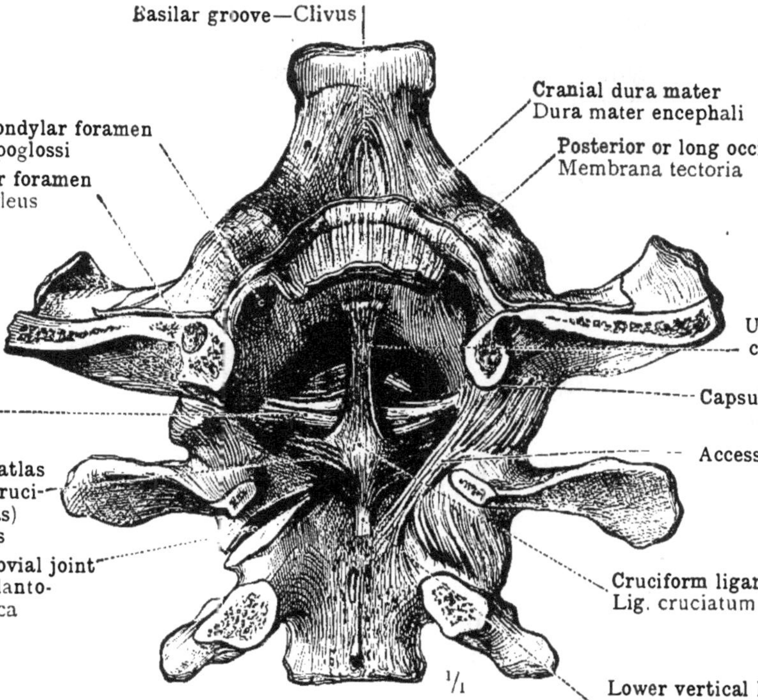

FIG. 419.—CRUCIFORM LIGAMENT OF THE ATLAS; LATERAL OR ALAR ODONTOID OR CHECK LIGAMENTS OCCIPITO-ATLANTAL AND ATLANTO-AXIAL SYNOVIAL JOINTS, THE RIGHT CLOSED, THE LEFT OPEN.

The cranial dura mater and the posterior or long occipito-axial ligament[1] have been cut transversely in the basilar groove and turned upwards.

[1] See note to p. 177.

[2] *Accessory occipito-axial ligament.* This ligament is not mentioned by the author, though it is well shown in Fig. 419. The accessory ligament is a bundle of fibres strengthening the capsule of the occipito-atlantal joint at its postero-internal angle. It runs downwards and inwards from the back of the occipital condyle to the body of the axis near the base of the odontoid process.—TR.

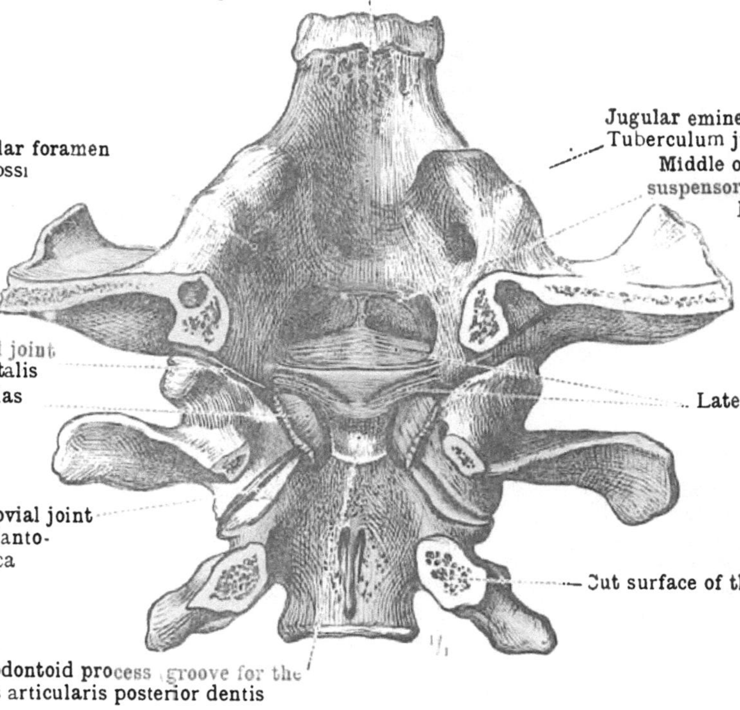

FIG. 420.—LATERAL OR ALAR ODONTOID OR CHECK LIGAMENTS. MIDDLE ODONTOID LIGAMENT OR SUSPENSORY LIGAMENT OF THE AXIS.

The transverse ligament of the atlas has been divided in the middle and the parts have been turned outwards; the dura mater and the posterior or long occipito-axial ligament have been entirely removed.

THE ATLAS AND THE AXIS WITH THE ANTERIOR PORTION OF THE OCCIPITAL BONE SEEN FROM BEHIND, A SECTION HAVING BEEN MADE SIMILAR TO THAT IN THE PREPARATION SHOWN IN FIG. 414.

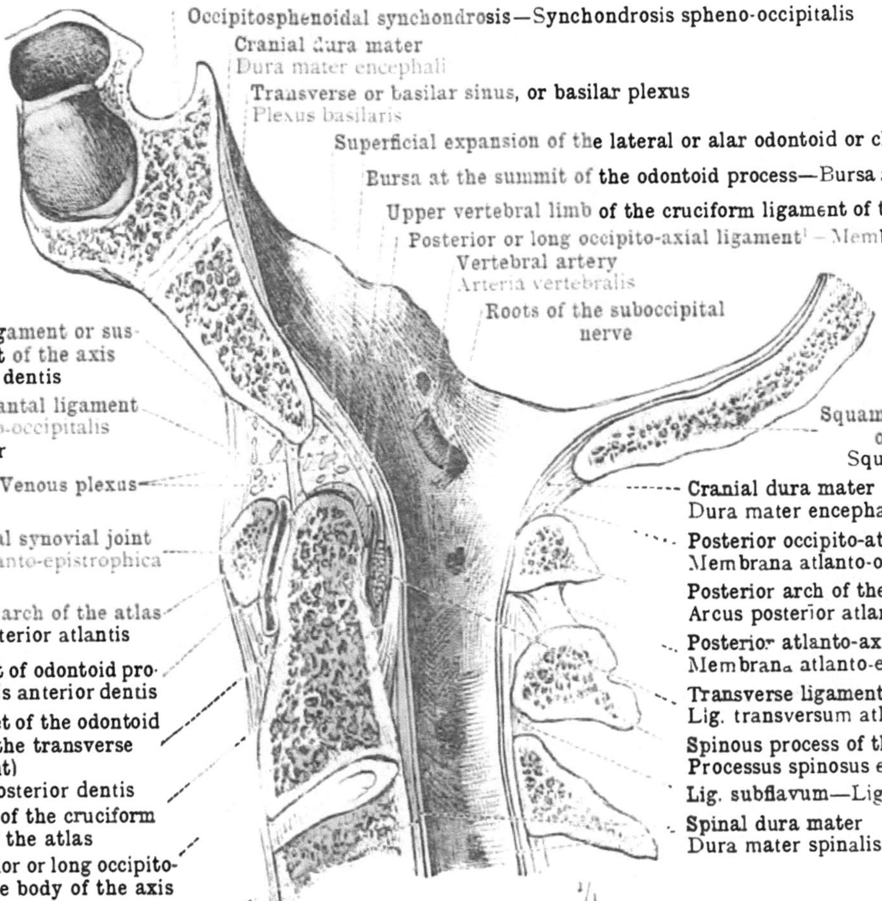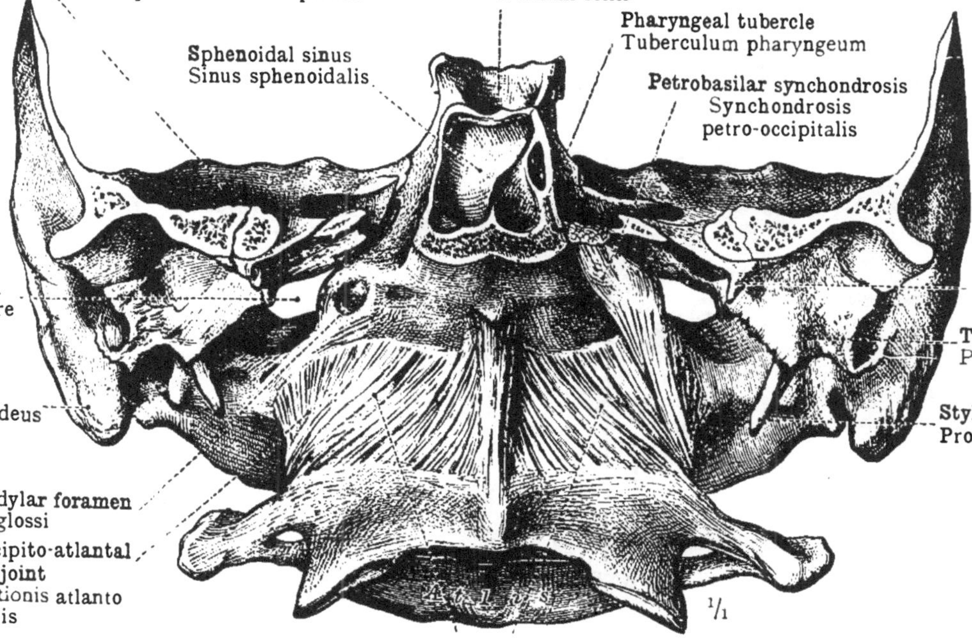

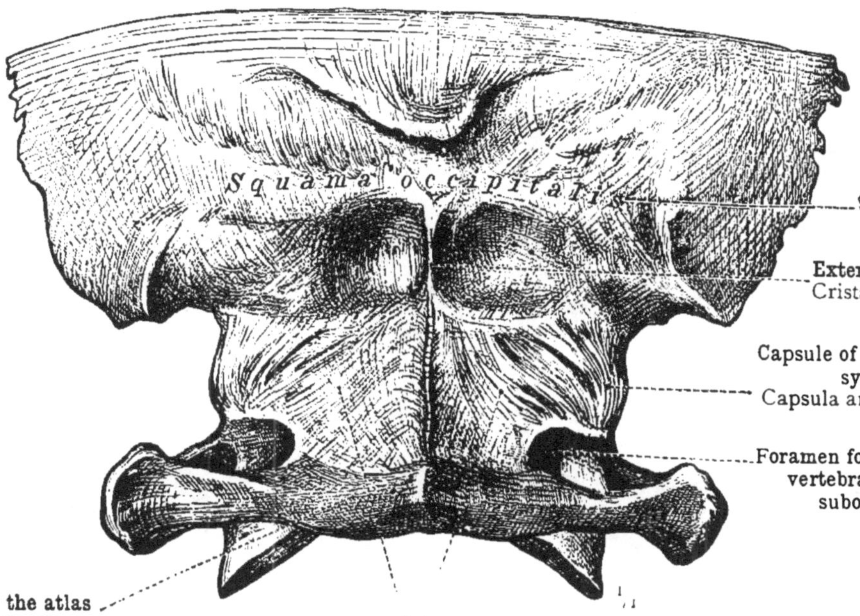

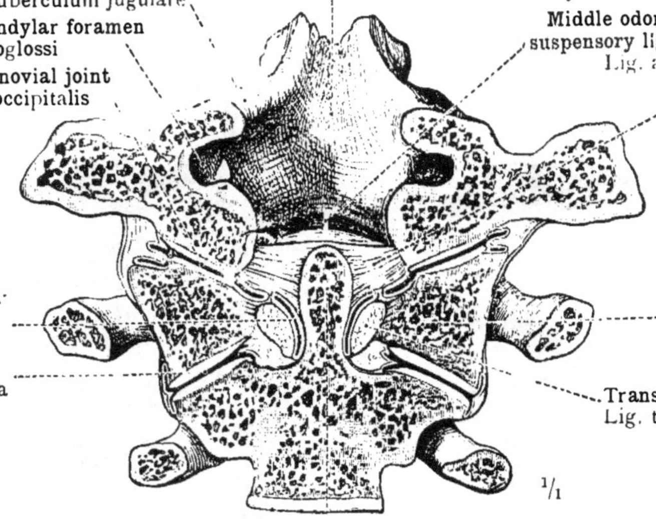

FIG. 421.—OCCIPITO-ATLANTAL AND ATLANTO-AXIAL ARTICULATIONS IN FRONTAL SECTION. LATERAL OR ALAR ODONTOID OR CHECK LIGAMENTS AND MIDDLE ODONTOID LIGAMENT OR SUSPENSORY LIGAMENT OF THE AXIS.

The section passes through the middle of the posterior condylar foramina, and divides the summit of the antero-posterior curve of the occipital condyles.

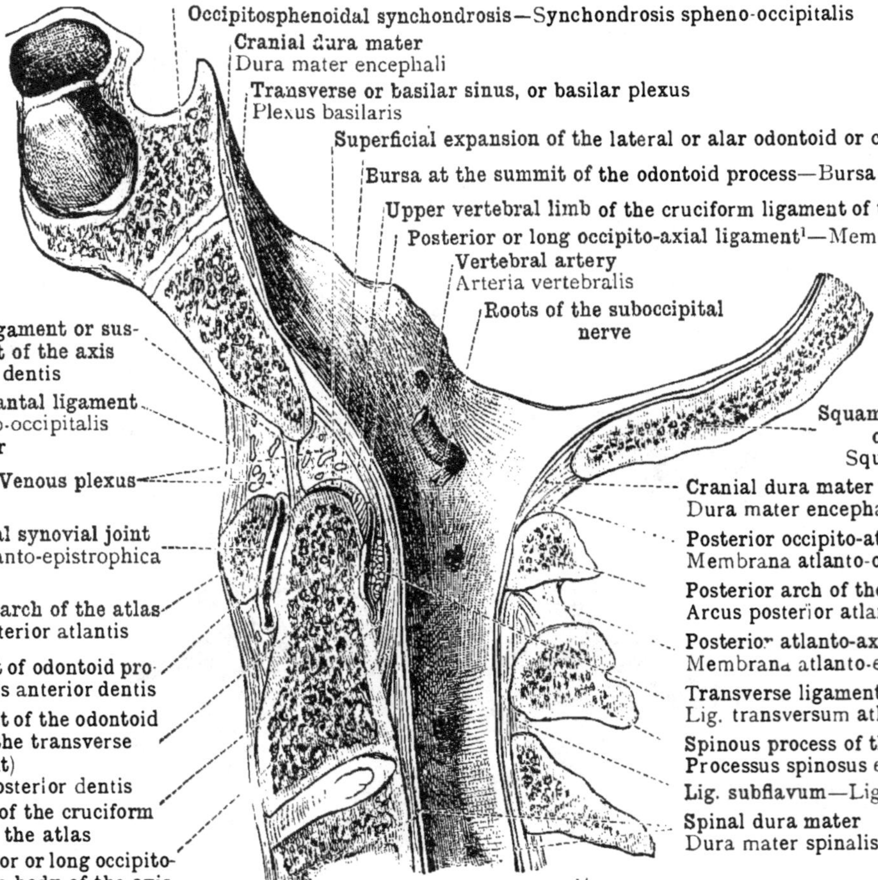

See note to p. 177.

FIG. 422.—ARTICULATIONS AND LIGAMENTS OF THE ODONTOID PROCESS. STRATIFORM ARRANGEMENT OF THE CRUCIFORM LIGAMENT OF THE ATLAS, THE POSTERIOR OR LONG OCCIPITO-AXIAL LIGAMENT, AND THE DURA MATER. SPHENO-OCCIPITAL SYNCHONDROSIS. (MEDIAN SECTION THROUGH THE POSTERIOR PORTION OF THE BASE OF THE CRANIUM AND THE THREE UPPERMOST CERVICAL VERTEBRÆ.)

Articulationes atlanto-occipitalis et atlanto-epistrophica—Occipito-atlantal and atlanto-axial

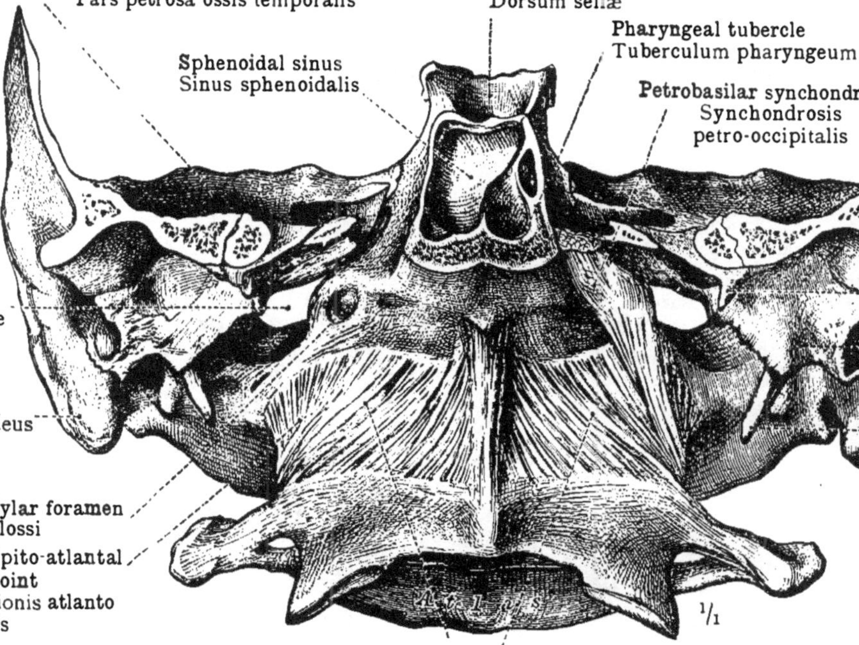

FIG. 423.—ANTEP OR OCCIPITO-ATLANTAL LIGAMENT AND PETROBASILAR SYNCHONDROSIS. (THE ATLAS WITH THE POSTERIOR PORTION OF THE BASE OF THE SKULL, SEEN FROM BEFORE.)

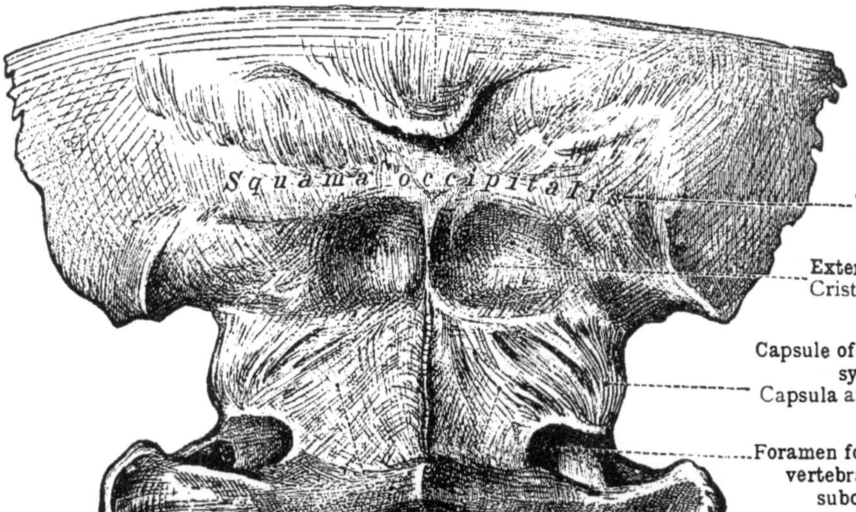

FIG. 424.—POSTERIOR OCCIPITO-ATLANTAL LIGAMENT. (THE ATLAS WITH THE OCCIPITAL BONE, SEEN FROM BEHIND.)

Articulatio atlanto-occipitalis—Occipito-atlantal articulation.

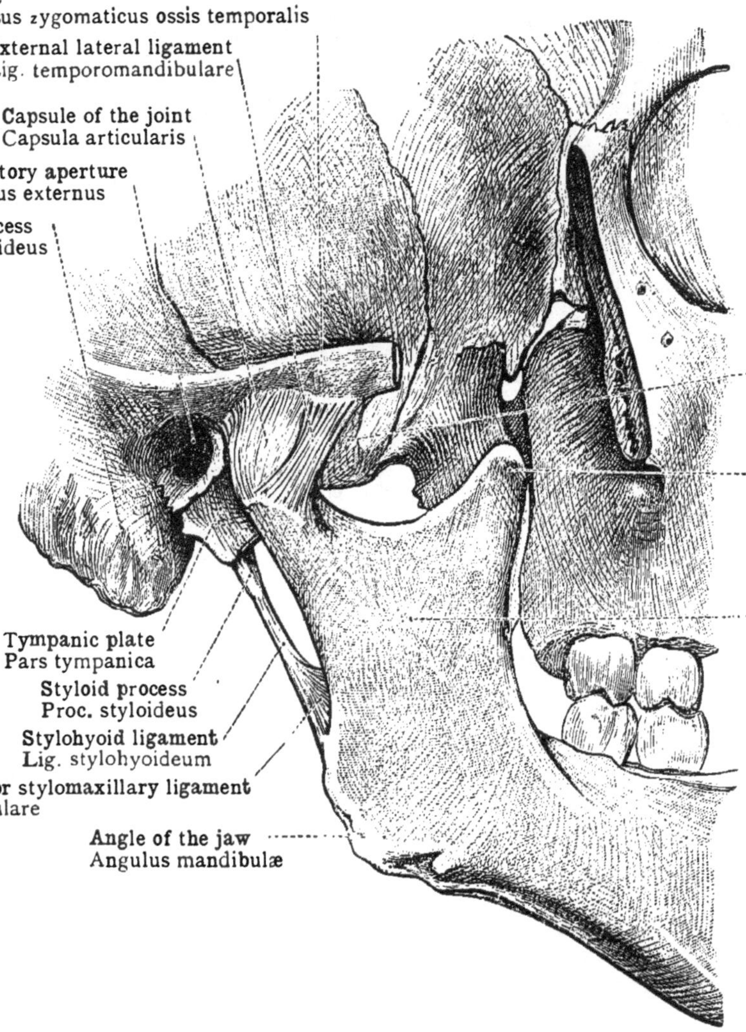

FIG. 425.—ARTICULATIO MANDIBULARIS, TEMPOROMANDIBULAR OR TEMPOROMAXILLARY ARTICULATION: LIGAMENTA TEMPOROMANDIBULARE ET STYLOMANDIBULARE, EXTERNAL LATERAL AND STYLOMANDIBULAR OR STYLOMAXILLARY LIGAMENTS. LIGAMENTUM STYLOHYOIDEUM, STYLOHYOID LIGAMENT. (RIGHT TEMPOROMANDIBULAR OR TEMPOROMAXILLARY ARTICULATION, SEEN FROM THE OUTER SIDE.)

Articulatio mandibularis—Temporomandibular or temporomaxillary articulation.

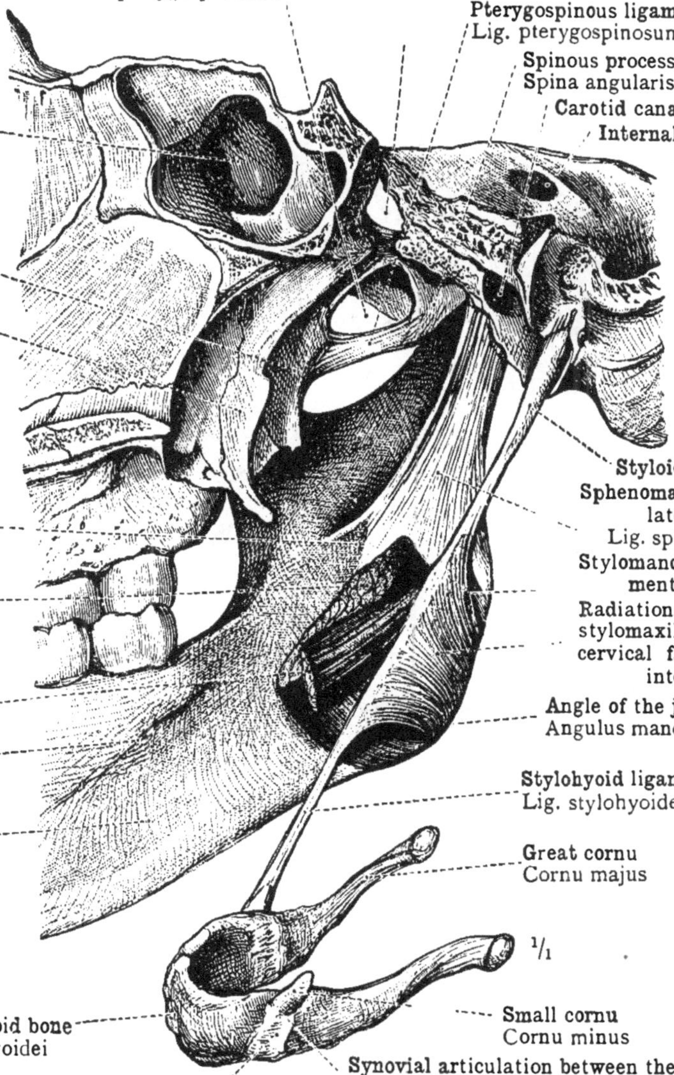

FIG. 426.—ARTICULATIO MANDIBULARIS, TEMPOROMANDIBULAR OR TEMPOROMAXILLARY ARTICULATION. LIGAMENTA SPHENOMANDIBULARE ET STYLOMANDIBULARE, SPHENOMANDIBULAR OR INTERNAL LATERAL AND STYLOMANDIBULAR OR STYLOMAXILLARY LIGAMENT. RELATIONS OF THE STYLOMANDIBULAR OR STYLOMAXILLARY LIGAMENT TO STYLOGLOSSUS AND INTERNAL PTERYGOID MUSCLES. LIGAMENTUM PTERYGOSPINOSUM, PTERYGOSPINOUS LIGAMENT. (THE POSTERIOR PART OF THE FACIAL PORTION OF THE SKULL WITH THE ADJOINING PORTION OF THE BASE OF THE SKULL, DIVIDED SAGITALLY SOMEWHAT TO THE LEFT OF THE MEDIAN PLANE.)

The basilar and condylar portions of the occipital bone have been removed.

Articulatio mandibularis—Temporomandibular or temporomaxillary articulation.

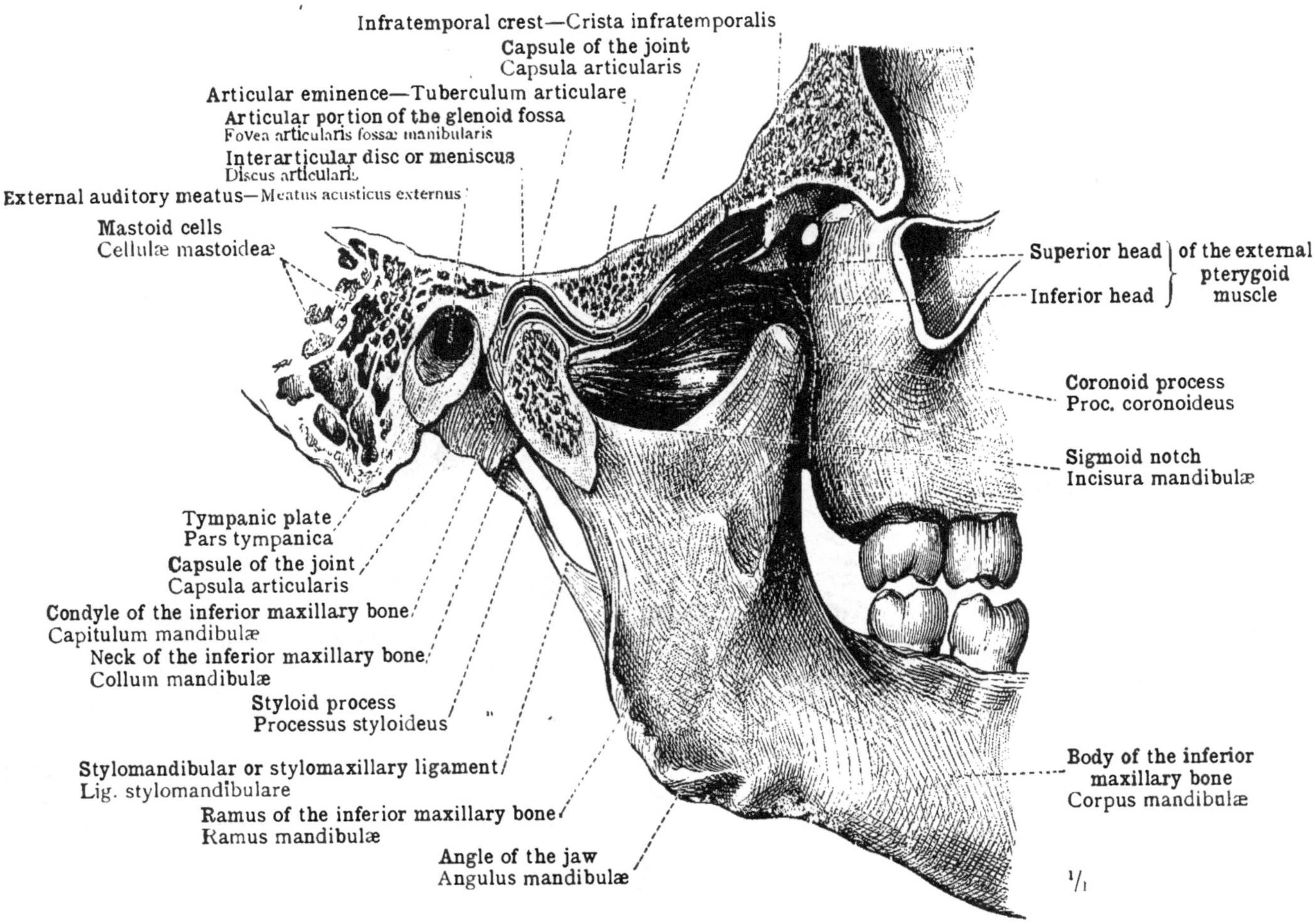

FIG. 427.—ARTICULATIO MANDIBULARIS, TEMPOROMANDIBULAR OR TEMPOROMAXILLARY ARTICULATION DISCUS ARTICULARIS, INTERARTICULAR DISC OR MENISCUS, AND LIGAMENTUM STYLOMANDIBULARE, STYLOMANDIBULAR OR STYLOMAXILLARY LIGAMENT. RELATIONS OF THE SUPERIOR HEAD OF THE EXTERNAL PTERYGOID MUSCLE TO THE ANTERIOR WALL OF THE CAPSULAR LIGAMENT AND TO THE INTERARTICULAR DISC OR MENISCUS. (RIGHT TEMPOROMANDIBULAR OR TEMPOROMAXILLARY ARTICULATION, DIVIDED IN A PLANE NEARLY APPROACHING THE SAGITTAL; THE INTERNAL PORTION BEING FIGURED.)

The section runs somewhat obliquely forwards and inwards.

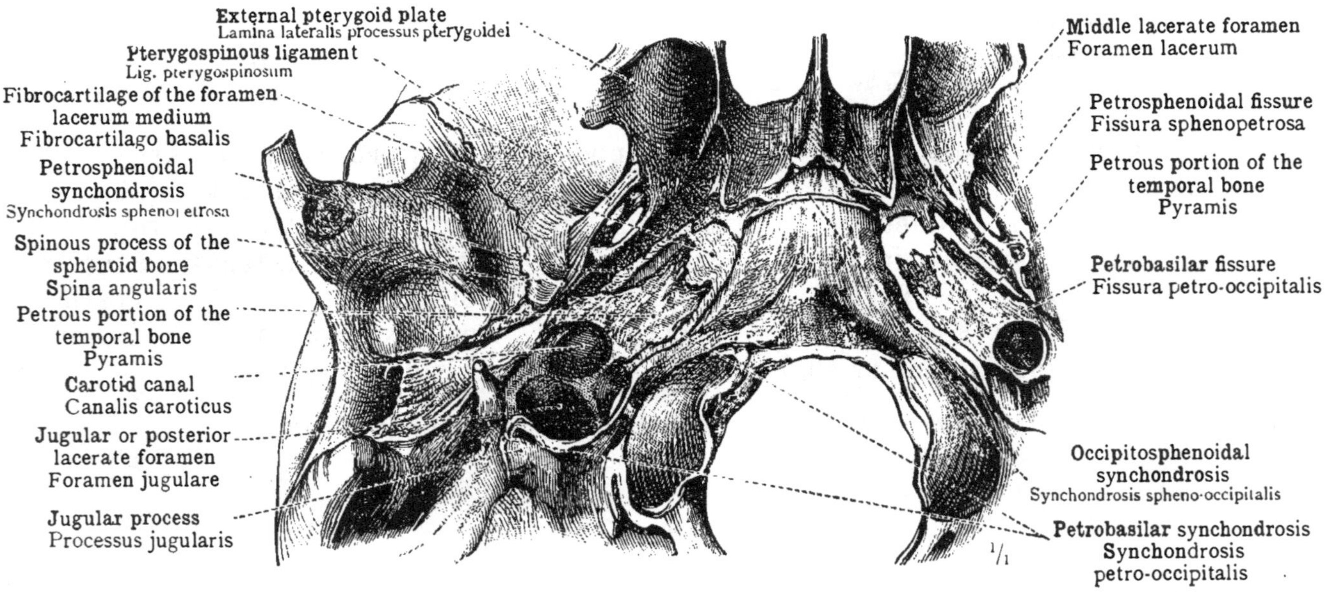

FIG. 428.—FIBROCARTILAGO BASALIS; FIBROCARTILAGE OF THE FORAMEN LACERUM MEDIUM: SYNCHONDROSES SPHENOPETROSA, PETRO-OCCIPITALIS, ET SPHENO-OCCIPITALIS; PETROSPHENOIDAL, PETROBASILAR, AND OCCIPITOSPHENOIDAL SYNCHONDROSES: LIGAMENTUM PTERYGOSPINOSUM; PTERYGOSPINOUS LIGAMENT. (THE MIDDLE PORTION OF THE BASE OF THE SKULL, SEEN FROM BELOW.)

JUNCTURÆ OSSIUM EXTREMITATUM, SUPERIORIS ET INFERIORIS

THE ARTICULATIONS OF THE SUPERIOR AND INFERIOR EXTREMITIES

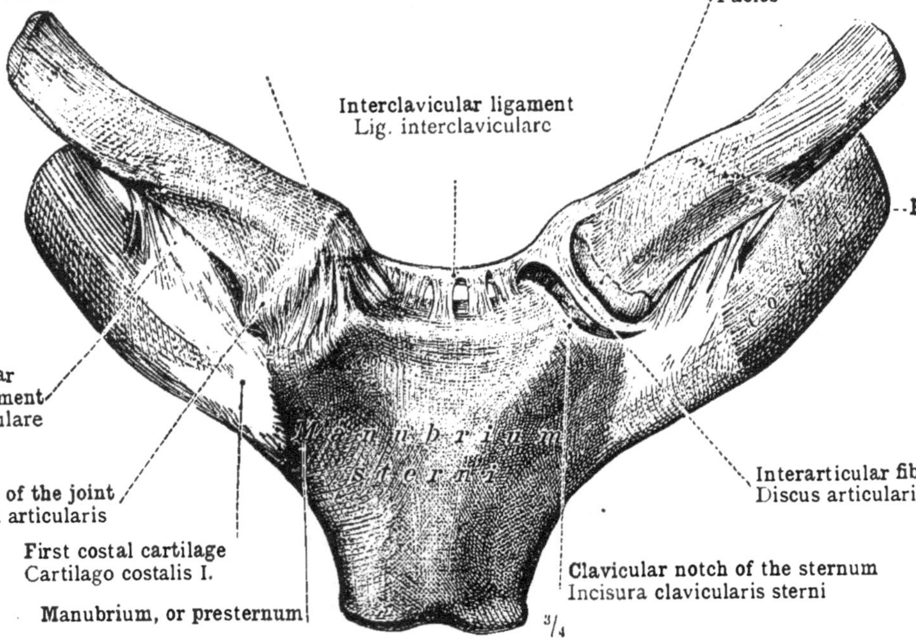

Fig. 429.—Articulatio Sternoclavicularis, Sternoclavicular Articulation: Capsula Articularis, Capsule of the Joint; Discus Articularis, Interarticular Fibrocartilage; Ligamenta Interclaviculare et Costoclaviculare, Interclavicular and Costoclavicular or Rhomboid Ligaments.

The left sternoclavicular articulation has been opened by the removal of the anterior wall of the capsular ligament.

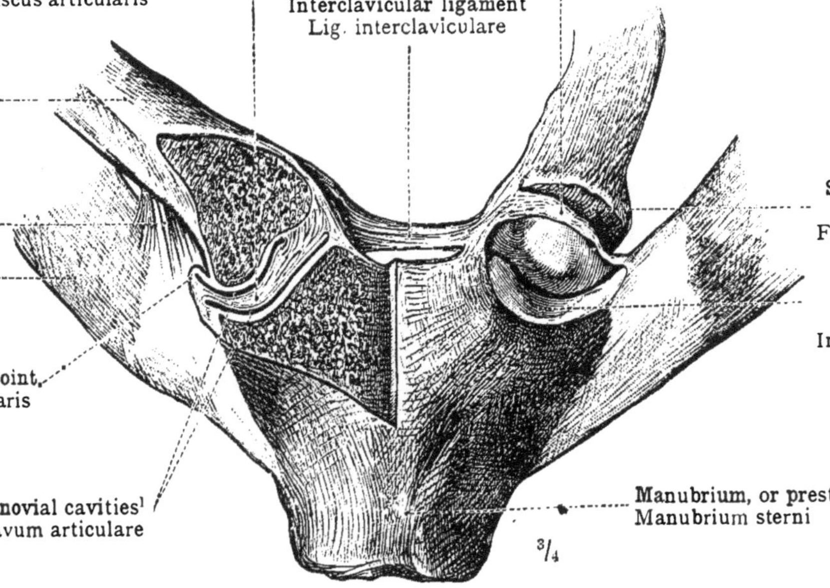

[1] The interarticular fibrocartilage is occasionally defective in the centre, and in rare cases even entirely wanting; there is then only one synovial cavity.—Tr.

Fig. 430.—Articulatio Sternoclavicularis, Sternoclavicular Articulation: Discus et Capsula Articularis, Interarticular Fibrocartilage and Capsular Ligament; Cavum Articulare, Synovial Cavity or Cavities; Ligamenta Interclaviculare et Costoclaviculare, Interclavicular and Costoclavicular or Rhomboid Ligaments.

The right sternoclavicular articulation has been divided by a frontal section; in the left, the capsule has been removed and the clavicle has been drawn backwards.

Sternoclavicular Articulation, seen from Before.

Articulationes et ligamenta cinguli extremitatis superioris—Articulations and ligaments of the shoulder-girdle.

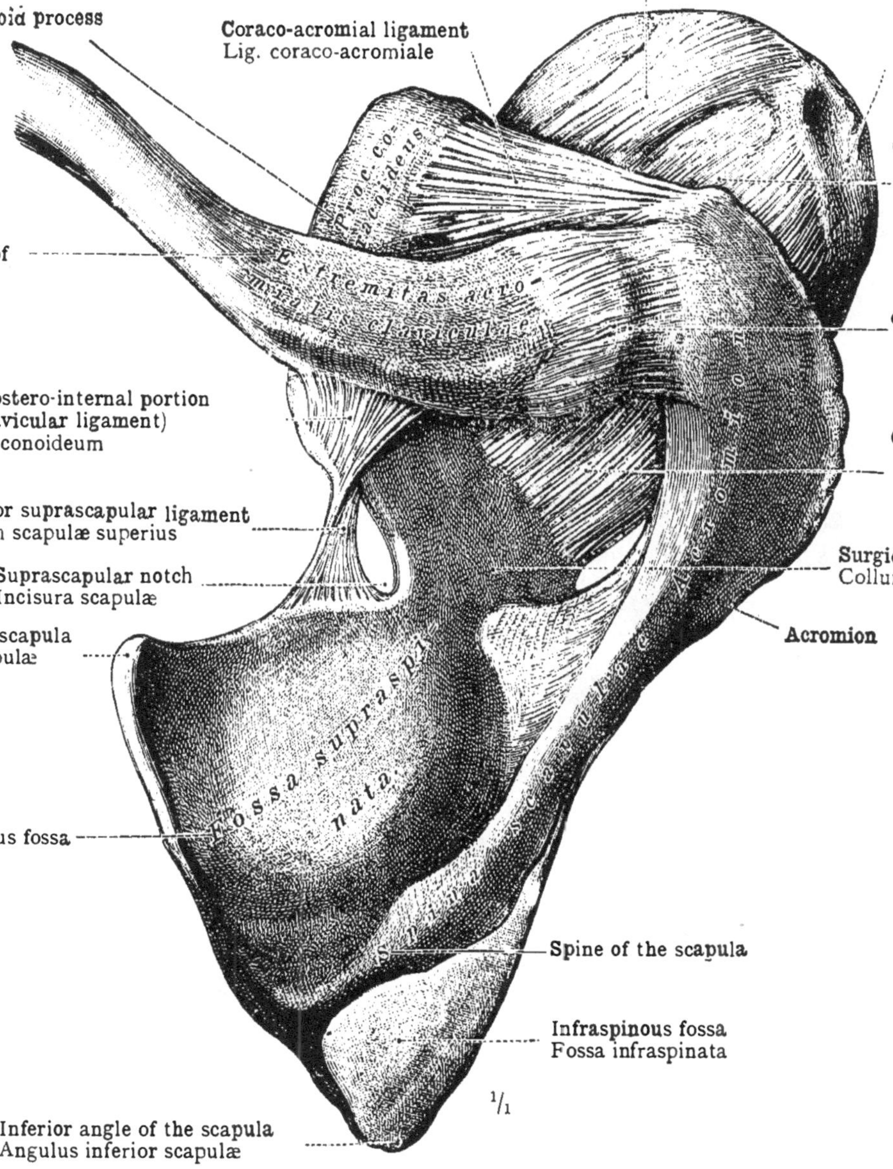

FIG. 431.—LIGAMENTA ACROMIOCLAVICULARE ET CORACOCLAVICULARE, SUPERIOR ACROMIOCLAVICULAR LIGAMENT AND CORACOCLAVICULAR LIGAMENT (CONOID PORTION); LIGAMENTA CORACO-ACROMIALE ET TRANSVERSUM SCAPULÆ SUPERIUS, CORACO-ACROMIAL AND SUPRASCAPULAR LIGAMENTS. (THE RIGHT SCAPULA WITH THE ACROMIAL HALF OF THE CLAVICLE AND THE SHOULDER-JOINT, SEEN FROM ABOVE.)

Articulationes et ligamenta cinguli extremitatis superioris—Articulations and ligaments of the shoulder-girdle.

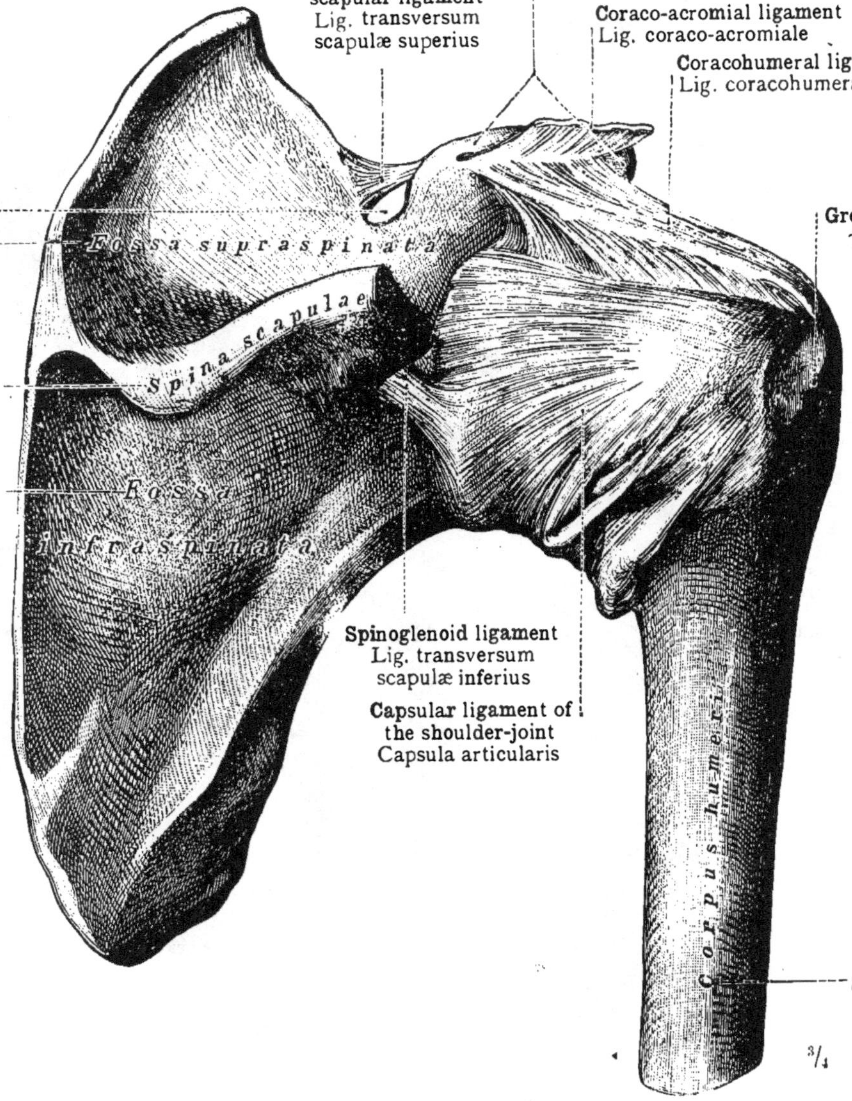

FIG. 432.—ARTICULATIO HUMERI, SHOULDER-JOINT: CAPSULA ARTICULARIS, CAPSULAR LIGAMENT; LIGAMENTUM CORACOHUMERALE, CORACOHUMERAL LIGAMENT; LIGAMENTUM TRANSVERSUM SCAPULÆ SUPERIUS ET LIGAMENTUM TRANSVERSUM SCAPULÆ INFERIUS, CORACOSCAPULAR OR SUPRASCAPULAR LIGAMENT AND SPINOGLENOID LIGAMENT. (THE RIGHT SHOULDER-JOINT, SEEN FROM BEHIND.)

The acromion has been sawn off, and the coracoid extremity of the coraco-acromial ligament has been turned upwards.

Articulatio humeri—Shoulder-joint.

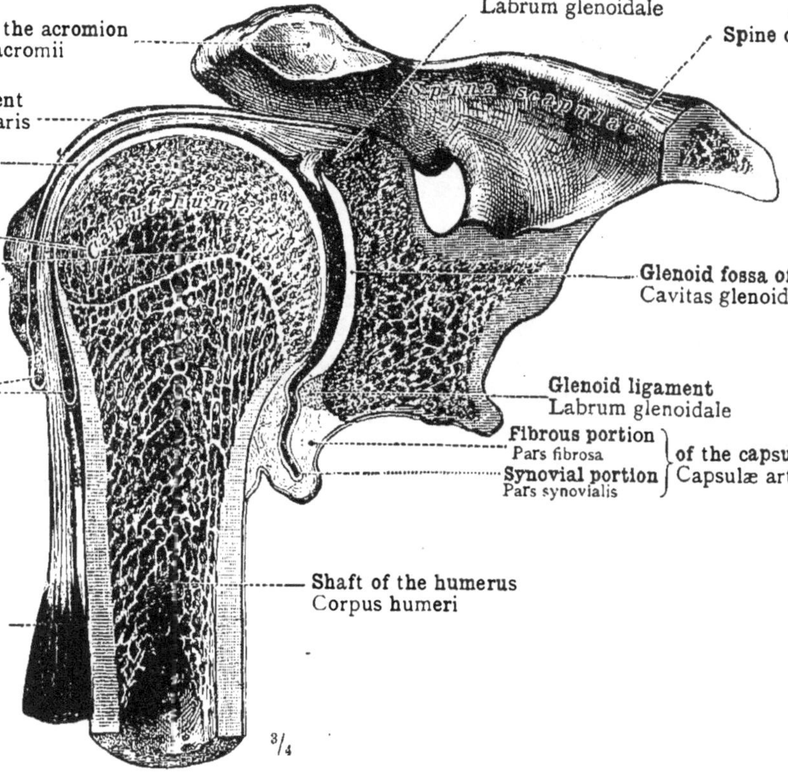

FIG. 433.—ARTICULATIO HUMERI, SHOULDER-JOINT: LABRUM GLENOIDALE, GLENOID LIGAMENT; RELATIONS OF THE TENDON OF THE LONG HEAD OF THE BICEPS MUSCLE AND OF THE EPIPHYSIAL DISC TO THE SYNOVIAL CAVITY OF THE ARTICULATION. (THE RIGHT SHOULDER-JOINT IN FRONTAL SECTION; POSTERIOR HALF.)

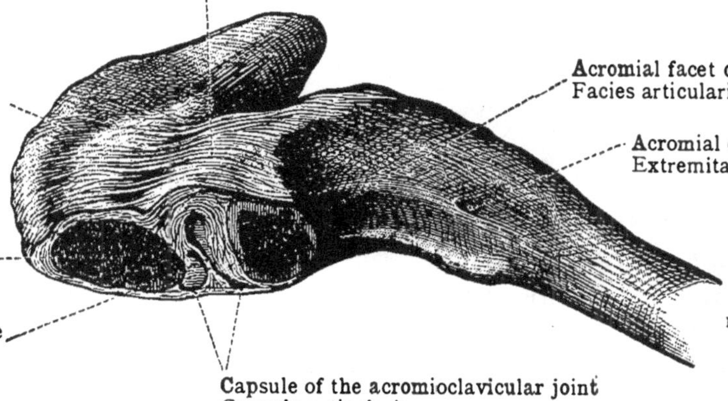

FIG. 434.—ARTICULATIO ACROMIOCLAVICULARIS, ACROMIOCLAVICULAR JOINT: DISCUS ARTICULARIS, INTERARTICULAR FIBROCARTILAGE; LIGAMENTUM ACROMIOCLAVICULARE, SUPERIOR ACROMIOCLAVICULAR LIGAMENT. (THE RIGHT ACROMIOCLAVICULAR ARTICULATION IN FRONTAL SECTION; POSTERIOR PORTION.)

Articulatio humeri—Shoulder-joint. Articulatio acromioclavicularis—Acromioclavicular articulation.

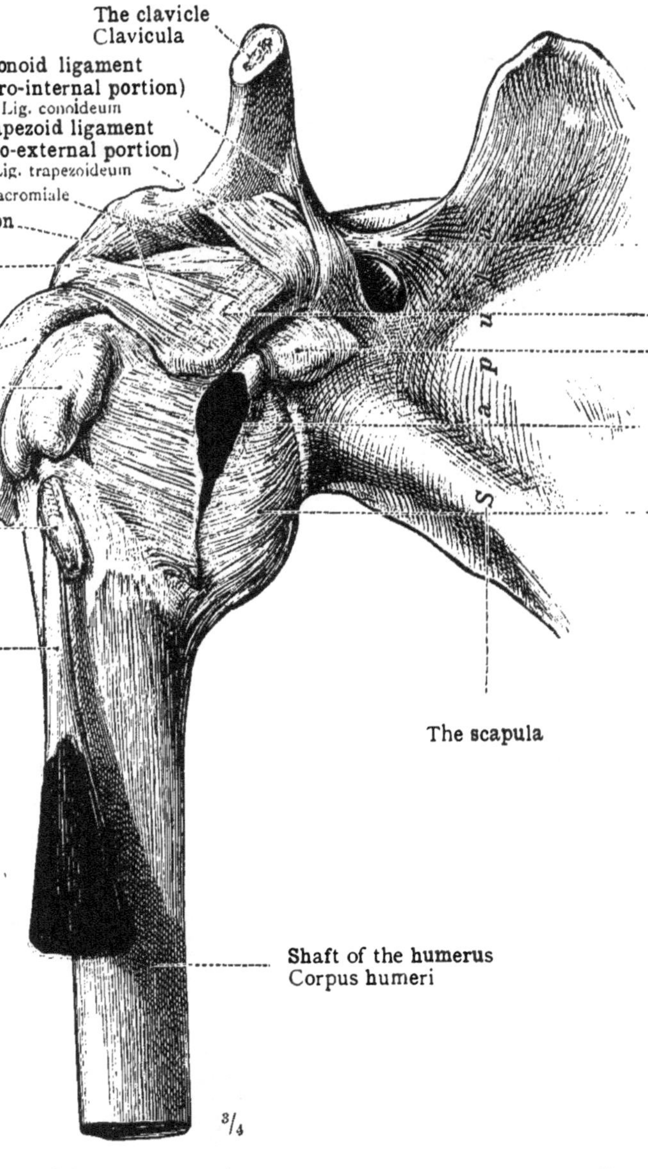

FIG. 435.—ARTICULATIONES HUMERI ET ACROMIOCLAVICULARIS, THE SHOULDER-JOINT AND THE STERNOCLAVICULAR ARTICULATION: BURSA MUSCULI SUBSCAPULARIS ET BURSA SUBDELTOIDEA, BURSA OF THE SUBSCAPULARIS MUSCLE AND SUBDELTOID OR SUBACROMIAL BURSA; VAGINA MUSCOSA INTERTUBERCULARIS, SYNOVIAL SHEATH OF THE BICIPITAL GROOVE; LIGAMENTA CORACOCLAVICULARE, CORACO-ACROMIALE, ET TRANSVERSUM SCAPULÆ SUPERIUS; THE CORACOCLAVICULAR (CONOID AND TRAPEZOID), CORACO-ACROMIAL, AND CORACOSCAPULAR OR SUPRASCAPULAR LIGAMENT. (RIGHT SHOULDER-JOINT, INJECTED WITH TALLOW; THE ACROMIAL EXTREMITY OF THE CLAVICLE HAS BEEN DRAWN UPWARDS. SEEN FROM BEFORE.)

Articulatio humeri—Shoulder-joint.

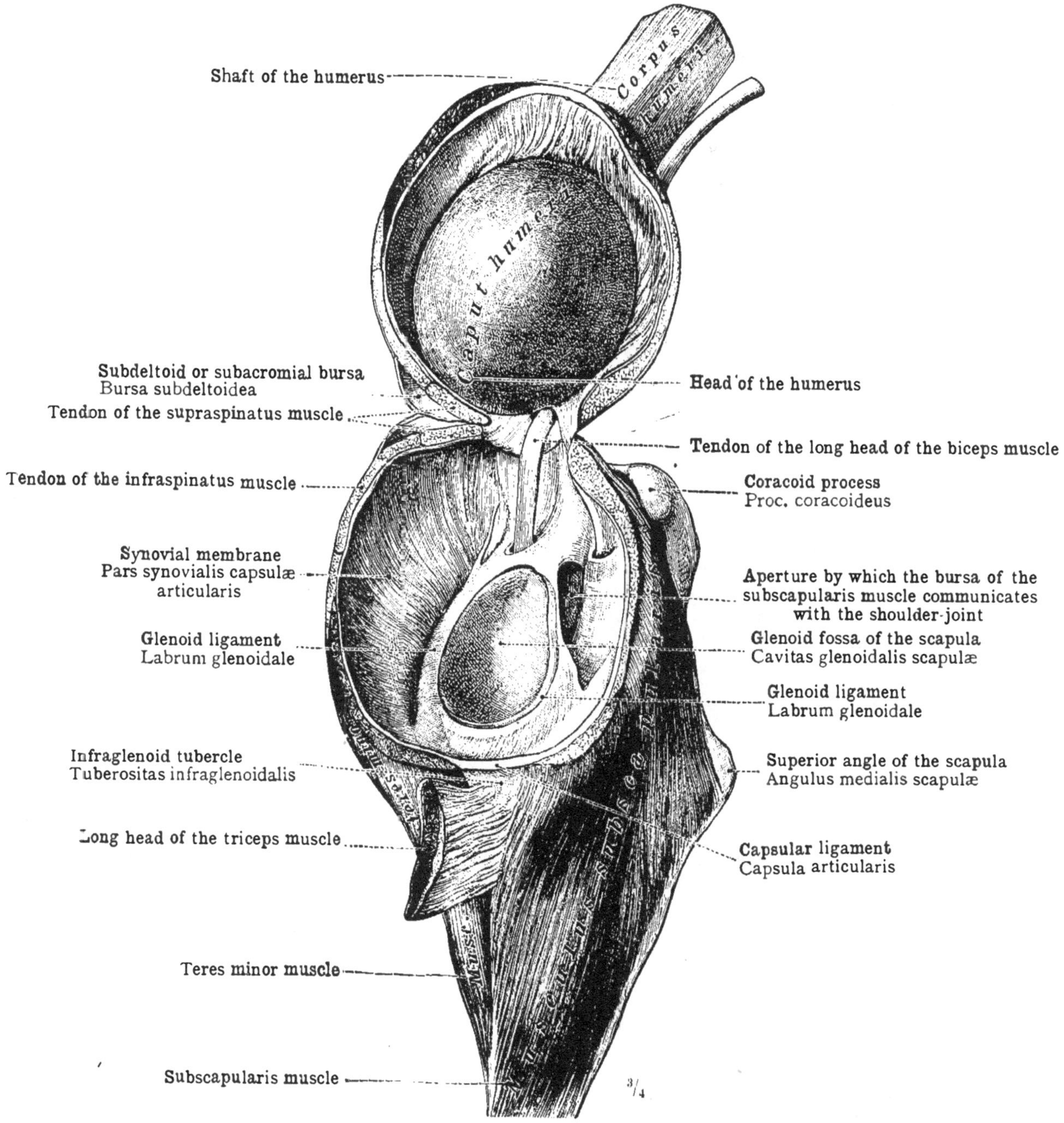

FIG. 436.—ARTICULATIO HUMERI, SHOULDER-JOINT: INTRACAPSULAR PORTION OF THE TENDON OF THE LONG HEAD OF THE BICEPS MUSCLE; LABRUM GLENOIDALE, GLENOID LIGAMENT; APERTURE OF COMMUNICATION OF THE BURSA OF THE SUBSCAPULARIS MUSCLE WITH THE SHOULDER-JOINT; RELATIONS OF THE TENDONS OF THE SCAPULAR MUSCLES WITH THE CAPSULE OF THE SHOULDER-JOINT. (RIGHT SHOULDER-JOINT FROM THE OUTER SIDE)

After tallow had been injected into the joint and allowed to harden, the capsular ligament and the surrounding scapular muscles were divided by a circular incision midway between their attachments to the scapula and the humerus, a strip of the capsule, however, being left undivided, where the tendon of the long head of the biceps muscle passes through the joint. The humerus with the distal half of the capsule has been turned upwards.

Articulatio humeri—Shoulder-joint.

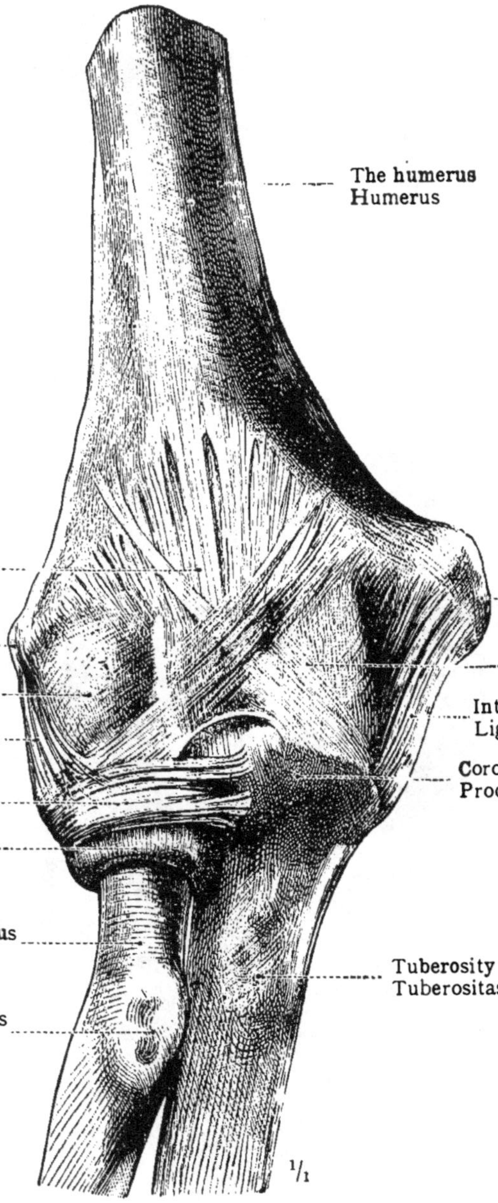

[1] Projection of the synovial membrane of the elbow-joint, which membrane, after passing downwards between the vertical articular surface of the head of the radius and the inner surface of the orbicular ligament, forms a circular pouch or sac below this ligament around the neck of the radius.—TR.

FIG. 437.—ARTICULATIO CUBITI, ELBOW-JOINT: CAPSULA ARTICULARIS, CAPSULE OF THE JOINT; LIGAMENTA COLLATERALIA, LATERAL LIGAMENTS; LIGAMENTUM ANNULARE RADII, ANNULAR OR ORBICULAR LIGAMENT OF THE RADIUS; *RECESSUS SACCIFORMIS (*see note above*). (RIGHT ELBOW-JOINT, UNOPENED; ANTERIOR OR PALMAR ASPECT.)

The *recessus sacciformis has been injected with tallow.

Articulatio cubiti—Elbow-joint.

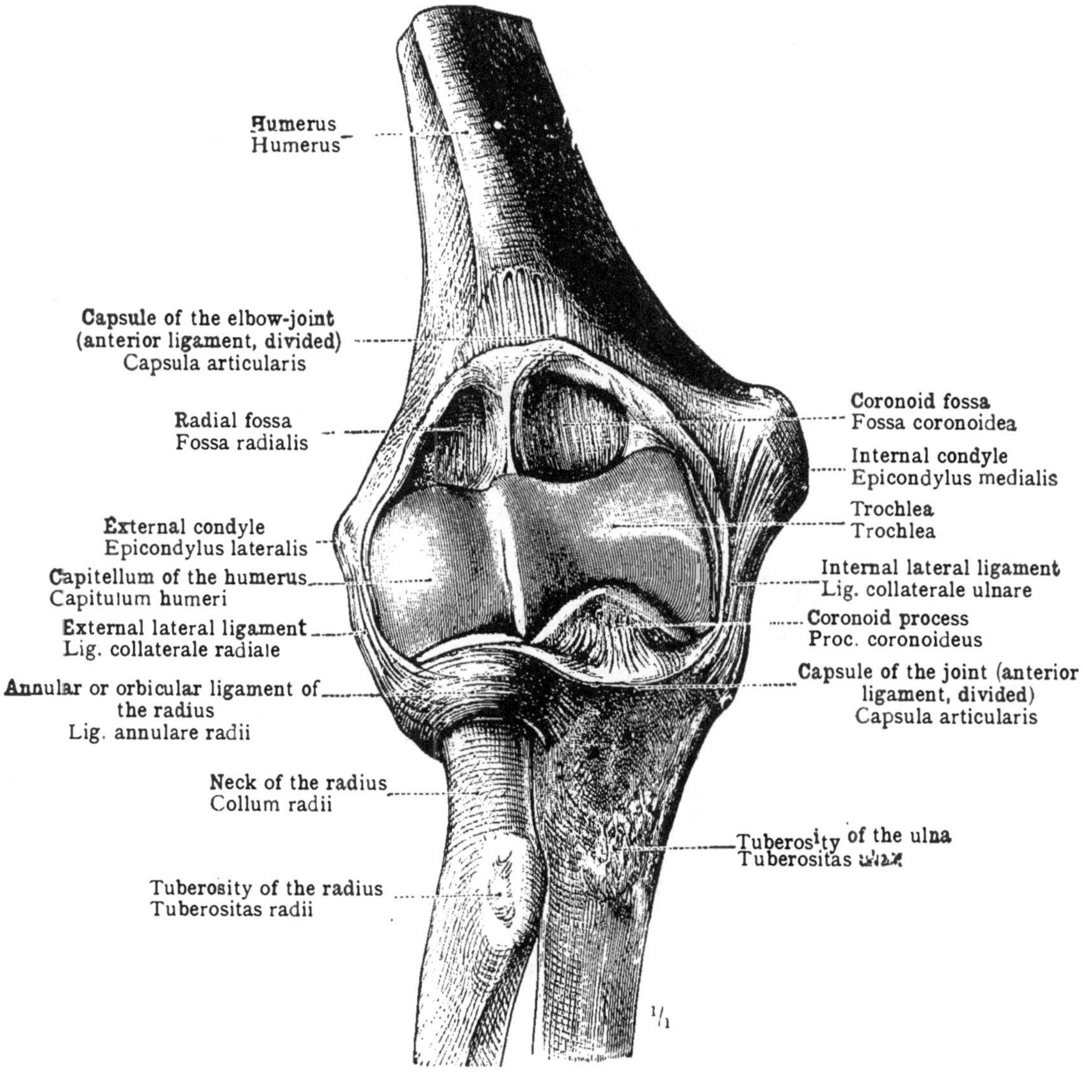

FIG. 438.—ARTICULATIO CUBITI, ELBOW-JOINT; ATTACHMENT OF THE CAPSULE TO THE ANTERIOR SURFACES OF THE HUMERUS AND THE ULNA (ANTERIOR LIGAMENT); LIGAMENTA COLLATERALIA, LATERAL LIGAMENTS; LIGAMENTUM ANNULARE RADII, ANNULAR OR ORBICULAR LIGAMENT OF THE RADIUS. (RIGHT ELBOW-JOINT; ANTERIOR OR PALMAR ASPECT.)

The capsule has been divided above and below, close to its attachment to the bones, and between the lateral ligaments (*i.e.*, the greater portion of the anterior ligament has been removed); the cut ends of the anterior ligament have been folded back against the bones. The *recessus sacciformis see note on previous page—has been removed.

Articulatio cubiti Elbow-ioint.

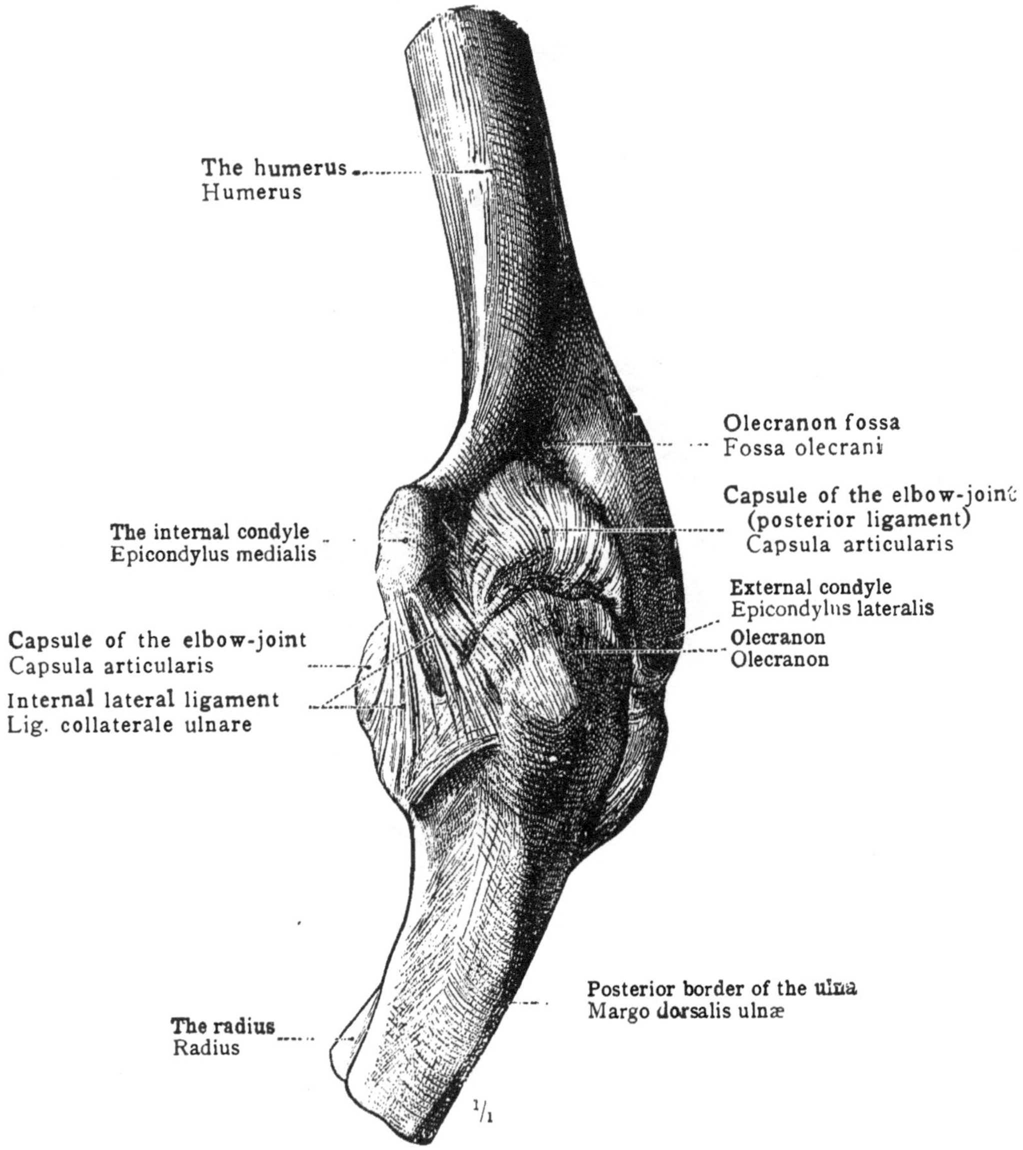

FIG. 439.—ARTICULATIO CUBITI, ELBOW-JOINT: CAPSULA ARTICULARIS, CAPSULE OF THE JOINT; LIGAMENTUM COLLATERALE ULNARE, INTERNAL LATERAL LIGAMENT. (RIGHT ELBOW-JOINT; POSTERO-INTERNAL ASPECT.)

Articulatio cubiti—Elbow-joint.

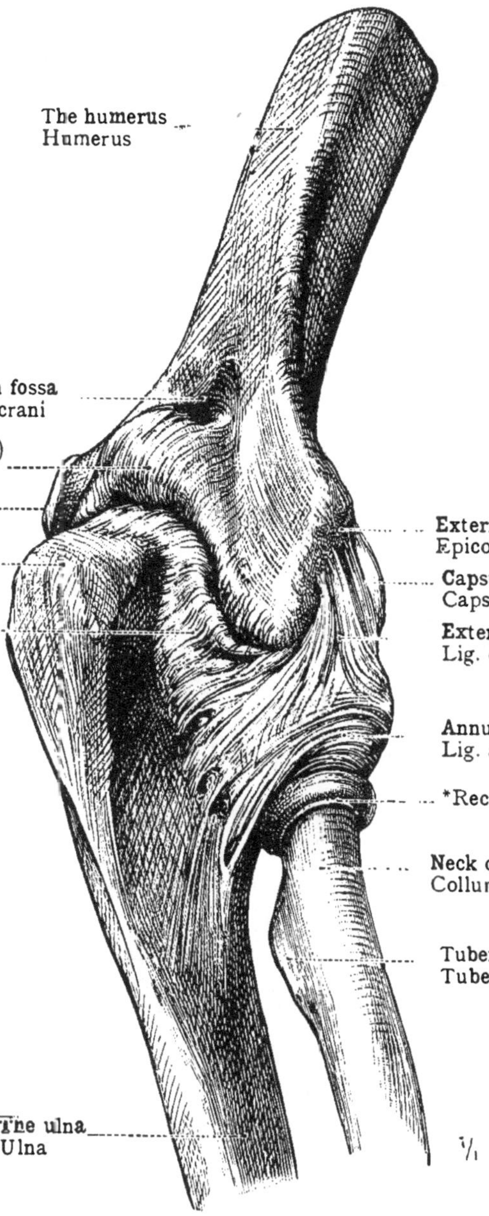

[1] See note to p. 204.

FIG. 440.—ARTICULATIO CUBITI, ELBOW-JOINT: CAPSULA ARTICULARIS, CAPSULE OF THE JOINT; LIGAMENTUM COLLATERALE RADIALE, EXTERNAL LATERAL LIGAMENT; LIGAMENTUM ANNULARE RADII, ANNULAR OR ORBICULAR LIGAMENT OF THE RADIUS; *RECESSUS SACCIFORMIS. (RIGHT ELBOW-JOINT; POSTERO-EXTERNAL ASPECT.)

The *recessus sacciformis has been injected with tallow.

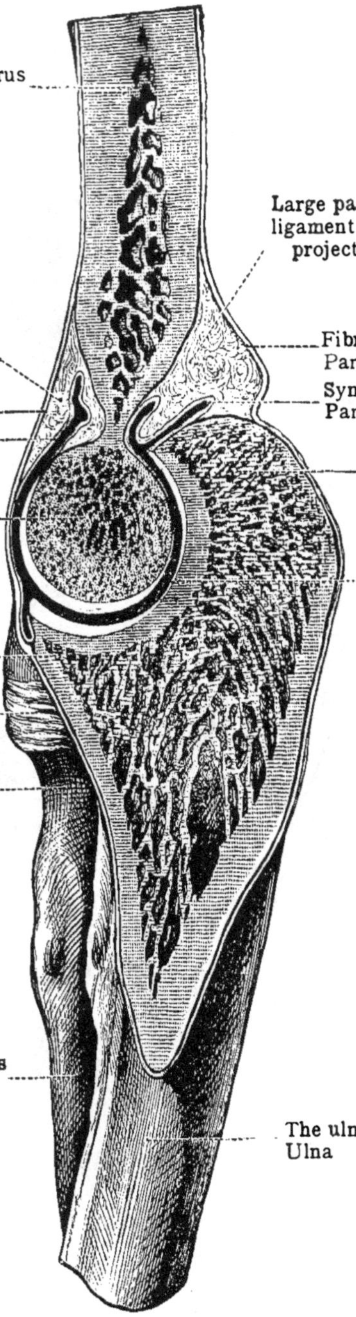

FIG. 441.—ARTICULATIO HUMERO-ULNARIS, HUMERO-ULNAR ARTICULATION. (SAGITTAL SECTION OF THE RIGHT ELBOW-JOINT ; THE RADIAL HALF IS FIGURED.)

The section passes through the trochlea and the great sigmoid cavity of the ulna, in a plane vertical to the axis of the trochlea.

Articulatio cubiti—Elbow-joint.

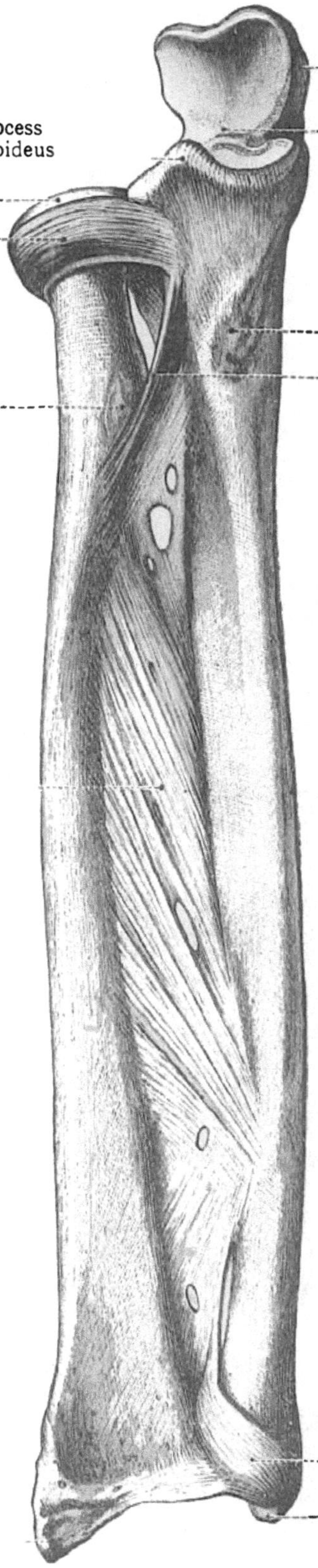

IG. 442.—ARTICULATIONES RADIO-ULNARES, PROXIMALIS ET DISTALIS; RADIO-ULNAR ARTICULATIONS, SUPERIOR AND INFERIOR: LIGAMENTUM ANNULARE RADII, ANNULAR OR ORBICULAR LIGAMENT OF THE RADIUS; MEMBRANA INTEROSSEA ANTIBRACHII, INTEROSSEOUS MEMBRANE OR LIGAMENT OF THE FOREARM. (THE BONES OF THE RIGHT FOREARM WITH THE RADIO-ULNAR LIGAMENTS; ANTERIOR OR PALMAR ASPECT.)

Articulations of the Bones of the Forearm.

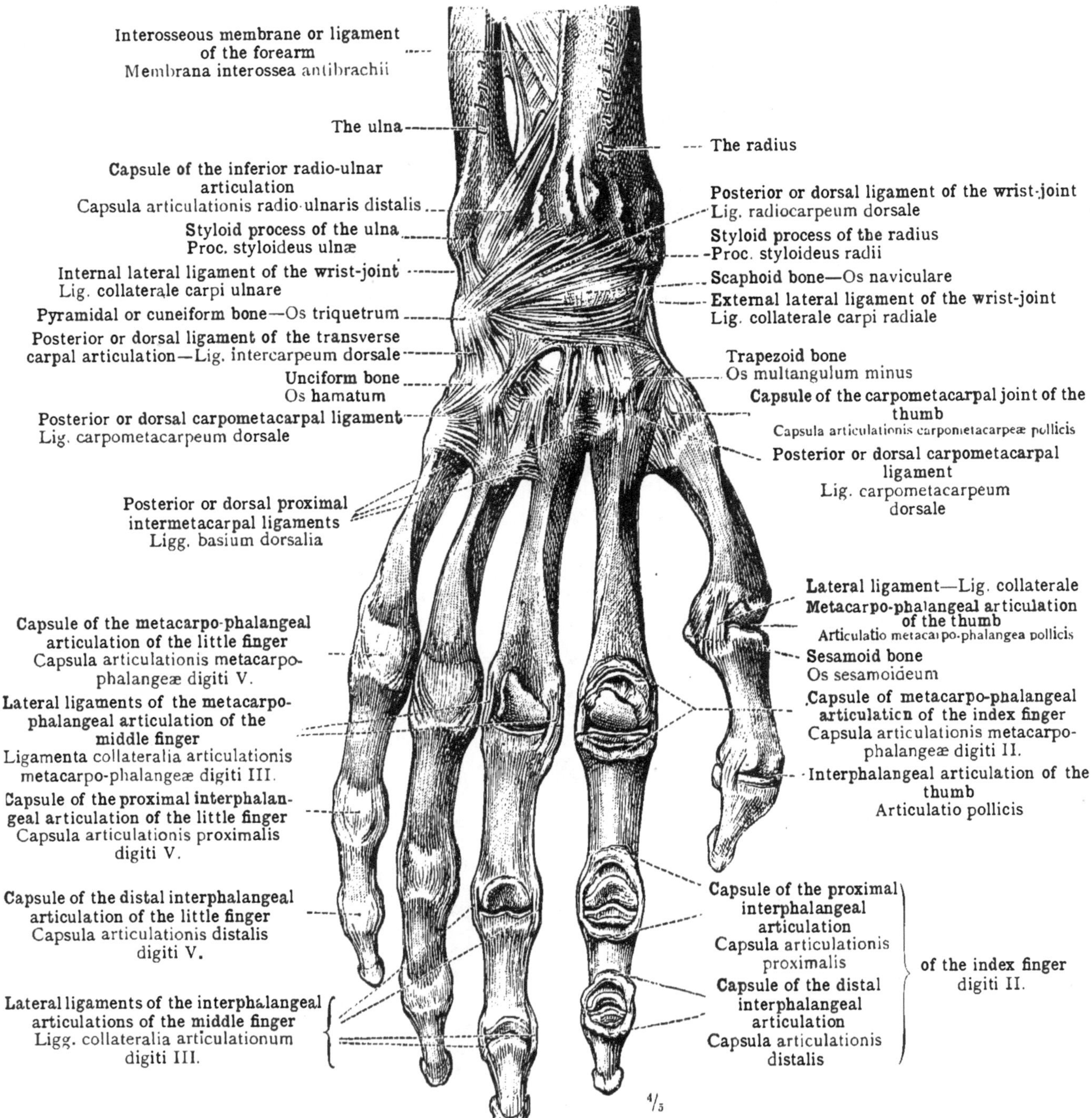

FIG. 443.—THE POSTERIOR OR DORSAL LIGAMENTS OF THE WRIST AND HAND: LIGAMENTA COLLATERALIA CARPI, LATERAL LIGAMENTS OF THE WRIST AND THE CARPUS; SUPERFICIAL POSTERIOR OR DORSAL LIGAMENTS OF CARPUS AND METACARPUS. THE CAPSULES AND THE LATERAL LIGAMENTS OF THE METACARPO-PHALANGEAL AND INTERPHALANGEAL ARTICULATIONS.

In the articulations of the index finger the posterior wall of the capsule has been divided transversely across the middle of the joint, and the ends have been turned upwards and downwards; in the articulations of the thumb and the middle finger the capsule has been divided only between the lateral ligaments, leaving these intact; in the articulations of the ring and little fingers the capsule has not been opened.

Articulationes manus et digitorum—Articulations of the hand and fingers.

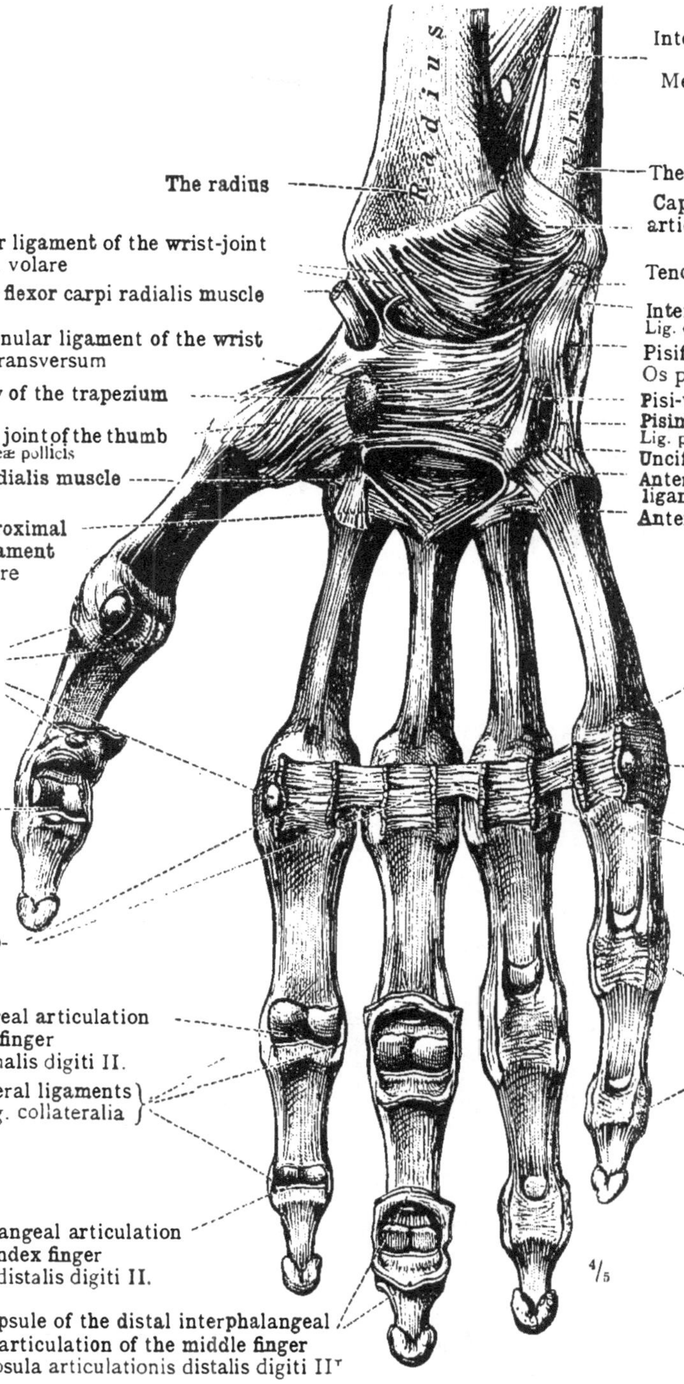

[1] These are fibrous plates rather than ligaments properly so called, and, being thickened into fibrocartilage at each side along their attachments to the lateral metacarpo-phalangeal ligaments, they are grooved on the palmar surfaces for the flexor tendon. Macalister calls them *glenoid* ligaments. It is in the lateral fibrocartilaginous portions of these plates that the sesamoid bones of the metacarpo-phalangeal joint of the thumb, and occasionally of some of the other fingers, are developed.—Tr.

FIG. 444.—THE ANTERIOR OR PALMAR LIGAMENTS OF THE WRIST AND HAND: THE SUPERFICIAL LIGAMENTS OF THE CARPUS AND THE METACARPUS; THE CAPSULES AND LIGAMENTS OF THE METACARPO-PHALANGEAL AND THE INTERPHALANGEAL ARTICULATIONS. LIGAMENTUM CARPI TRANSVERSUM, ANTERIOR ANNULAR LIGAMENT OF THE WRIST; CANALIS CARPI, CANAL OF THE CARPUS BENEATH THE ANTERIOR ANNULAR LIGAMENT (FOR THE TRANSMISSION OF THE FLEXOR TENDONS). RELATIONS OF THE TENDONS OF THE FLEXOR CARPI ULNARIS AND FLEXOR CARPI RADIALIS MUSCLE TO THE ANTERIOR OR PALMAR CARPAL AND METACARPAL LIGAMENTS. LIGAMENTA ACCESSORIA VOLARIA, ANTERIOR OR PALMAR METACARPO-PHALANGEAL LIGAMENTS; LIGAMENTA CAPITULORUM TRANSVERSA, TRANSVERSE METACARPAL LIGAMENT (ANTERIOR OR PALMAR DISTAL INTERMETACARPAL LIGAMENTS). OSSA SESAMOIDEA, SESAMOID BONES.

In the interphalangeal articulations of the index finger the anterior portions of the capsules between the lateral ligaments have been entirely cut away; in those of the middle finger the capsules have been divided transversely across the middle of the joint and the divided halves of the anterior ligament turned upwards and downwards; in the interphalangeal articulation of the thumb the anterior portion of the capsule has been divided along its attachment to the distal phalanx and the lateral ligaments, and, together with the sesamoid bones embedded in it on each side, has been turned upwards; in the remaining joints the capsule has been left intact.

Articulationes manus et digitorum—Articulations of the hand and fingers.

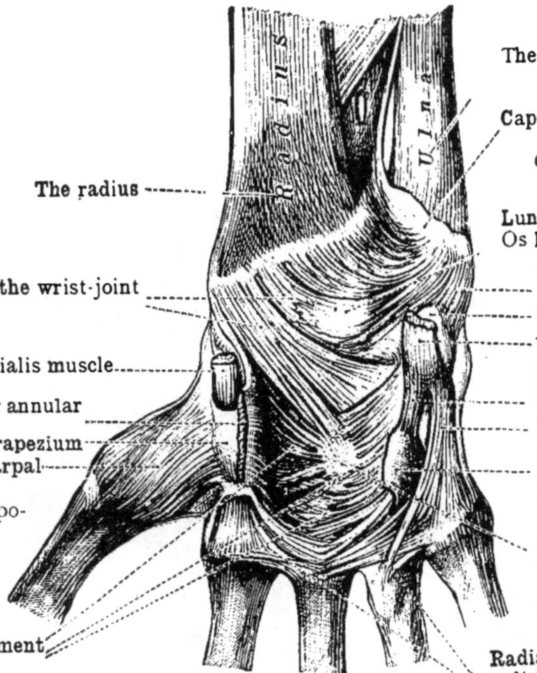

FIG. 445.—THE ANTERIOR OR PALMAR LIGAMENTS OF THE RIGHT CARPUS, SHOWN BY THE REMOVAL OF THE ANTERIOR ANNULAR LIGAMENT OF THE WRIST: LIGAMENTUM RADIOCARPEUM VOLARE, ANTERIOR OR PALMAR LIGAMENT OF THE WRIST-JOINT; LIGAMENTUM CARPI RADIATUM, ANTERIOR OR RADIATE LIGAMENT OF THE CARPUS.

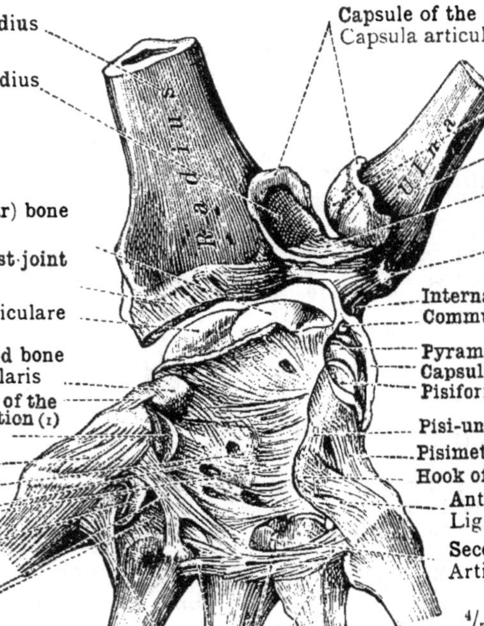

(1) Lig. intercarpeum volare. [Connecting the tuberosities of the scaphoid bone and the trapezium.—TR.]
(2) Capsula articulationis carpometacarpeæ pollicis (3) Os capitatum (4) Lig. carpi radiatum (5) Lig. collaterale carpi ulnare (6) Capsula articulationis ossis pisiformis

FIG. 446.—THE ANTERIOR OR PALMAR LIGAMENTS OF THE INTERCARPAL (TRANSVERSE CARPAL) AND CARPOMETACARPAL ARTICULATIONS, AFTER THE ANTERIOR ANNULAR LIGAMENT OF THE WRIST AND THE TENDONS OF THE FLEXOR CARPI RADIALIS AND FLEXOR CARPI ULNARIS HAVE BEEN ENTIRELY REMOVED.

The radiocarpal and distal radio-ulnar articulations have been opened, the triangular fibrocartilage and the internal lateral ligament of the wrist-joint being left intact; the bones of the forearm have been separated from one another and from the carpus; the pisipyramidal articulation, the carpometacarpal articulations of the thumb and the ring finger, and the second intermetacarpal articulation, have been partially opened.

Articulatio manus—Articulations of the hand.

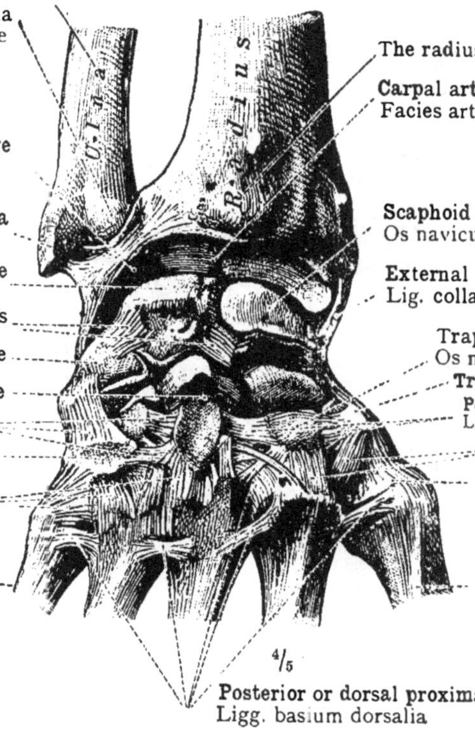

FIG. 447.—THE SHORT POSTERIOR OR DORSAL LIGAMENTS OF THE TRANSVERSE CARPAL ARTICULATION, AND OF THE CARPOMETACARPAL AND INTERMETACARPAL ARTICULATIONS. (THE RIGHT CARPUS WITH THE DISTAL EXTREMITIES OF THE BONES OF THE FOREARM AND THE PROXIMAL EXTREMITIES OF THE METACARPAL BONES.)

The distal radio-ulnar articulation and the radiocarpal and transverse carpal articulations have been opened by the removal of the posterior ligaments, and the bones of the forearm have been drawn a little upwards and away from the carpus.

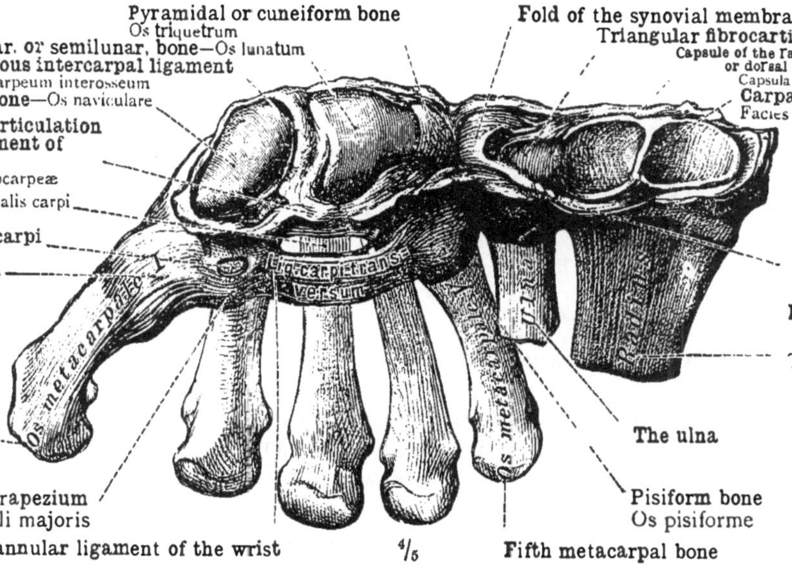

FIG. 448.—THE ARTICULAR SURFACES AND THE ATTACHMENTS OF THE CAPSULE OF THE RADIOCARPAL ARTICULATION OR WRIST-JOINT; CANALIS CARPI, THE CANAL OF THE CARPUS. (THE RIGHT CARPUS WITH THE METACARPAL BONES; ANTERO-SUPERIOR ASPECT.)

The distal extremities of the bones of the forearm have been turned to the ulnar side, after division of the capsule of the wrist-joint with the exception of the internal lateral ligament.

Articulatio manus—Articulations of the hand.

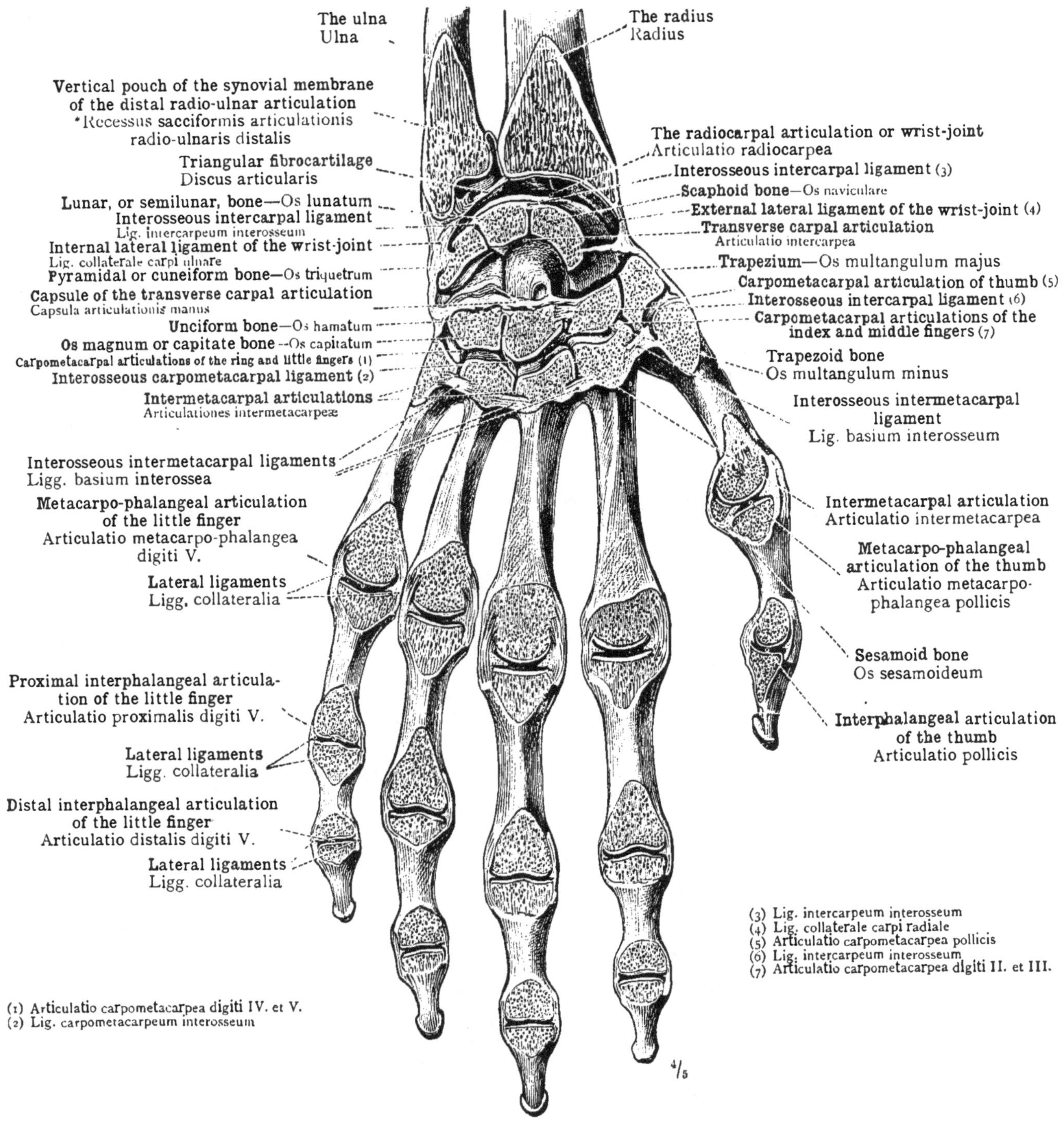

FIG. 449.—ARTICULATIO RADIO-ULNARIS DISTALIS, DISTAL RADIO-ULNAR ARTICULATION. ARTICULATIO MANUS, ARTICULATIONS OF THE HAND: ARTICULATIONES RADIOCARPEA ET INTERCARPEA, RADIOCARPAL ARTICULATION OR WRIST-JOINT AND TRANSVERSE CARPAL ARTICULATION. ARTICULATIONES CARPOMETACARPEÆ, CARPOMETACARPAL ARTICULATIONS; ARTICULATIONES INTERMETACARPEÆ, INTERMETACARPAL ARTICULATIONS. ARTICULATIONES METACARPO-PHALANGEÆ, METACARPO-PHALANGEAL ARTICULATIONS; ARTICULATIONES DIGITORUM MANUS, INTERPHALANGEAL ARTICULATIONS OF THE FINGERS. (THE SKELETON OF THE RIGHT HAND WITH THE DISTAL EXTREMITIES OF THE BONES OF THE FOREARM; POSTERIOR OR DORSAL ASPECT.)

The articulations are all opened by a section in the frontal plane: and whereas in the fingers this plane passes through the joints from side to side, dividing the lateral ligaments; in the thumb, owing to the opposition of this member, the plane of section passes through the joints in a dorsopalmar direction, and divides the dorsal and palmar ligaments.

Articulationes manus et digitorum—Articulations of the hand and fingers.

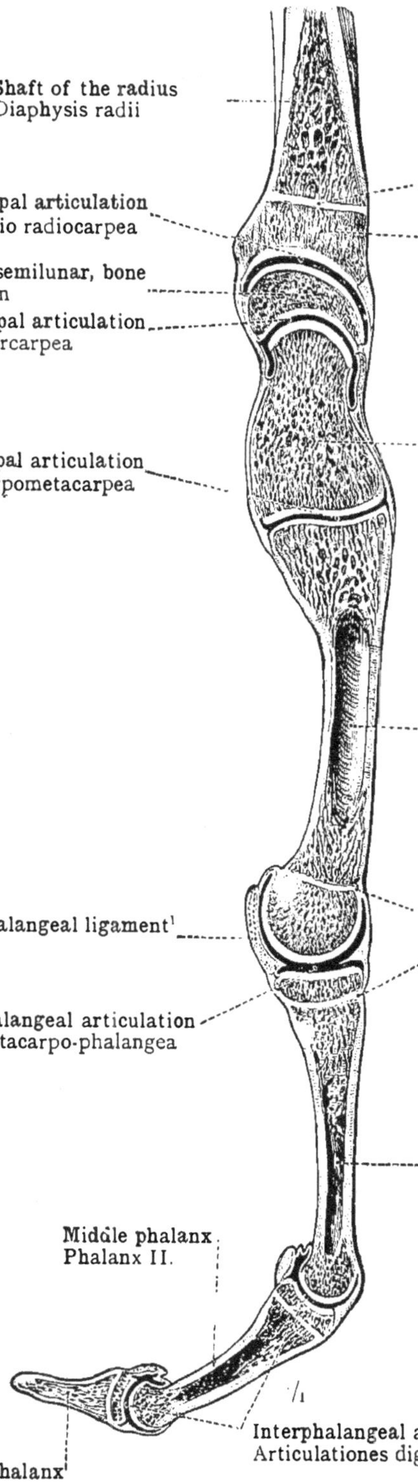

[1] See note on p. 211.

FIG. 450.—THE ARTICULATIONS OF THE HAND, SEEN IN SAGITTAL OR DORSOPALMAR SECTION, SHOWING THEIR RELATIONS TO THE EPIPHYSIAL DISCS. (THE RADIAL PORTION OF THE DIVIDED RIGHT HAND OF A YOUTH AGED SEVENTEEN YEARS.)

The section traverses the distal extremity of the radius, the carpus, and the metacarpal bone an phalanges of the middle finger.

Articulationes manus et digitorum—Articulations of the hand and fingers.

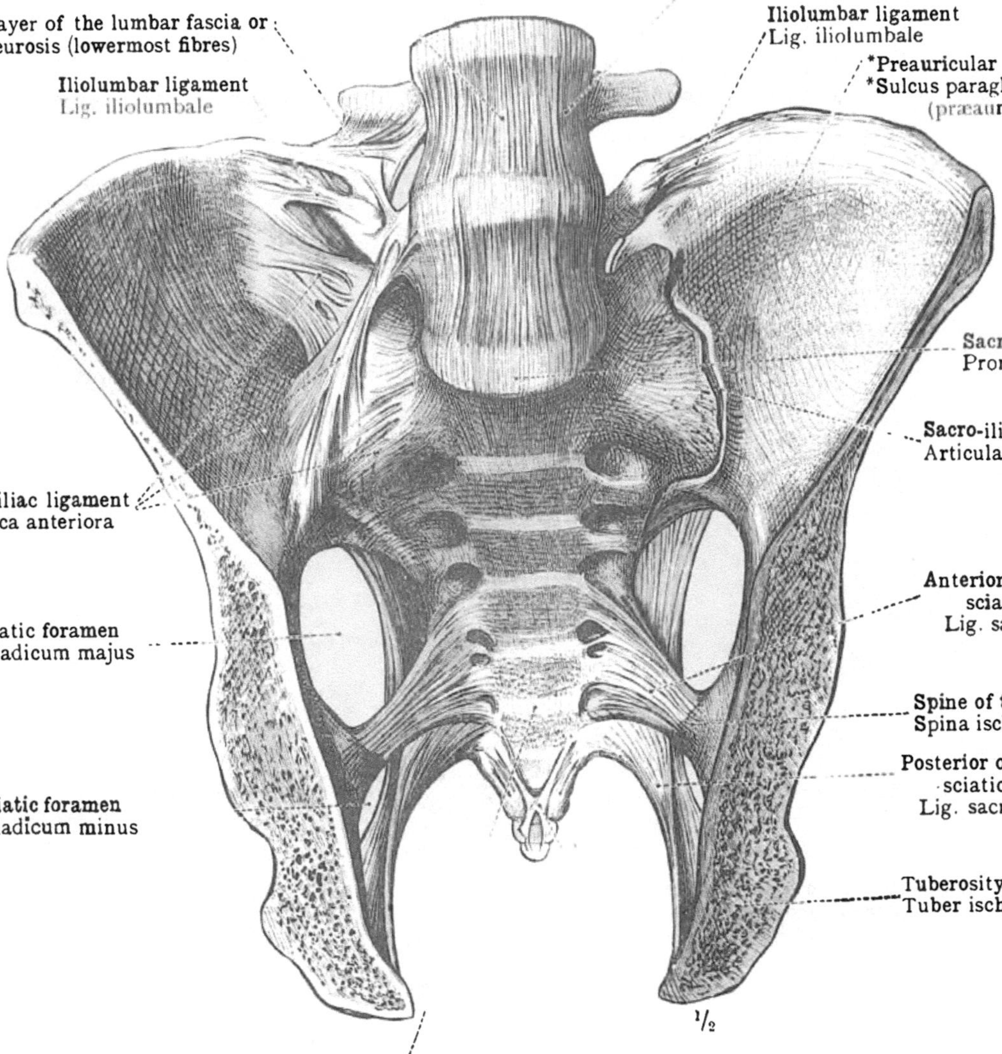

[1] Intervertebral disc of the sacrococcygeal articulation.—TR.

FIG. 451.—ARTICULATIO SACRO-ILIACA, SACRO-ILIAC ARTICULATION: LIGAMENTA SACRO-ILIACA ANTERIORA, ANTERIOR SACRO-ILIAC LIGAMENT; LIGAMENTUM ILIOLUMBALE, ILIOLUMBAR LIGAMENT. LIGAMENTA SACROSPINOSUM ET SACROTUBEROSUM, SMALL OR ANTERIOR AND GREAT OR POSTERIOR SACROSCIATIC LIGAMENTS. FORAMINA ISCHIADICA MAJUS ET MINUS, GREAT AND SMALL SACROSCIATIC FORAMINA. (THE PELVIS WITH THE FOURTH AND FIFTH LUMBAR VERTEBRÆ, IN FRONTAL SECTION; POSTERIOR HALF, SEEN FROM BEFORE.)

The ligaments of the right sacro-iliac articulation are intact; those of the left articulation have been removed.

Articulationes et ligamenta cinguli extremitatis interioris—Articulations and ligaments of the pe vic girdle.

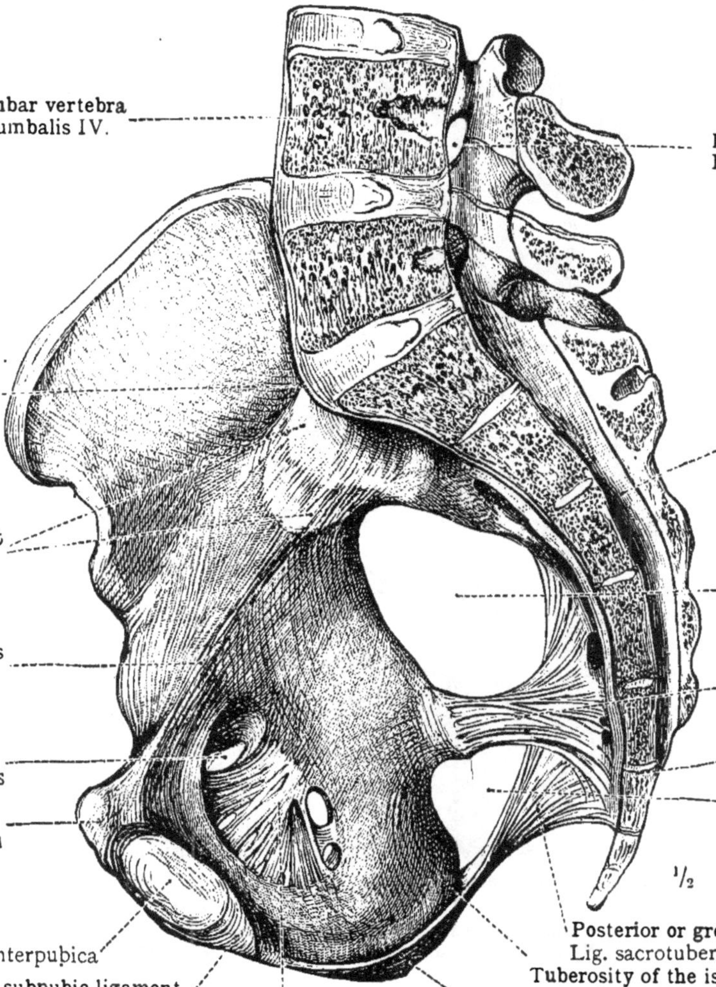

[1] See note on p. 216.

Fig. 452.—Ligamenta Sacrotuberosum et Sacrospinosum, Posterior or Great and Anterior or Small Sacrosciatic Ligaments; Foramina Ischiadica, Sacrosciatic Foramina. Membrana Obturatoria, Obturator Membrane or Ligament; Canalis Obturatorius, Obturator Canal. Articulatio Sacro-iliaca, Sacro-iliac Articulation. (The Right Half of a Pelvis divided in the Median Plane; seen from the Inner Side.)

Articulationes et ligamenta cinguli extremitatis inferioris—Articulations and ligaments of the pelvic girdle.

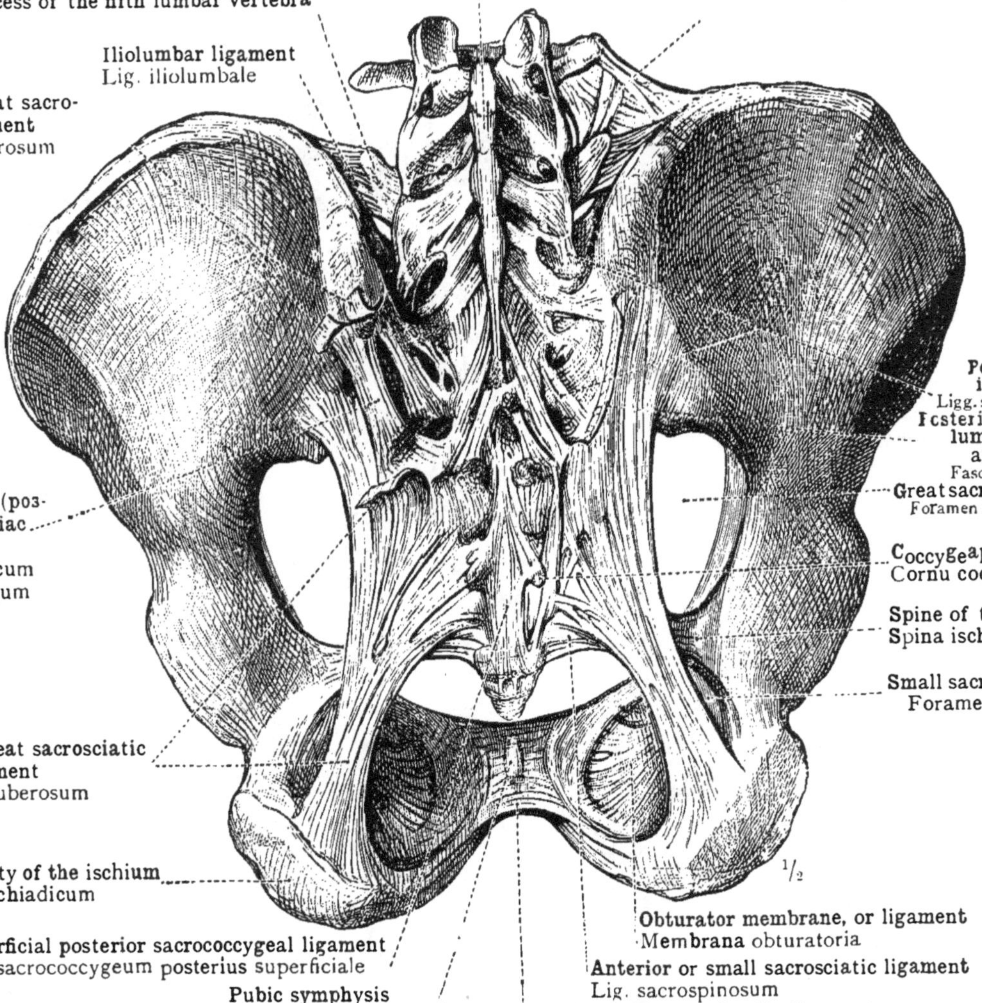

[1] Macalister and some other English anatomists agree with Toldt in naming this ligament the *interosseous* sacro-iliac ligament. That name is, however, misapplied, since the fibres of the ligament do not connect two closely adjacent parallel articular surfaces. True interosseous fine fibres are occasionally found connecting corresponding parts of the auricular surfaces of the sacrum and the ilium.—Tr.

FIG. 453.—POSTERIOR LIGAMENTS OF THE PELVIC GIRDLE: LIGAMENTUM SACROTUBEROSUM, POSTERIOR OR GREAT SACROSCIATIC LIGAMENT, AND ITS RELATION TO THE POSTERIOR LAYER OF THE LUMBAR APONEUROSIS. FORAMINA ISCHIADICA, SACROSCIATIC FORAMINA. LIGAMENTUM SACRO-ILIACUM POSTERIUS LONGUM, LONG OR OBLIQUE (POSTERIOR) SACRO-ILIAC LIGAMENT; LIGAMENTA SACRO-ILIAC INTEROSSEA, POSTERIOR SACRO-ILIAC LIGAMENT (*see note above*); LIGAMENTUM ILIOLUMBALE, ILIOLUMBAR LIGAMENT. (THE PELVIS WITH THE FOURTH AND FIFTH LUMBAR VERTEBRÆ; SEEN FROM BEHIND.)

On the right side, the posterior layer of the lumbar aponeurosis has been divided close to its continuation into the posterior or great sacrosciatic ligament, and turned outwards; on the left side, this superficial portion of the posterior or great sacrosciatic ligament has been cut across, and the divided ends have been turned upwards and downwards. The lowermost fibres of the middle layer of the lumbar aponeurosis have on the right side been left intact, but on the left side entirely removed.

Articulationes et ligamenta cinguli extremitatis inferioris—Articulations and ligaments of the pelvic girdle.

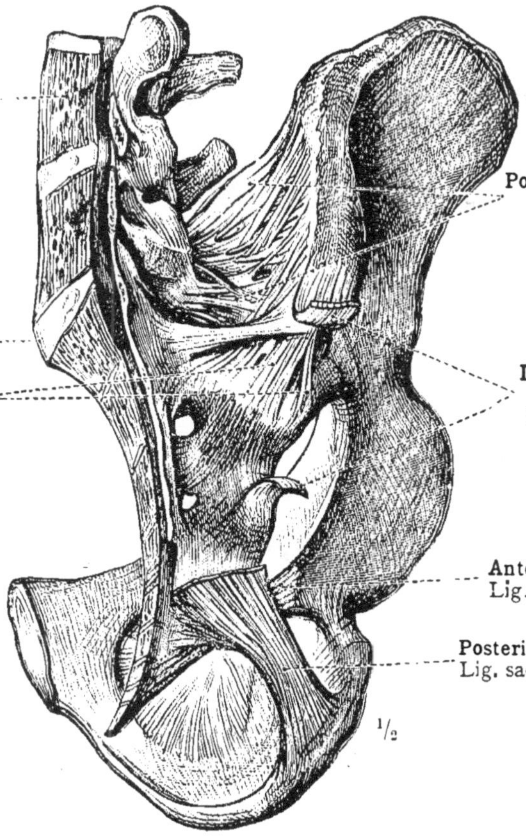

FIG. 454.—DEEP POSTERIOR LIGAMENTS OF THE SACRO-ILIAC ARTICULATION: LIGAMENTA SACRO-ILIACA INTEROSSEA, POSTERIOR SACRO-ILIAC LIGAMENTS; LIGAMENTUM SACRO-ILIACUM POSTERIUS BREVE, POSTERIOR (SHORT) SACRO-ILIAC LIGAMENT. (THE RIGHT HALF OF A PELVIS DIVIDED IN THE MEDIAN PLANE; POSTERO-INTERNAL ASPECT.)

The upper portion of the posterior or great sacrosciatic ligament has been removed; the long or oblique (posterior) sacro-iliac ligament has been divided transversely in the middle, and the ends have been turned upwards and downwards.

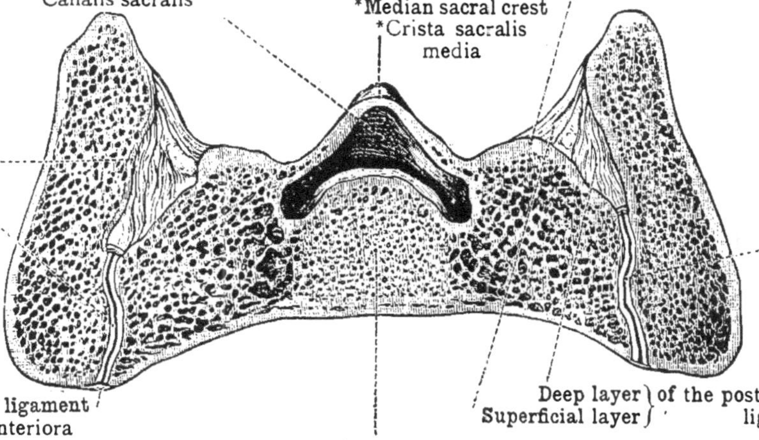

FIG. 455.—HORIZONTAL SECTION THROUGH THE SACRO-ILIAC ARTICULATION; UPPER SURFACE OF LOWER SEGMENT: SUPERFICIAL AND DEEP LAYERS OF THE POSTERIOR SACRO-ILIAC LIGAMENT.

The section was made in a plane at right angles to the long axis of the pelvis, and passes through the middle of the body of the first sacral vertebra.

1 This forms part of the *posterior sacro-iliac ligament* of English anatomists. See note on p. 218.—TR. 2 See note on p. 218.

Articulationes et ligamenta cinguli extremitatis inferioris—Articulations and ligaments of the pelvic girdle.

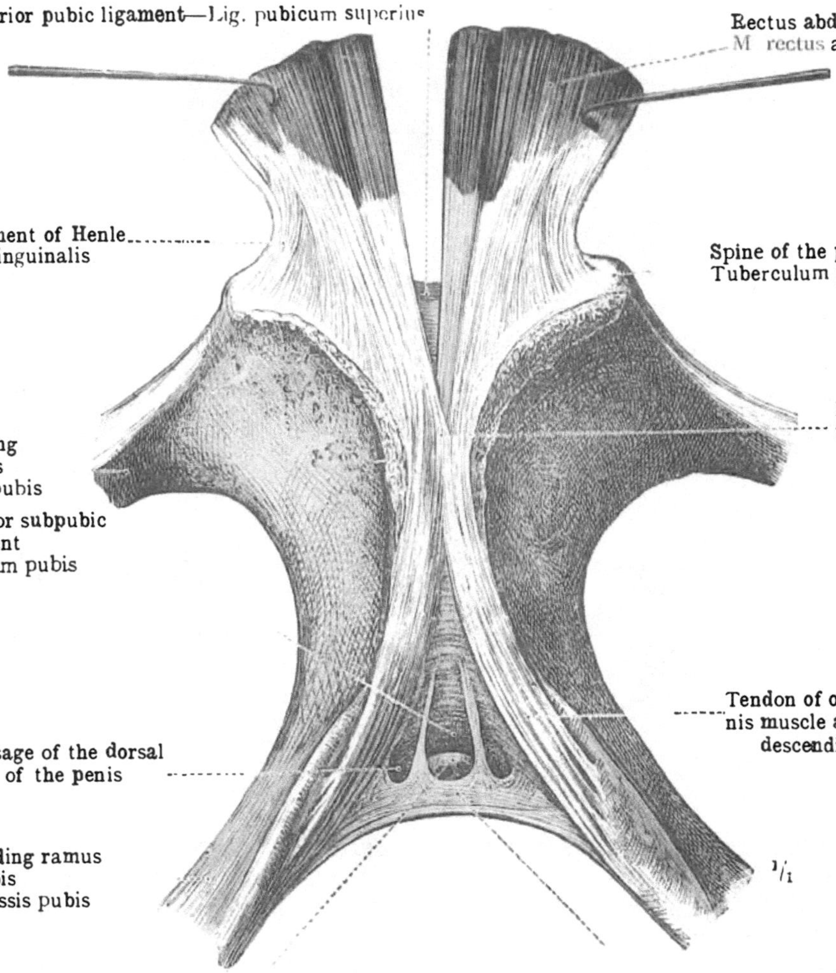

FIG. 456.—SYMPHYSIS OSSIUM PUBIS, PUBIC SYMPHYSIS: LIGAMENTUM PUBICUS SUPERIUS, SUPERIOR PUBIC LIGAMENT; LIGAMENTUM ARCUATUM PUBIS, INFERIOR PUBIC OR SUBPUBIC LIGAMENT; LIGAMENTUM TRANSVERSUM PELVIS, TRANSVERSE LIGAMENT OF THE PELVIS. THE ORIGIN OF THE TENDONS OF THE RECTUS ABDOMINIS MUSCLES FROM THE PUBIS, AND THE RELATION OF THESE TENDONS TO THE PUBIC SYMPHYSIS. (THE ANTERIOR ASPECT OF THE PUBIC SYMPHYSIS.)

The lower extremities of the rectus abdominis muscles have been pulled a little apart.

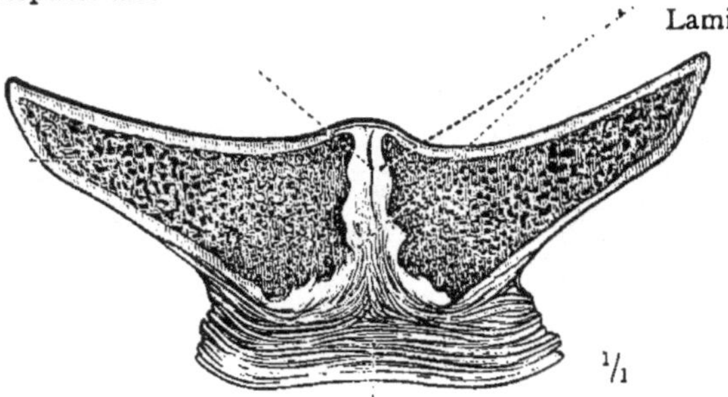

[1] The *anterior pubic ligament* is not mentioned by the author. It consists of two parts, a superficial and a deep. The *deep part*, which is not shown in any of the figures, is made up of fibres passing transversely from bone to bone in front of the interpubic disc; the fibres of the *superficial part* are oblique, interlace freely, and are mainly derived from the tendons of the external oblique and rectus muscles of the abdomen, as well as from those of the superficial adductors of the thigh. These interlacing tendinous fibres of the superficial part of the anterior pubic ligament are shown in both the figures on this page.—TR.

[2] This ligament is a portion of the deep perineal fascia or triangular ligament of the urethra. The name of transverse ligament of the pelvis, which is rarely used in England, was given to it by Henle.—TR.

FIG. 457.—HORIZONTAL SECTION THROUGH THE PUBIC SYMPHYSIS OF A NULLIPAROUS WOMAN AGED TWENTY-ONE YEARS; UPPER SURFACE OF LOWER SEGMENT: LAMINA FIBROCARTILAGINEA INTERPUBICA, INTERPUBIC DISC; FISSURE IN THE INTERPUBIC DISC. RE-INFORCEMENT OF THE INTERPUBIC ARTICULATION BY THE INTERLACING ON ITS ANTERIOR SURFACE OF THE FIBRES OF THE TENDONS OF ORIGIN OF THE RECTUS ABDOMINIS MUSCLES AND THE TENDONS OF INSERTION OF THE EXTERNAL OBLIQUE MUSCLES.

The plane of section lies in the upper half of the symphysis.

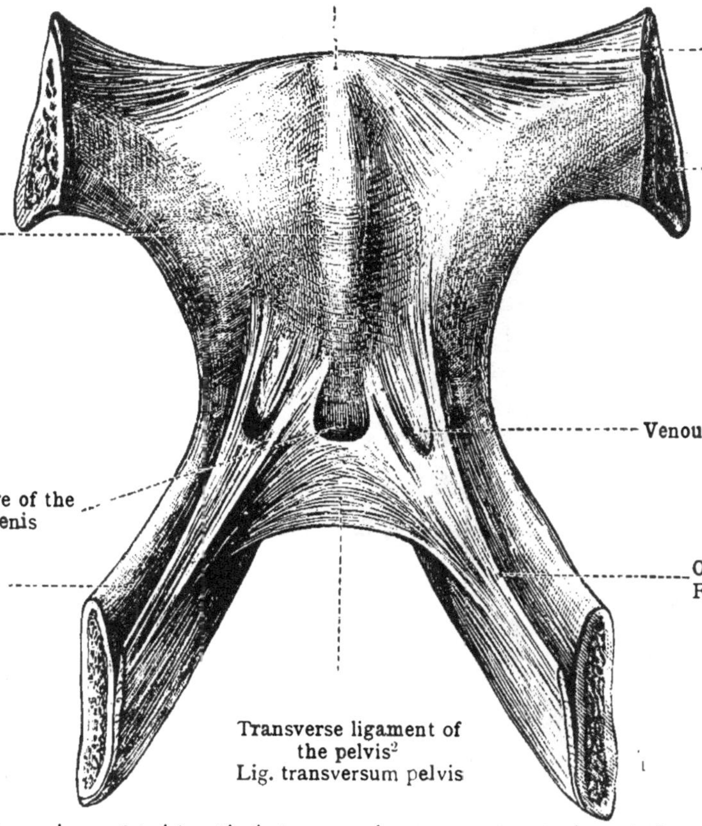

[1] The slight posterior prominence of the interpubic disc has not received any name from English anatomists. A few transverse fibres connect the pubic bones in this region, forming the *posterior pubic ligament*, which is not mentioned by Toldt.—TR.

[2] See note [2] on p. 220.

FIG. 458.—SYMPHYSIS OSSIUM PUBIS, PUBIC SYMPHYSIS: TORUS PUBICUS, POSTERIOR PROMINENCE OF THE INTERPUBIC DISC; LIGAMENTUM TRANSVERSUM PELVIS, TRANSVERSE LIGAMENT OF THE PELVIS (*see note* [2] *above*), WITH THE VENOUS FORAMINA; CONNEXIONS OF THE TRANSVERSE LIGAMENT OF THE PELVIS WITH THE OBTURATOR FASCIA. (THE PUBIC SYMPHYSIS SEEN FROM BEHIND.)

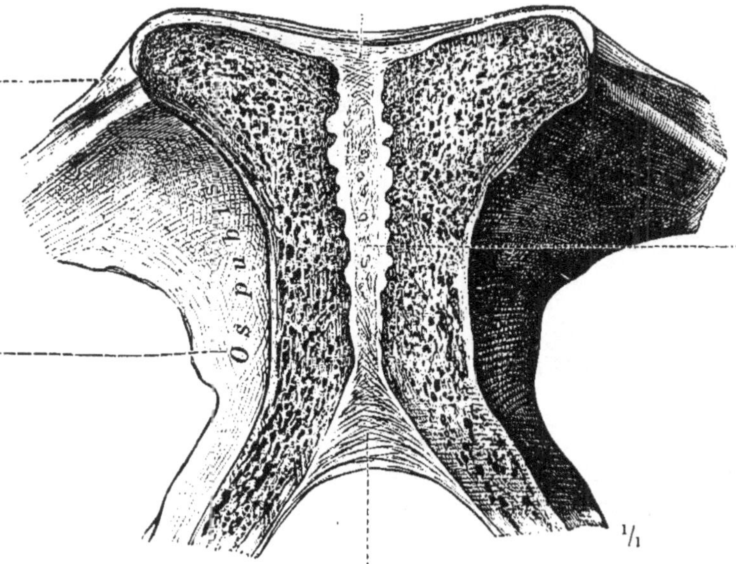

FIG. 459.—SYMPHYSIS OSSIUM PUBIS, PUBIC SYMPHYSIS: LAMINA FIBROCARTILAGINEA INTERPUBICA, INTERPUBIC DISC; LIGAMENTUM PUBICUM SUPERIUS, SUPERIOR PUBIC LIGAMENT; LIGAMENTUM ARCUATUM PUBIS, INFERIOR PUBIC OR SUBPUBIC LIGAMENT. (THE PUBIC SYMPHYSIS IN FRONTAL SECTION; ANTERIOR SURFACE OF POSTERIOR SEGMENT.)

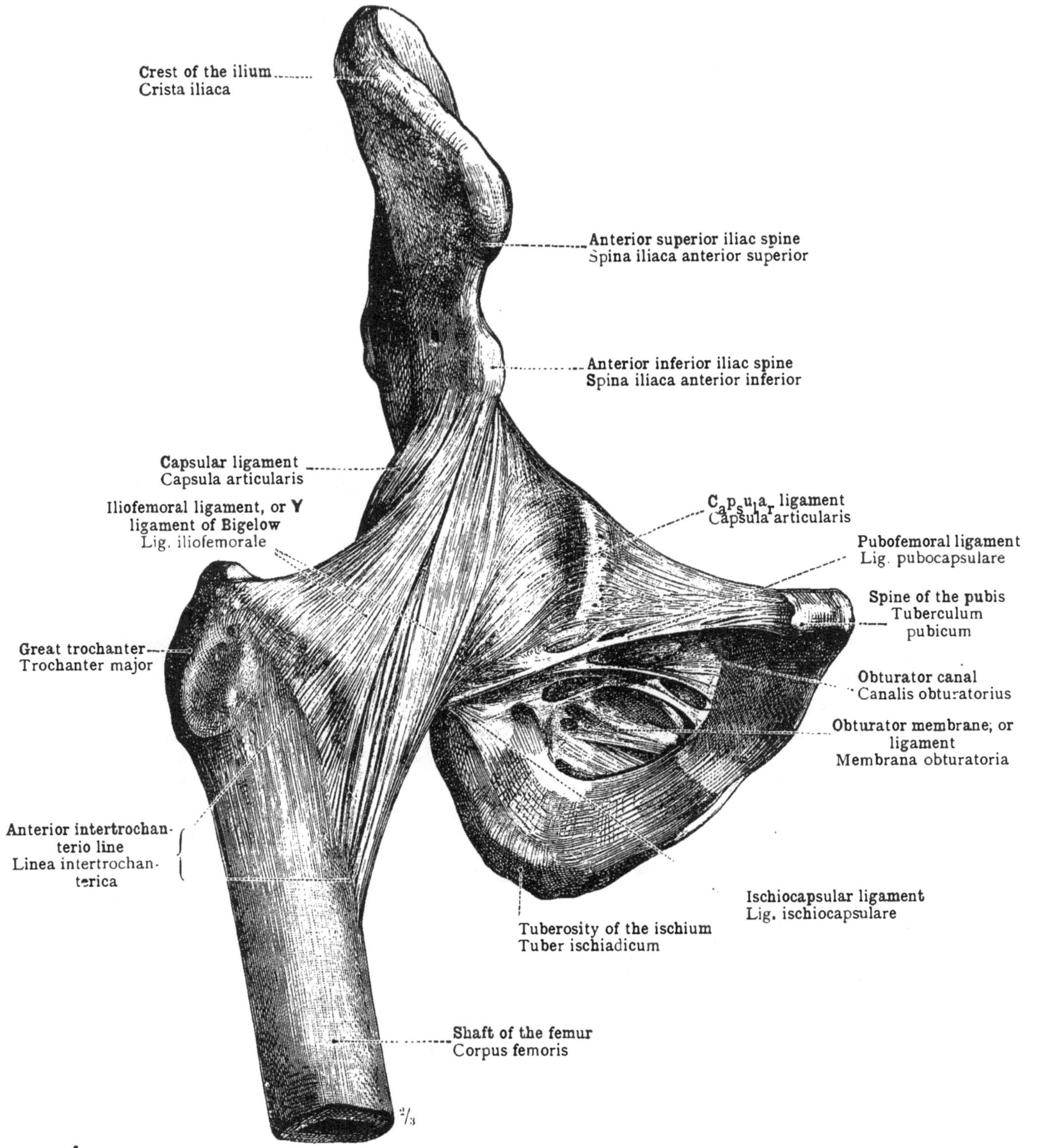

FIG. 460.—ARTICULATIO COXÆ, THE HIP-JOINT: LIGAMENTUM ILIOFEMORALE, ILIOFEMORAL LIGAMENT, OR Y LIGAMENT OF BIGELOW; LIGAMENTUM PUBOCAPSULARE, PUBOFEMORAL LIGAMENT, AND ITS RELATIONS TO THE OBTURATOR MEMBRANE. (THE RIGHT HIP-JOINT, SEEN FROM BEFORE.)

Articulatio coxæ.–The hip-joint.

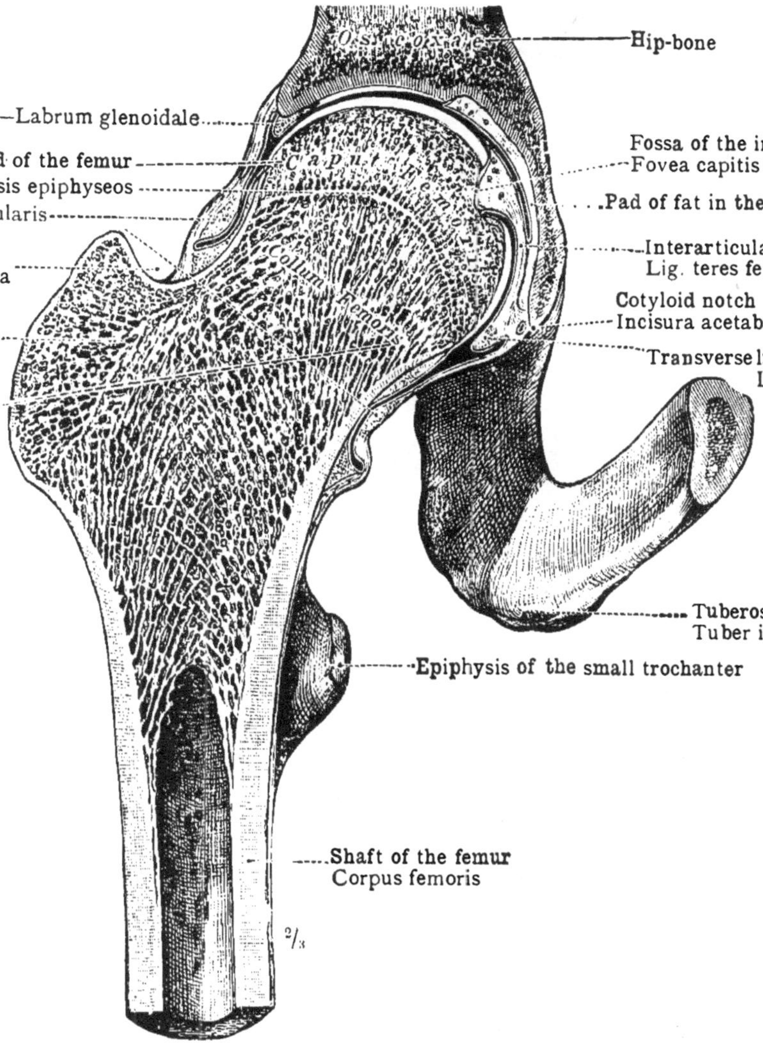

FIG. 461.—ARTICULATIO COXÆ, THE HIP-JOINT: CAPSULA ARTICULARIS, CAPSULAR LIGAMENT; ZONA ORBICULARIS, THE CIRCULARLY DISPOSED FIBRES OF THE CAPSULAR LIGAMENT, FORMING A BAND ROUND THE NECK OF THE FEMUR, WHICH IS MOST DISTINCT BEHIND AND BELOW. RELATION OF THE EPIPHYSIAL DISC OF THE HEAD OF THE FEMUR TO THE HIP-JOINT. (THE RIGHT HIP-JOINT IN FRONTAL SECTION; ANTERIOR SURFACE OF POSTERIOR SEGMENT.)

The section passes through the middle of the cotyloid notch and of the fossa of the interarticular ligament.

Articulatio coxæ—The hip-joint.

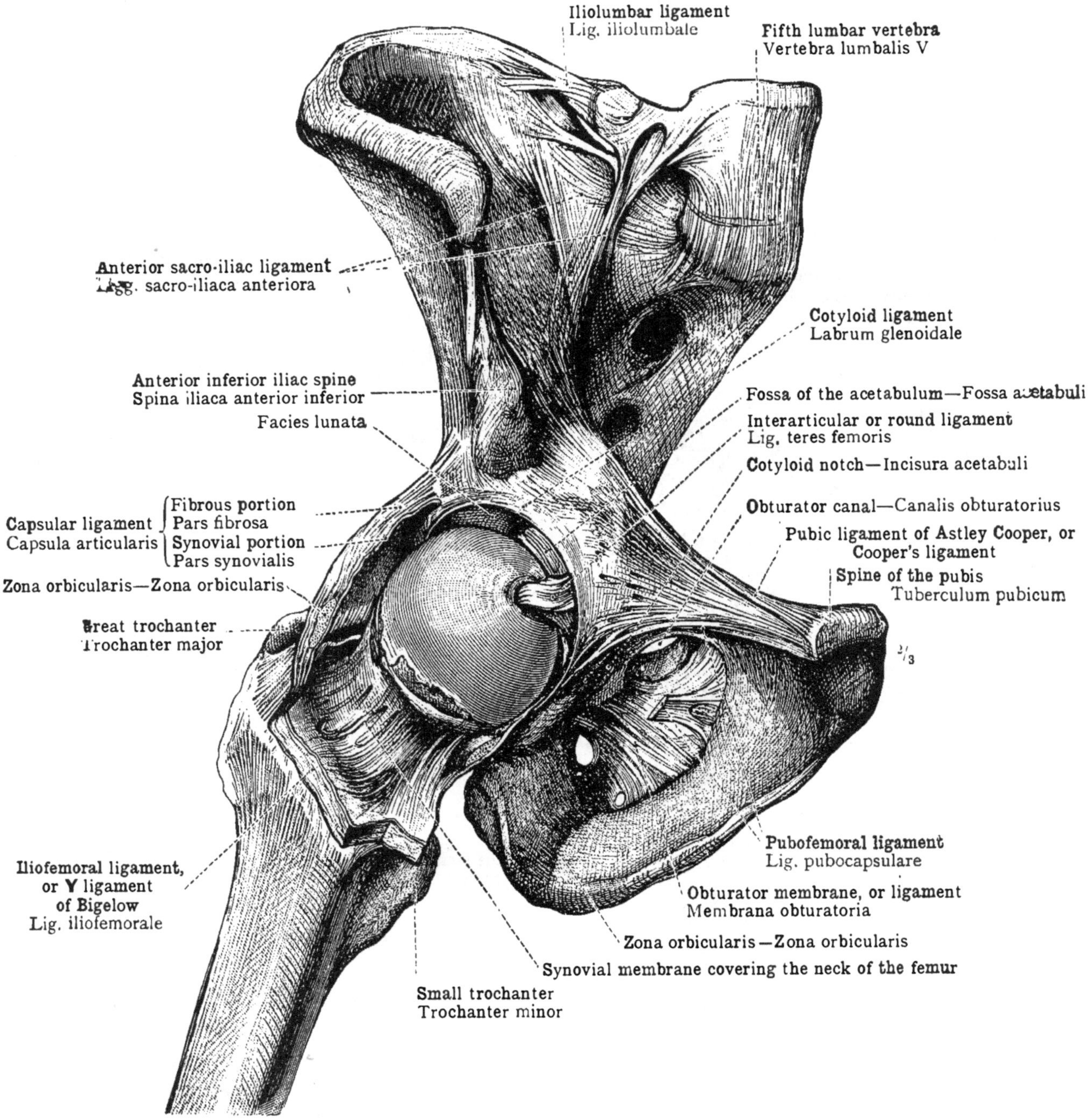

FIG. 462.—ARTICULATIO COXÆ, THE HIP-JOINT; LIGAMENTUM TERES FEMORIS INTERARTICULAR OR ROUND LIGAMENT OF THE HIP-JOINT[1]; LABRUM GLENOIDALE, COTYLOID LIGAMENT; CAPSULA ARTICULARIS, CAPSULAR LIGAMENT OF THE HIP-JOINT; REFLECTION OF THE SYNOVIAL MEMBRANE OF THE HIP-JOINT FROM THE INNER SURFACE OF THE CAPSULAR LIGAMENT ON TO THE NECK OF THE FEMUR; ZONA ORBICULARIS, CIRCULAR BAND OF THE CAPSULAR LIGAMENT ROUND THE NECK OF THE FEMUR.[2] (THE RIGHT HIP-JOINT SEEN FROM BEFORE.)

The anterior wall of the capsular ligament has been removed, except for a narrow band at its distal attachment, which has been turned outwards. The head of the femur has been slightly withdrawn from its socket in a downward and outward direction.

[1] Perhaps most frequently known in England by its Latin name, *ligamentum teres*.
[2] Also frequently known in England by its Latin name, *zona orbicularis*.

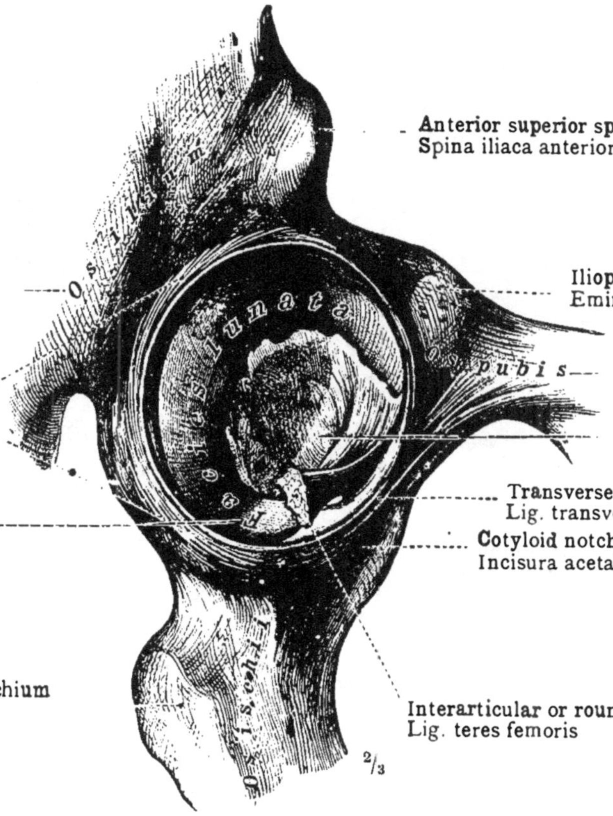

FIG. 463.—ARTICULATIO COXÆ, THE HIP-JOINT: THE ACETABULUM; LABRUM GLENOIDALE ET LIGAMENTUM TRANSVERSUM ACETABULI, THE COTYLOID LIGAMENT AND THE TRANSVERSE LIGAMENT OF THE ACETABULUM. LIGAMENTUM TERES FEMORIS, THE INTERARTICULAR OR ROUND LIGAMENT. (VIEW OF THE INTERIOR OF THE SOCKET OF THE RIGHT HIP-JOINT.)

The interarticular or round ligament has been divided close to its attachment to the head of the femur.

Articulatio coxæ—The hip-joint.

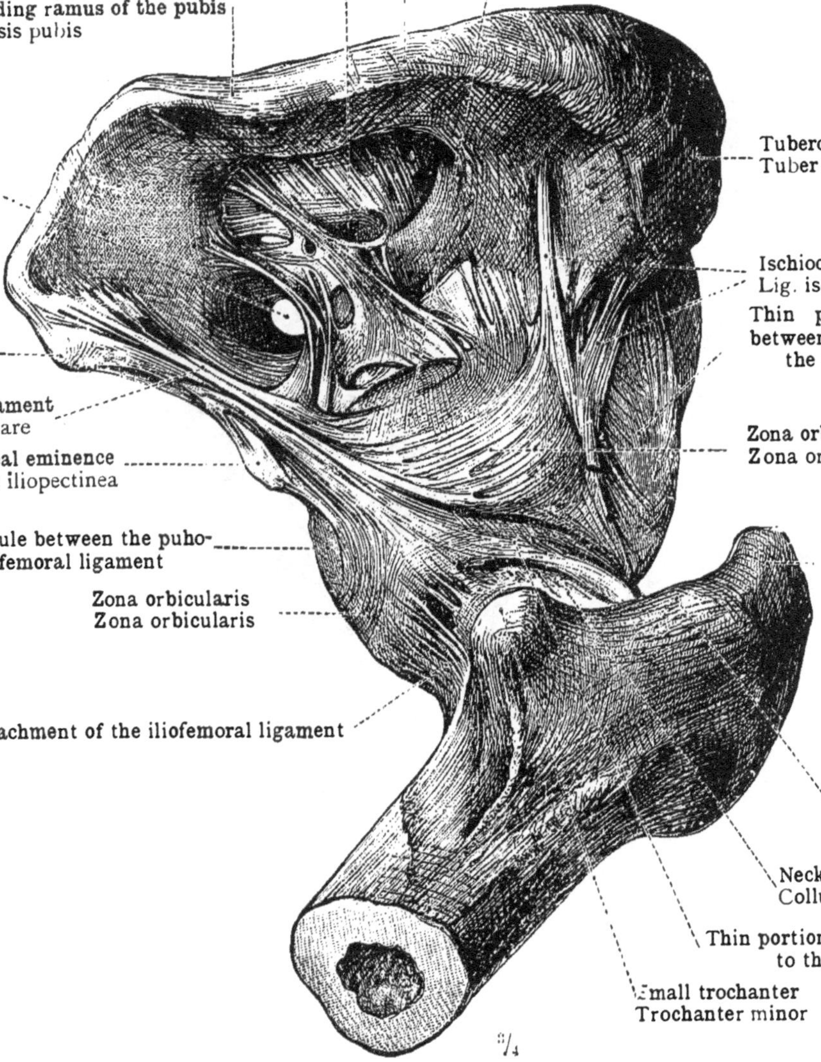

FIG. 464.—ARTICULATIO COXÆ, THE HIP-JOINT: CAPSULA ARTICULARIS, THE CAPSULAR LIGAMENT; ZONA ORBICULARIS (*see p.* 223), AND ITS RELATIONS TO THE PUBOFEMORAL AND ISCHIOCAPSULAR LIGAMENTS. MEMBRANA OBTURATORIA ET CANALIS OBTURATORIUS, OBTURATOR MEMBRANE OR LIGAMENT AND OBTURATOR CANAL. (THE POSTERO-INTERNAL SIDE OF THE RIGHT HIP-JOINT SEEN FROM BELOW.)

The articular cavity has been injected with tallow.

Articulatio coxæ—The hip-joint.

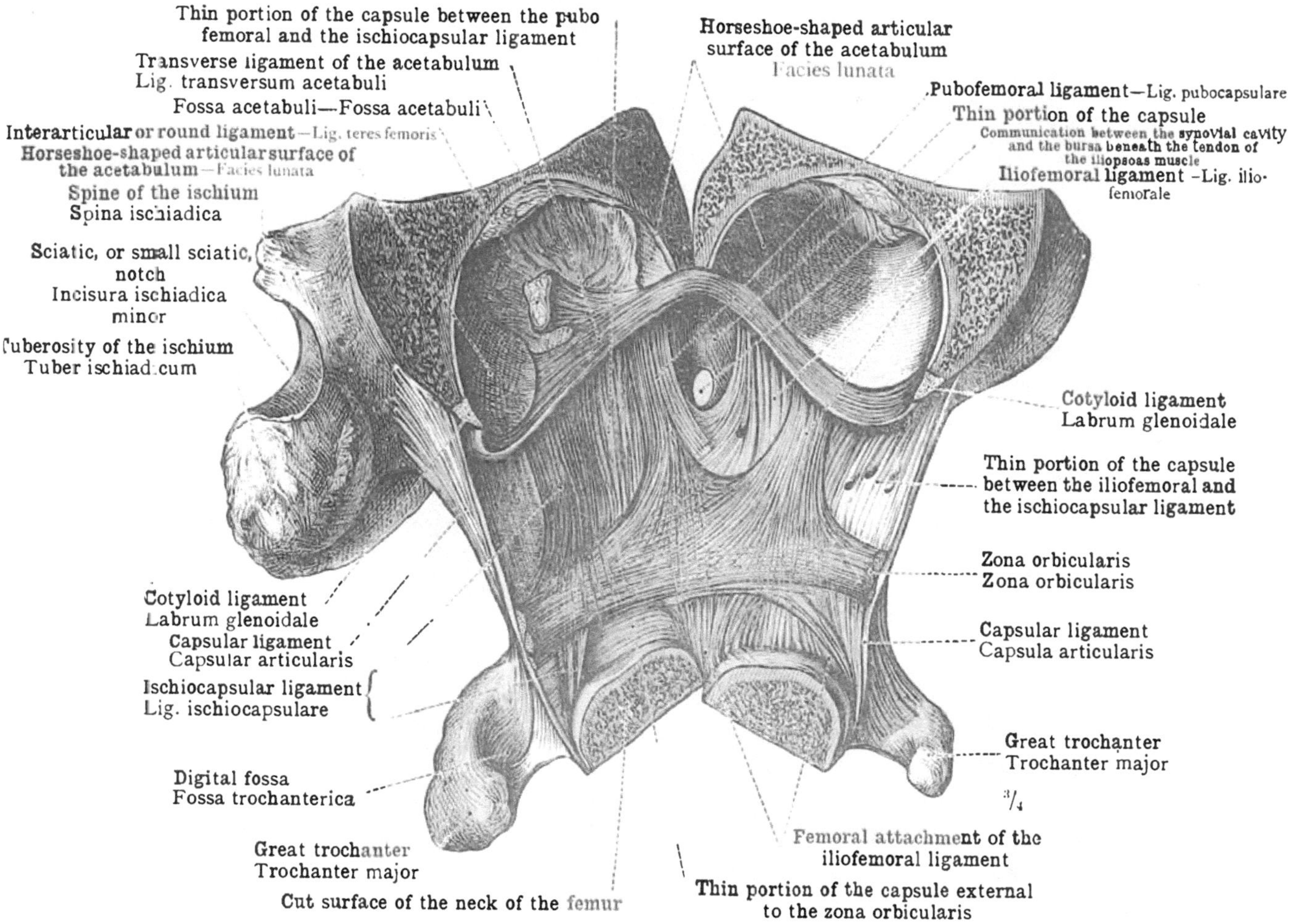

FIG. 465.—ARTICULATIO COXÆ, THE HIP-JOINT: *ZONA* ORBICULARIS (*see p.* 223), AND ITS RELATIONS TO THE ILIOFEMORAL, PUBOFEMORAL, AND ISCHIOCAPSULAR LIGAMENTS; THE THIN PORTIONS OF THE CAPSULE, AND THE COMMUNICATION BETWEEN THE SYNOVIAL CAVITY AND THE BURSA BENEATH THE TENDON OF THE ILIOPSOAS MUSCLE; THE ACETABULUM, WITH THE TRANSVERSE LIGAMENT OF THE ACETABULUM, AND THE INTERARTICULAR OR ROUND LIGAMENT.

After the capsule of the right hip-joint had been prepared from without, the joint was fully flexed; the capsule was then divided by a section in the direction of a line passing from the middle of the upper border of the great trochanter to the inner border of the iliopectineal eminence; the ilium was cut away except for that portion of the bone which contributes to the formation of the acetabulum, and the neck of the femur was sawn across just internal to the distal attachment of the capsule; the interarticular ligament was divided close to the head of the femur, and this latter, together with the intracapsular portion of the neck, was removed; the acetabulum and the remaining proximal portion of the femur were divided in two by a continuation of the section already made through the upper wall of the capsule; the two halves of the acetabulum and the head and neck of the femur were then opened out till the cut surfaces met at a very obtuse angle; so that the capsule and the cotyloid ligament were fully exposed from within. The synovial membrane was dissected off, and the inner surface of the capsule cleaned from fat and cellular tissue.

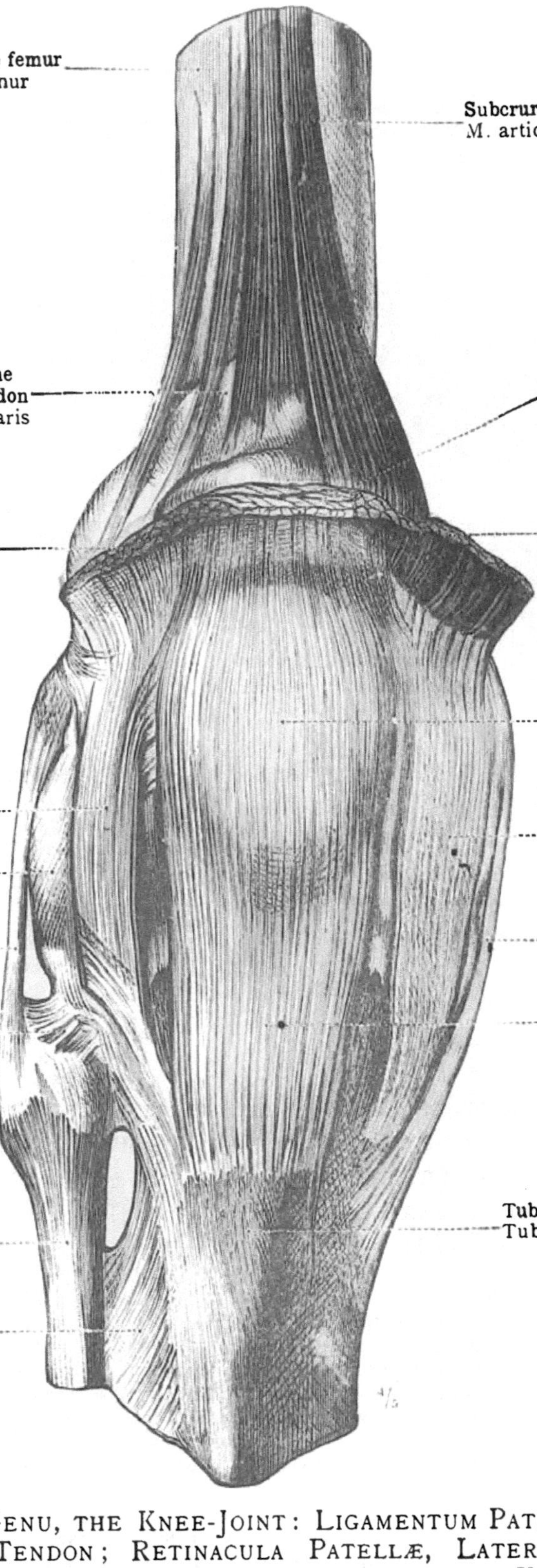

FIG. 466.—ARTICULATIO GENU, THE KNEE-JOINT: LIGAMENTUM PATELLÆ, PATELLAR LIGAMENT, OR INFRAPATELLAR TENDON; RETINACULA PATELLÆ, LATERAL PATELLAR LIGAMENTS; LIGAMENTA COLLATERALIA, LATERAL LIGAMENTS OF THE KNEE-JOINT. BURSA SUPRAPATELLARIS, THE BURSA BENEATH THE SUPRAPATELLAR TENDON; THE RELATION OF THE UNUSUALLY LARGE SUBCRUREUS MUSCLE TO THE CAPSULE OF THE KNEE-JOINT. ARTICULATIO TIBIOFIBULARIS, SUPERIOR TIBIOFIBULAR ARTICULATION: LIGAMENTA CAPITULI FIBULÆ, ANTERIOR SUPERIOR TIBIOFIBULAR LIGAMENT. (THE RIGHT KNEE-JOINT FROM BEFORE.)

The synovial cavity has been injected with tallow.

Articulatio genu—The knee-joint.

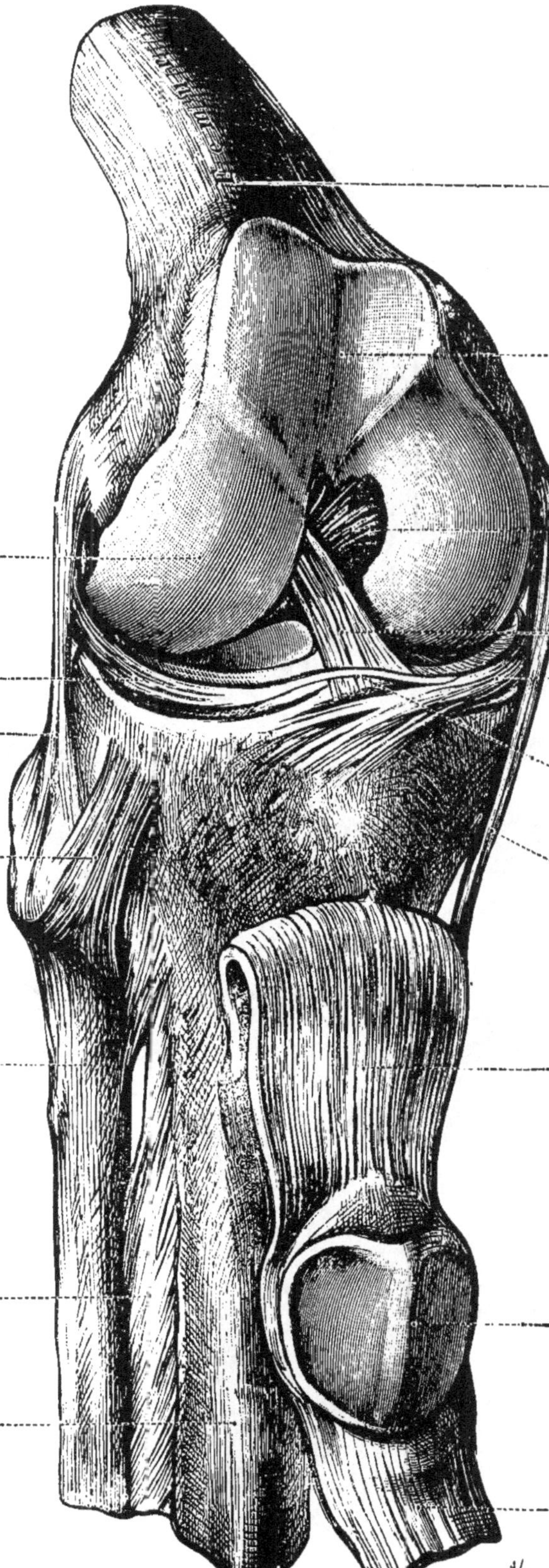

FIG. 467.—ARTICULATIO GENU, THE KNEE-JOINT: LIGAMENTA COLLATERALIA, LATERAL LIGAMENTS OF THE KNEE-JOINT; LIGAMENTA CRUCIATA, CRUCIAL LIGAMENTS; LIGAMENTUM PATELLÆ, PATELLAR LIGAMENT, OR INFRAPATELLAR TENDON. ARTICULATIO TIBIOFIBULARIS, SUPERIOR TIBIOFIBULAR ARTICULATION: LIGAMENTA CAPITULI FIBULÆ, ANTERIOR SUPERIOR TIBIOFIBULAR LIGAMENT. (THE RIGHT KNEE-JOINT SEEN FROM BEFORE AND WITHOUT.)

The capsular ligament has been removed from the front of the joint between the two lateral ligaments, and the patellar ligament has been turned downwards.

Articulatio genu—The knee-joint.

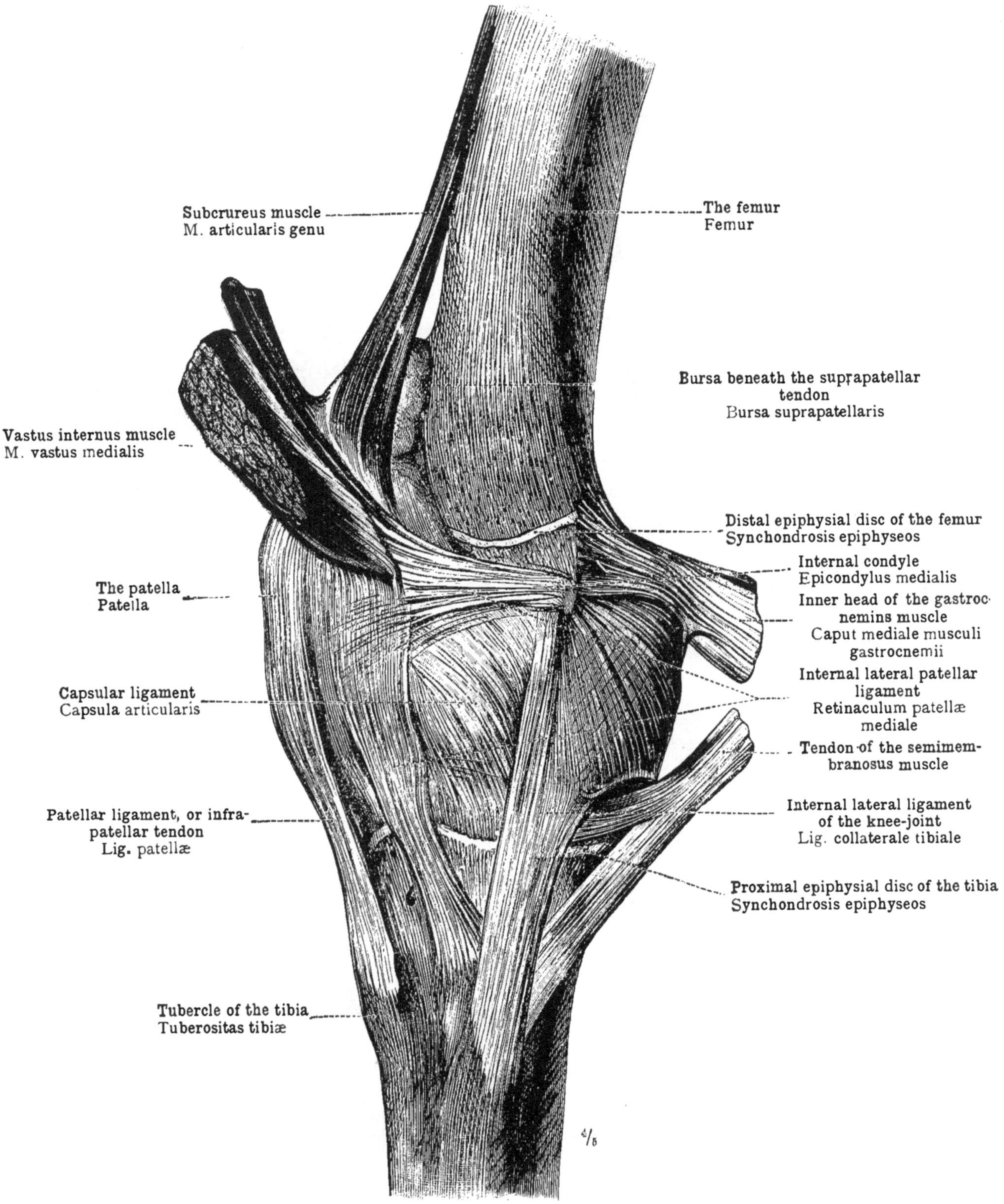

FIG. 468.—ARTICULATIO GENU, THE KNEE-JOINT: CAPSULA ARTICULARIS, CAPSULAR LIGAMENT, AND THE RELATIONS OF THE SUBCRUREUS MUSCLE TO THIS LIGAMENT; BURSA SUPRAPATELLARIS, THE BURSA BENEATH THE SUPRAPATELLAR TENDON. LIGAMENTUM COLLATERALE TIBIÆ, INTERNAL LATERAL LIGAMENT OF THE KNEE-JOINT; LIGAMENTUM PATELLÆ ET RETINACULUM PATELLÆ MEDIALE, PATELLAR LIGAMENT, OR INFRAPATELLAR TENDON, AND INTERNAL LATERAL PATELLAR LIGAMENT. RELATIONS OF THE EPIPHYSIAL DISCS TO THE ARTICULATION.

The same preparation as that of Fig. 466, seen from within.

Articulatio genu—The knee-joint.

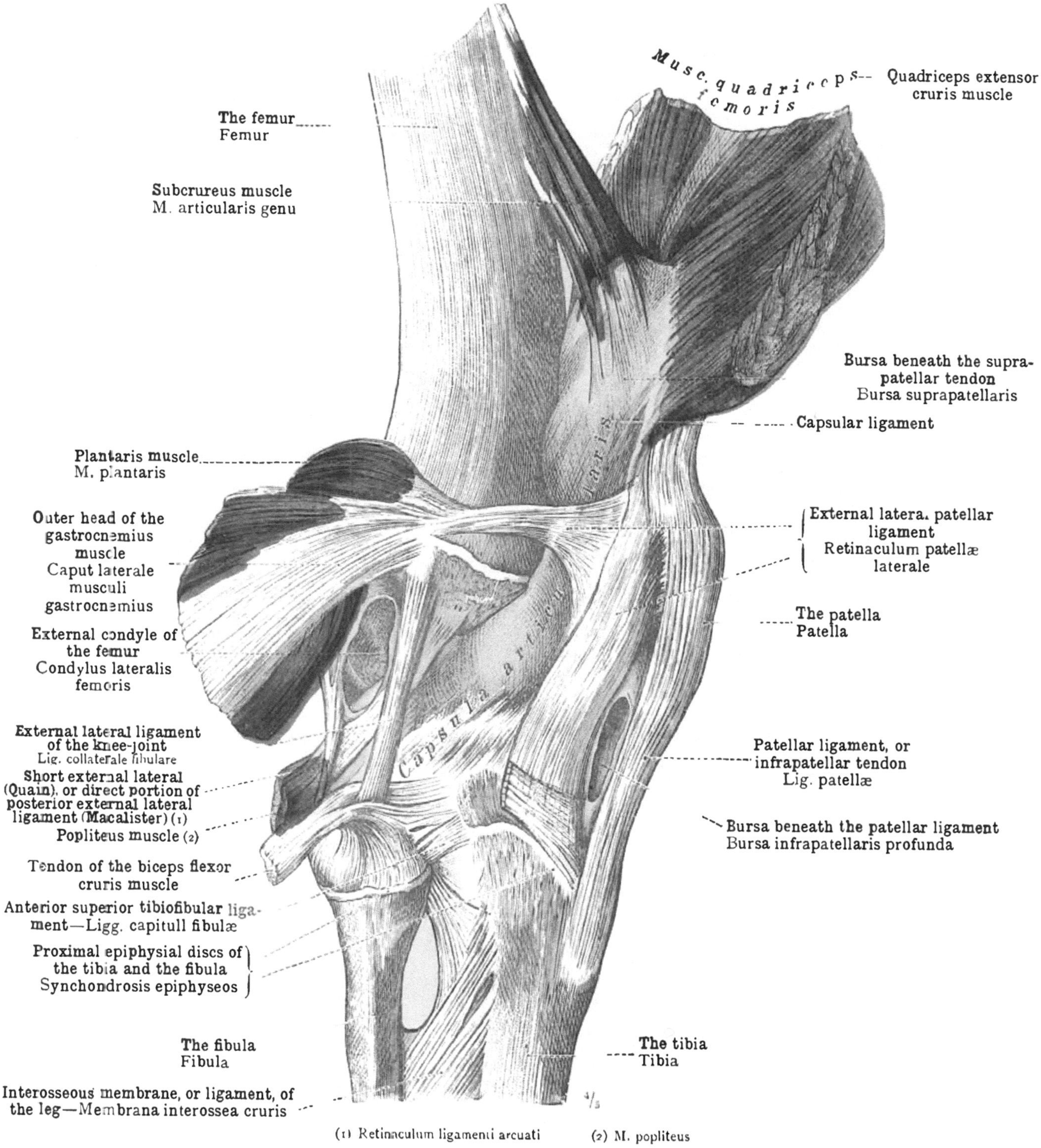

FIG. 469.—ARTICULATIO GENU, THE KNEE-JOINT: CAPSULA ARTICULARIS, CAPSULAR LIGAMENT; BURSA SUPRAPATELLARIS, AND THE RELATIONS OF THE QUADRICEPS EXTENSOR CRURIS MUSCLE TO THE SAME. LIGAMENTUM COLLATERALE FIBULARE, EXTERNAL LATERAL LIGAMENT OF THE KNEE-JOINT. LIGAMENTUM PATELLÆ ET RETINACULUM PATELLÆ LATERALE, PATELLAR LIGAMENT, OR INFRAPATELLAR TENDON, AND EXTERNAL LATERAL PATELLAR LIGAMENT; THE RELATIONS OF THE LATTER TO THE PLANTARIS MUSCLE AND TO THE OUTER HEAD OF THE GASTROCNEMIUS MUSCLE. BURSA INFRAPATELLARIS PROFUNDA, BURSA BENEATH THE PATELLAR LIGAMENT. ARTICULATIO TIBIOFIBULARIS, SUPERIOR TIBIOFIBULAR ARTICULATION. LIGAMENTA CAPITULI FIBULÆ, ANTERIOR SUPERIOR TIBIOFIBULAR LIGAMENT. RELATIONS OF THE EPIPHYSIAL DISCS TO BOTH THE JOINTS.

The same preparation as that of Figs. 466 and 468, seen from the outer side. The synovial cavity of the knee-joint has been opened behind the external lateral ligament of the knee-joint, and the bursa beneath the patellar ligament has also been opened.

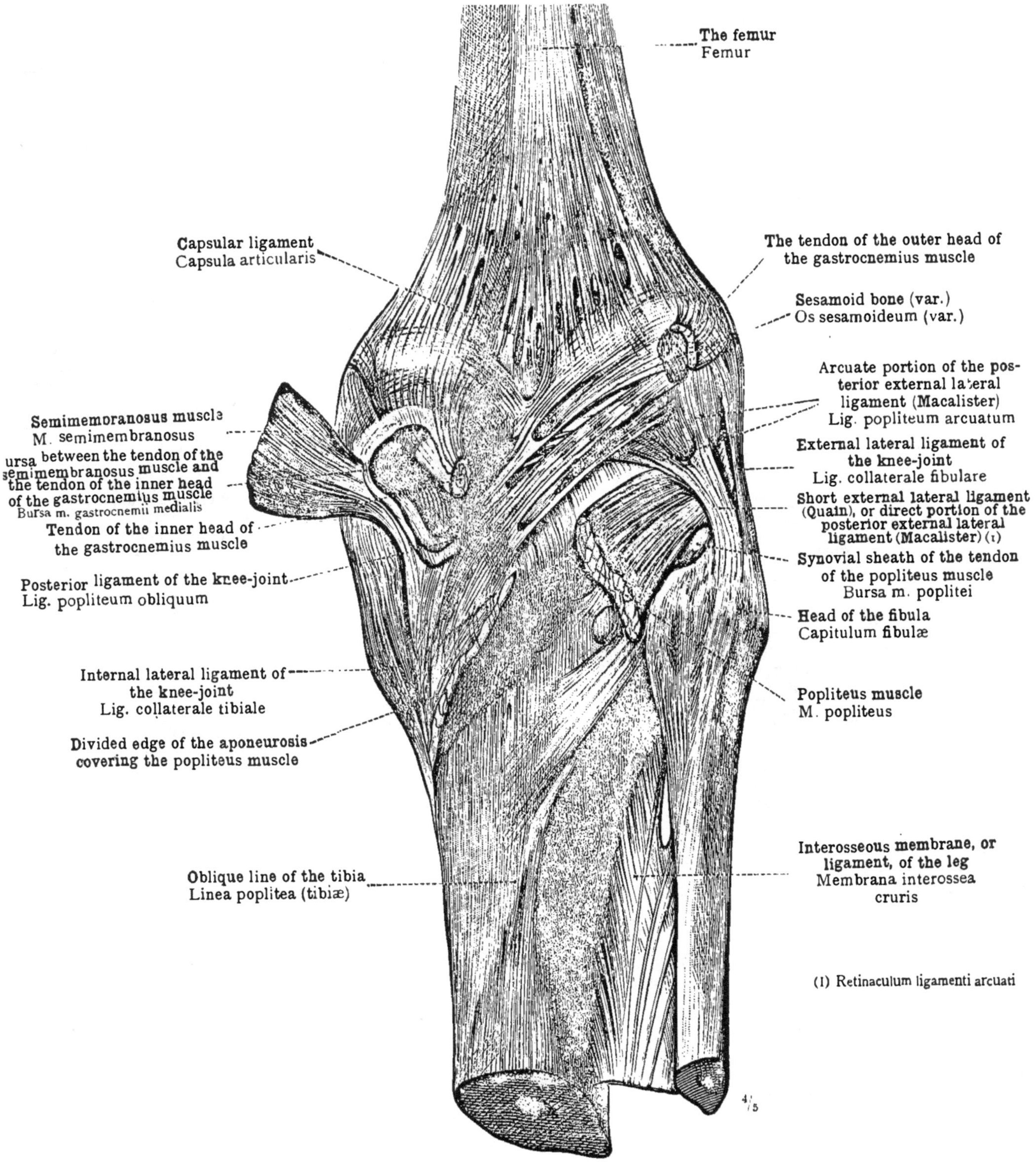

FIG. 470.—ARTICULATIO GENU, THE KNEE-JOINT: CAPSULA ARTICULARIS, CAPSULAR LIGAMENT; LIGAMENTUM POPLITEUM OBLIQUUM, POSTERIOR LIGAMENT OF THE KNEE-JOINT; RELATIONS OF THIS LIGAMENT TO THE TENDON OF THE SEMIMEMBRANOSUS MUSCLE AND TO THE OUTER HEAD OF THE GASTROCNEMIUS MUSCLE; LIGAMENTUM POPLITEUM ARCUATUM ET RETINACULUM LIGAMENTI ARCUATI, ARCUATE PORTION OF THE POSTERIOR EXTERNAL LATERAL LIGAMENT (MACALISTER), AND SHORT EXTERNAL LATERAL LIGAMENT (QUAIN), OR DIRECT PORTION OF THE POSTERIOR EXTERNAL LATERAL LIGAMENT (MACALISTER). BURSA MUSCULI GASTROCNEMII MEDIALIS, BURSA BETWEEN THE TENDON OF THE SEMIMEMBRANOSUS MUSCLE AND THE TENDON OF THE INNER HEAD OF THE GASTROCNEMIUS MUSCLE, COMMUNICATING WITH THE KNEE-JOINT AND HAVING A COMMON CAVITY WITH THE BURSA BETWEEN THE TENDON OF THE SEMIMEMBRANOSUS MUSCLE AND THE KNEE-JOINT. BURSA MUSCULI POPLITEI, SYNOVIAL SHEATH OF THE TENDON OF THE POPLITEUS MUSCLE. (THE RIGHT KNEE-JOINT, SEEN FROM BEHIND.)

Articulatio genu—The knee-joint.

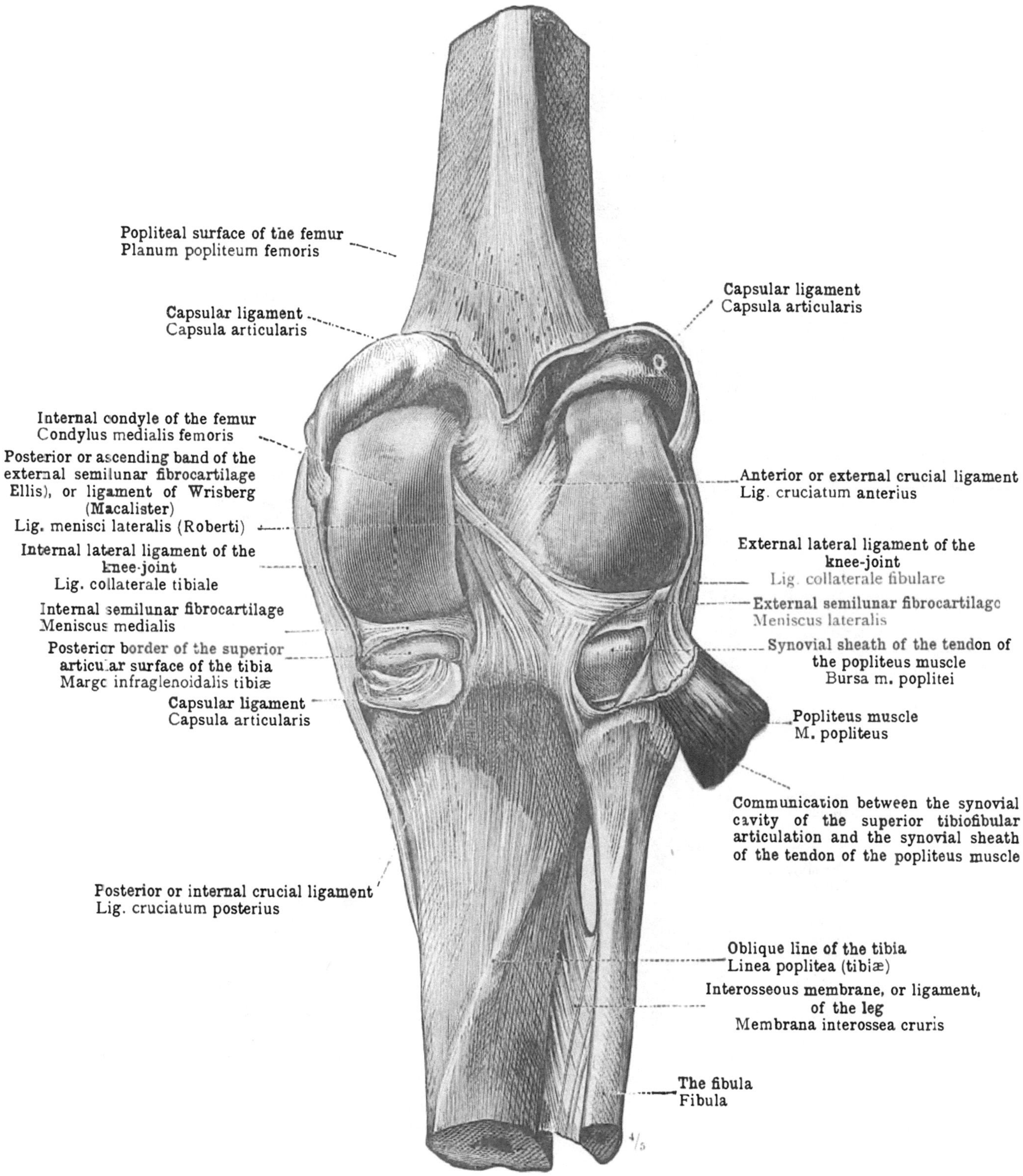

FIG. 471.—ARTICULATIO GENU, THE KNEE-JOINT: LIGAMENTA CRUCIATA, CRUCIAL LIGAMENTS, AND LIGAMENTUM MENISCI LATERALIS, POSTERIOR OR ASCENDING BAND OF THE EXTERNAL SEMILUNAR FIBROCARTILAGE (ELLIS) OR LIGAMENT OF WRISBERG (MACALISTER), (VARIETY[1]). COMMUNICATION OF THE SYNOVIAL SHEATH OF THE TENDON OF THE POPLITEUS MUSCLE WITH THE SYNOVIAL CAVITIES OF THE KNEE-JOINT AND OF THE SUPERIOR TIBIOFIBULAR ARTICULATION. (THE RIGHT KNEE-JOINT, SEEN FROM BEHIND.)

The posterior portion of the capsular ligament, between the external and internal lateral ligaments, has been removed, except for a strip left above close to the femoral attachment, which has been turned upwards; the synovial sheath of the tendon of the popliteus muscle has been opened at its inner side, and its posterior wall has been turned outwards with the tendon and the proximal portion of the popliteus muscle.

[1] Though this band is called a variety by Toldt, it is, in fact, usually present, but its situation varies; inasmuch as it passes, sometimes behind (as here), and sometimes before, and sometimes as a double band behind and before, the posterior or internal crucial ligament. Its strength and thickness varies much, but it is seldom entirely wanting.—TR.

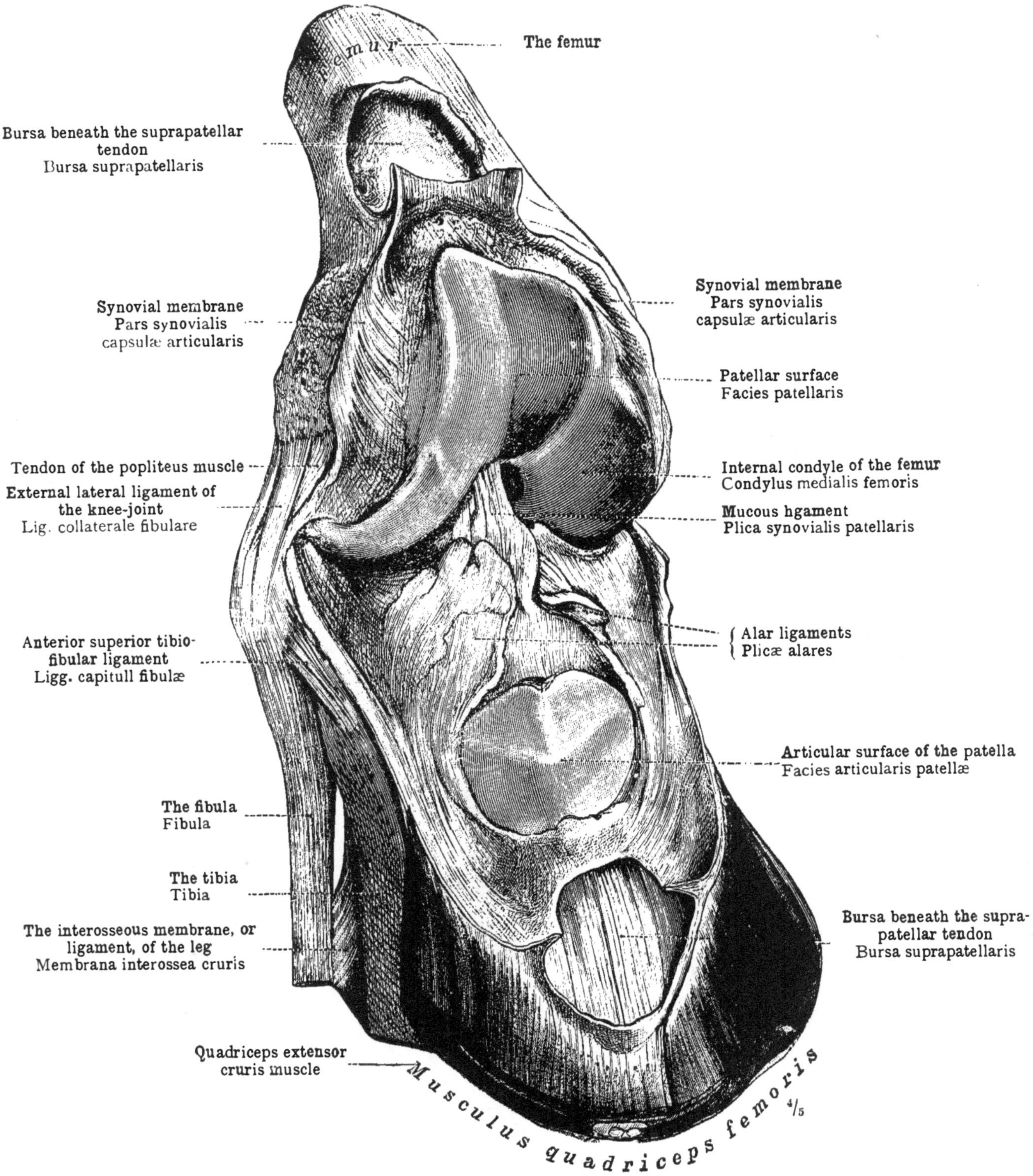

FIG. 472.—ARTICULATIO GENU, THE KNEE-JOINT: PARS SYNOVIALIS CAPSULÆ ARTICULARIS, SYNOVIAL MEMBRANE OF THE KNEE-JOINT; PLICA SYNOVIALIS PATELLARIS, MUCOUS LIGAMENT; PLICÆ ALARES, ALAR LIGAMENTS; BURSA SUPRAPATELLARIS, BURSA BENEATH THE SUPRAPATELLAR TENDON. (THE RIGHT KNEE-JOINT, SEEN FROM BEFORE AND WITHOUT.)

The joint was first injected, and the injected material allowed to solidify; the capsule of the joint was then prepared from without, the quadriceps extensor cruris muscle being left intact; subsequently the joint was opened by a section passing through the quadriceps muscle and the upper part of the front of the capsule from one lateral ligament to the other close to the attachment of the capsule to the femur, and the anterior wall of the joint together with the distal portion of the quadriceps extensor muscle was turned down. The quadriceps was divided at a somewhat higher level than the capsule, and the bursa beneath the suprapatellar tendon divided is the frontal plane, to show the communication of this bursa with the joint.

Articulatio genu—The knee-joint.

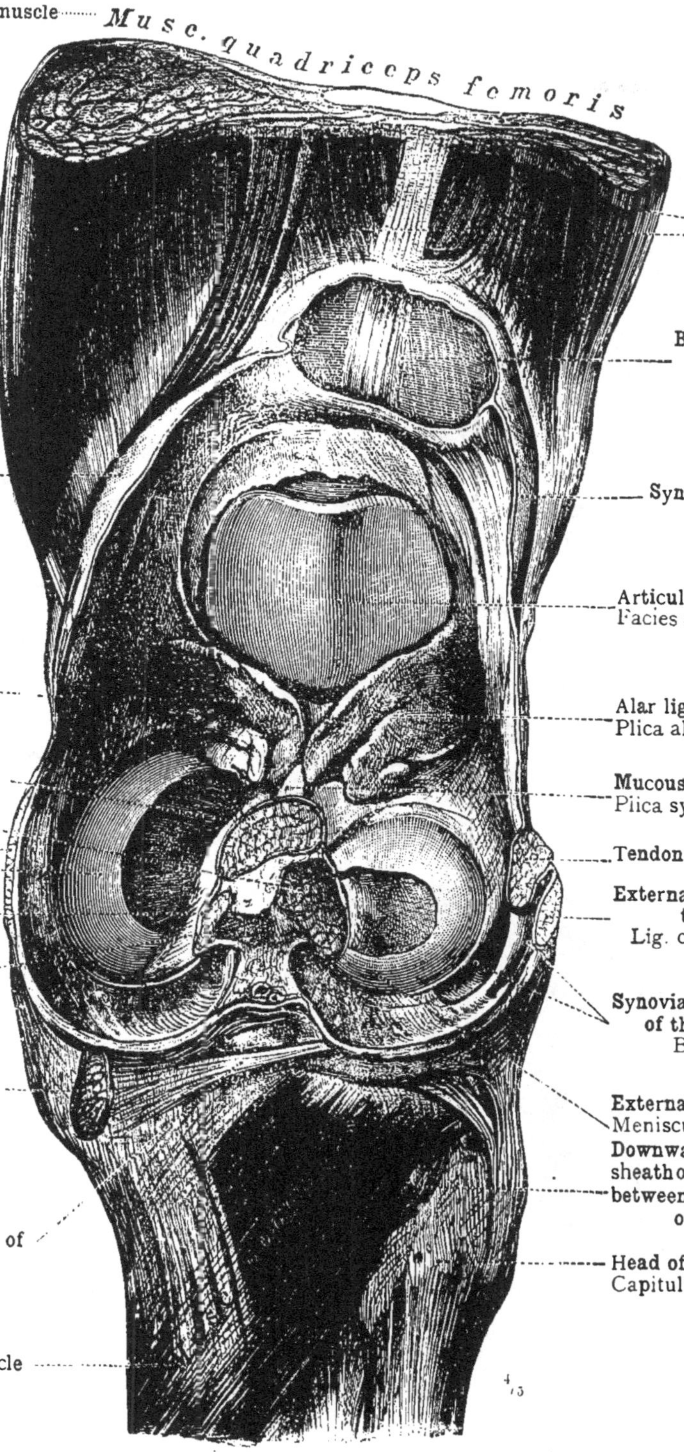

FIG. 473.—ARTICULATIO GENU, THE KNEE-JOINT: THE SEMILUNAR FIBROCARTILAGES, THE ALAR LIGAMENTS, AND THE MUCOUS LIGAMENT; THE INSERTION INTO THE SYNOVIAL MEMBRANE OF THE SUBCRUREUS MUSCLE; THE EXTENSION OF THE SYNOVIAL MEMBRANE OF THE KNEE-JOINT TO FORM THE SYNOVIAL SHEATH OF THE TENDON OF THE POPLITEUS MUSCLE AND THE BURSA BETWEEN THAT MUSCLE AND THE POSTERIOR SURFACE OF THE OUTER TUBEROSITY OF THE TIBIA, AND THE RELATION OF THE SYNOVIAL SHEATH OF THE TENDON TO THE EXTERNAL LATERAL LIGAMENT OF THE KNEE-JOINT. (THE PROXIMAL EXTREMITIES OF THE BONES OF THE LEG WITH THE ANTERIOR WALL OF THE CAPSULE OF THE KNEE-JOINT SEEN FROM BEHIND.)

After the joint had been injected, and the injected material allowed to solidify, the capsule of the joint was prepared from without, the quadriceps extensor cruris muscle being left intact; the lateral ligaments and the tendon of the popliteus muscle were then divided, and the capsule was opened behind and on either side at a higher level than the semilunar cartilages, and was divided in front along the line of its reflection on to the anterior surface of the femur; after division of the crucial ligaments, the femur was removed.

Articulatio genu—The knee-joint.

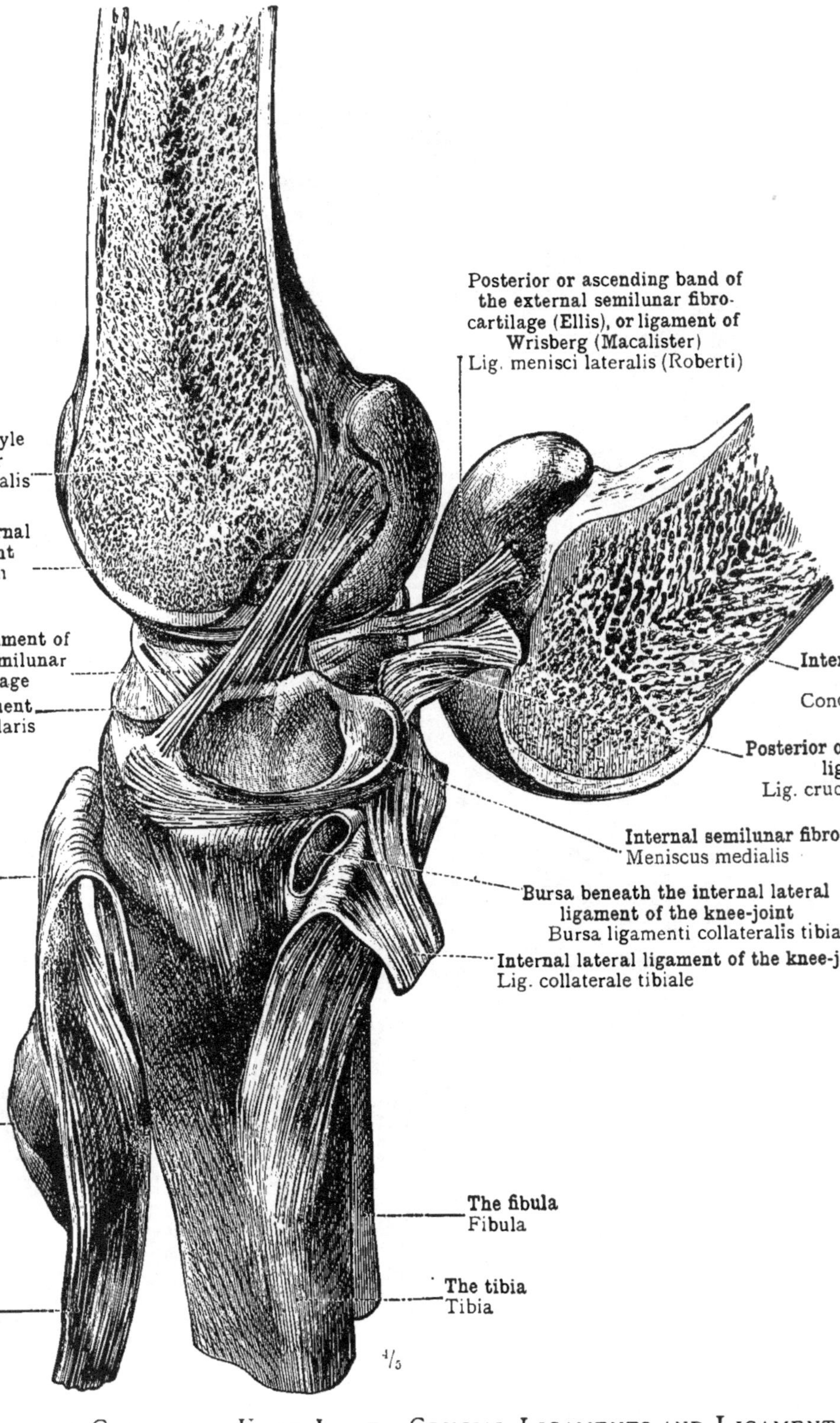

FIG. 474.—ARTICULATIO GENU, THE KNEE-JOINT: CRUCIAL LIGAMENTS AND LIGAMENT OF WRISBERG; BURSA BENEATH THE INTERNAL LATERAL LIGAMENT OF THE KNEE-JOINT. (THE RIGHT KNEE-JOINT SEEN FROM THE INNER SIDE.)

The capsule was removed, the patellar ligament and the internal lateral ligament were turned downwards: the femur was divided sagittally through the middle of the intercondylar fossa, and the external condyle placed in the position it occupies during extension of the knee-joint, while the internal condyle was turned backwards and rotated on its median axis to the extent of 180°.

Articulatio genu—The knee-joint.

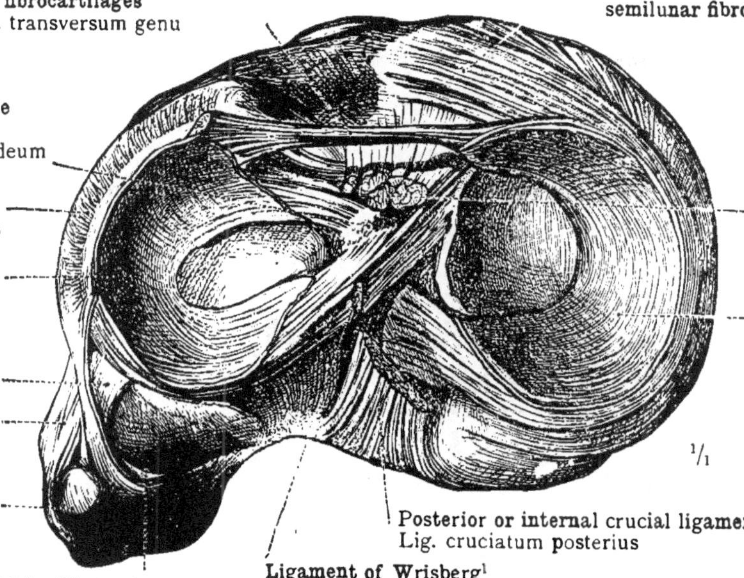

[1] See note to p. 233.

FIG. 475.—THE DISTAL ARTICULAR SURFACES OF THE KNEE-JOINT: THE INTERARTICULAR SEMILUNAR FIBROCARTILAGES, AND THE EXTENSION OF THE ANTERIOR EXTREMITIES OF THESE IN THE TRANSVERSE LIGAMENT OF THE SEMILUNAR FIBROCARTILAGES. THE COMMUNICATION BETWEEN THE SUPERIOR TIBIOFIBULAR ARTICULATION AND THE SYNOVIAL SHEATH OF THE TENDON OF THE POPLITEUS MUSCLE. (THE PROXIMAL EXTREMITY OF THE LEFT TIBIA WITH THE SEMILUNAR FIBROCARTILAGES AND THE HEAD OF THE FIBULA, SEEN FROM ABOVE.)

The capsule was divided above (proximal to) the semilunar fibrocartilages, the crucial ligaments were cut across, and the femur was removed.

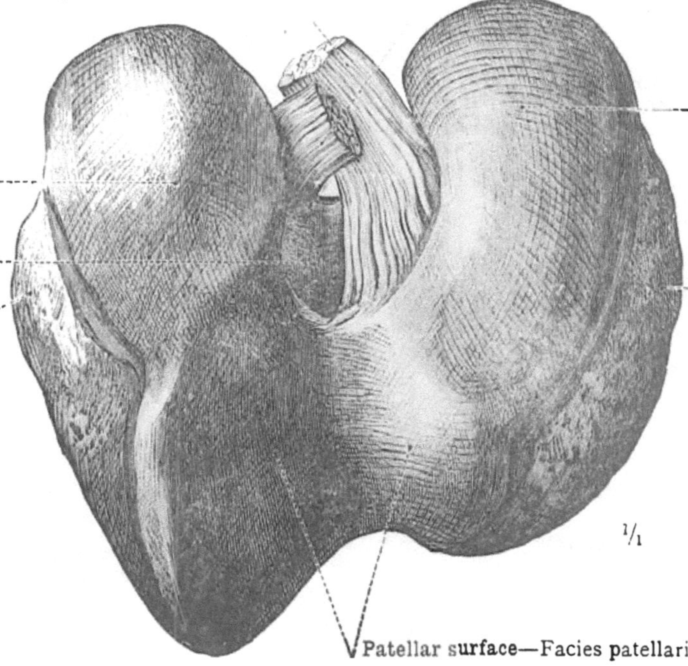

FIG. 476.—THE PROXIMAL ARTICULAR SURFACES OF THE KNEE-JOINT, AND THE FEMORAL ATTACHMENTS OF THE CRUCIAL LIGAMENTS.

The distal extremity of the femur removed from the preparation shown in Fig. 475, seen from below.

Articulatio genu—The knee-joint.

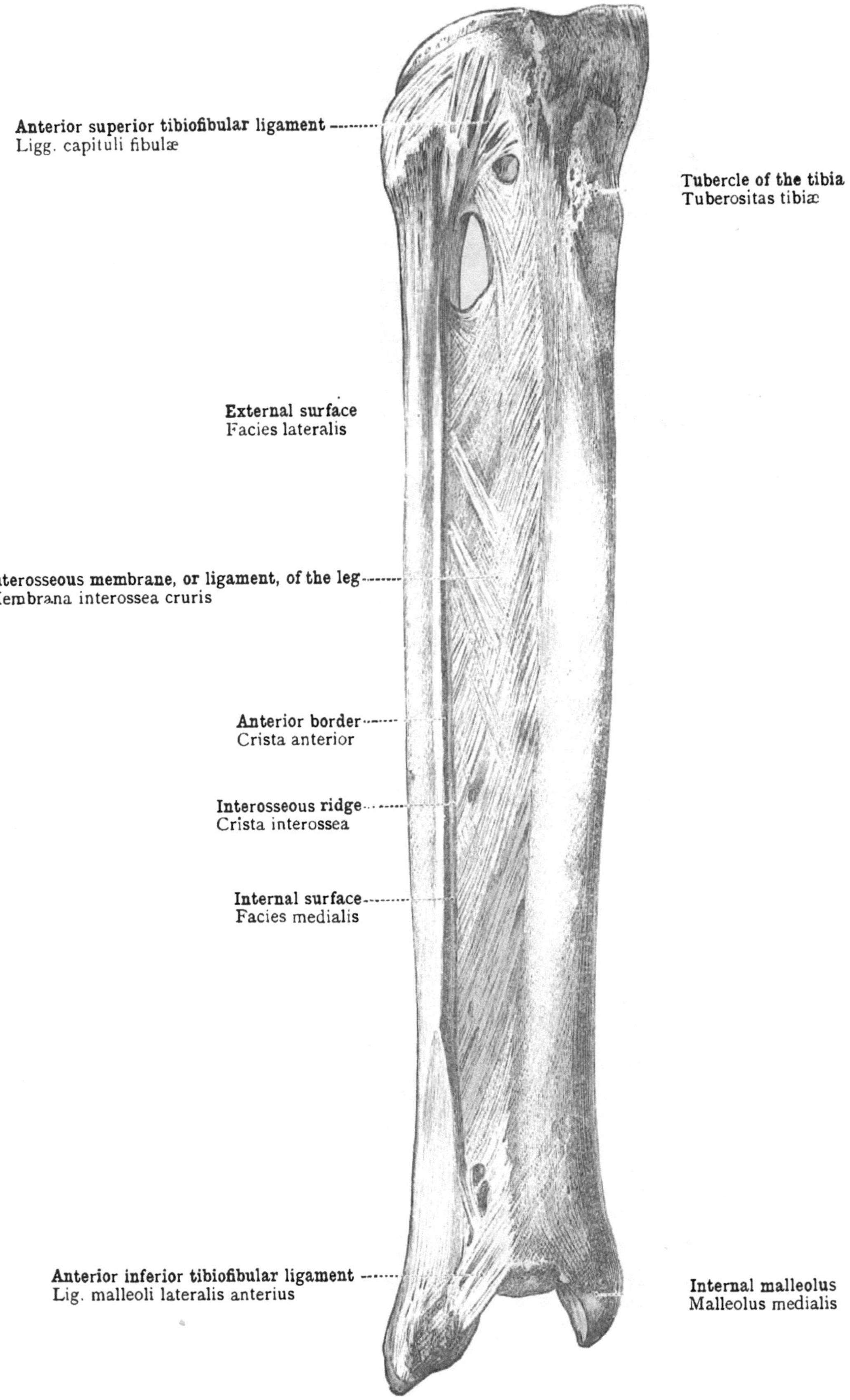

FIG. 477.—ARTICULATIO TIBIOFIBULARIS ET SYNDESMOSIS TIBIOFIBULARIS, THE TIBIOFIBULAR ARTICULATIONS. THE INTEROSSEOUS MEMBRANE, OR LIGAMENT, OF THE RIGHT LEG; THE ANTERIOR SUPERIOR AND ANTERIOR INFERIOR TIBIOFIBULAR LIGAMENTS. (SEEN FROM BEFORE.)

The Tibiofibular Articulations.

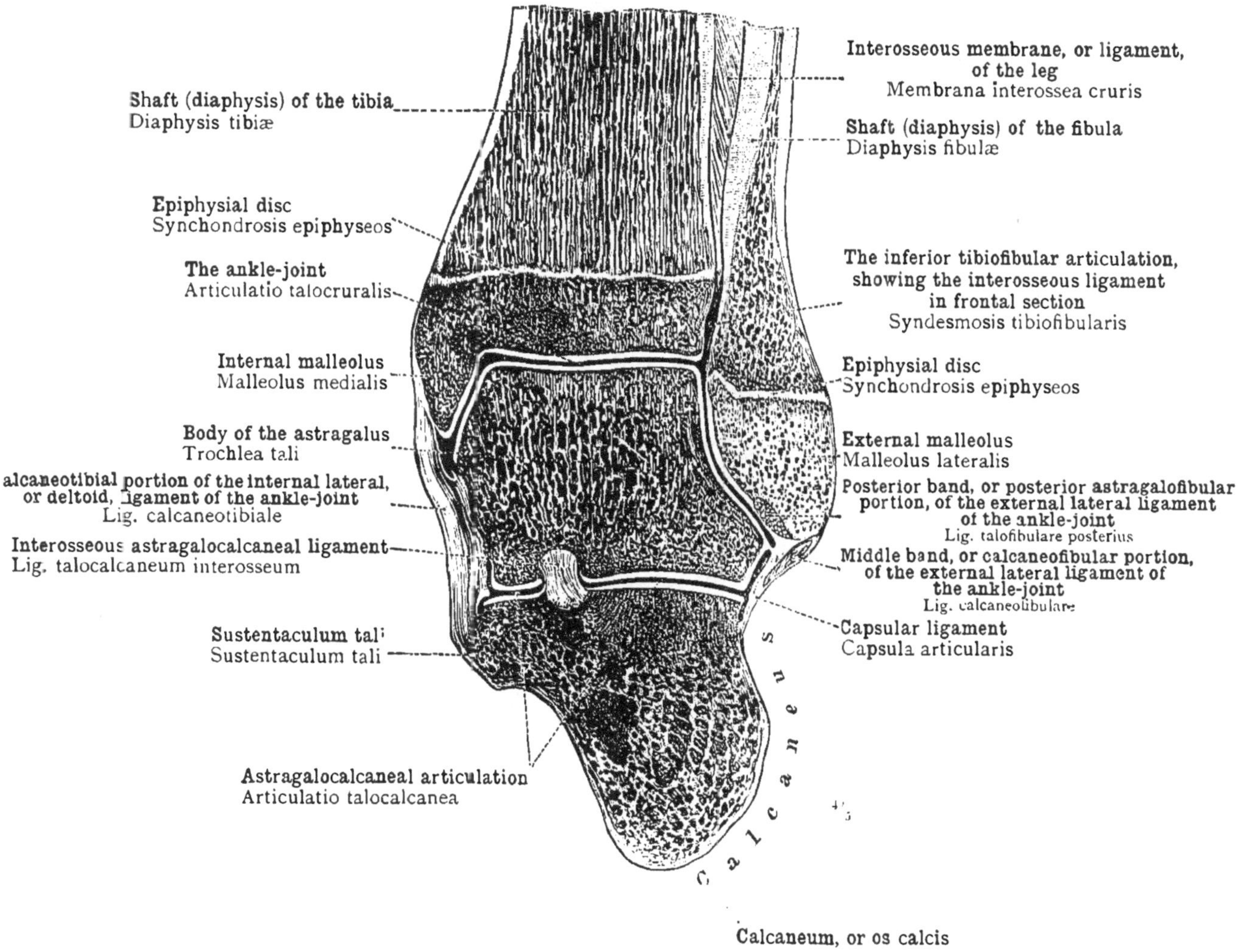

FIG. 478.—ARTICULATIONES TALOCRURALIS ET TALOCALCANEA, THE ANKLE-JOINT AND THE ASTRAGALOCALCANEAL ARTICULATION; SYNDESMOSIS TIBIOFIBULARIS, INFERIOR TIBIOFIBULAR ARTICULATION, SHOWING THE INTEROSSEOUS LIGAMENT. THE RELATIONS OF THE DISTAL EPIPHYSIAL DISCS OF THE TIBIA AND THE FIBULA TO THE ANKLE-JOINT. (THE ANKLE-JOINT AND THE ASTRAGALOCALCANEAL ARTICULATION OF THE RIGHT LEG, DIVIDED IN A VERTICAL PLANE CLOSELY APPROXIMATING THE FRONTAL PLANE; POSTERIOR SURFACE OF THE ANTERIOR SEGMENT.)

The plane of section passes through the lowermost parts of the lateral portions of the superior articular surface of the astragalus.

Articulationes pedis—The articulations of the foot.

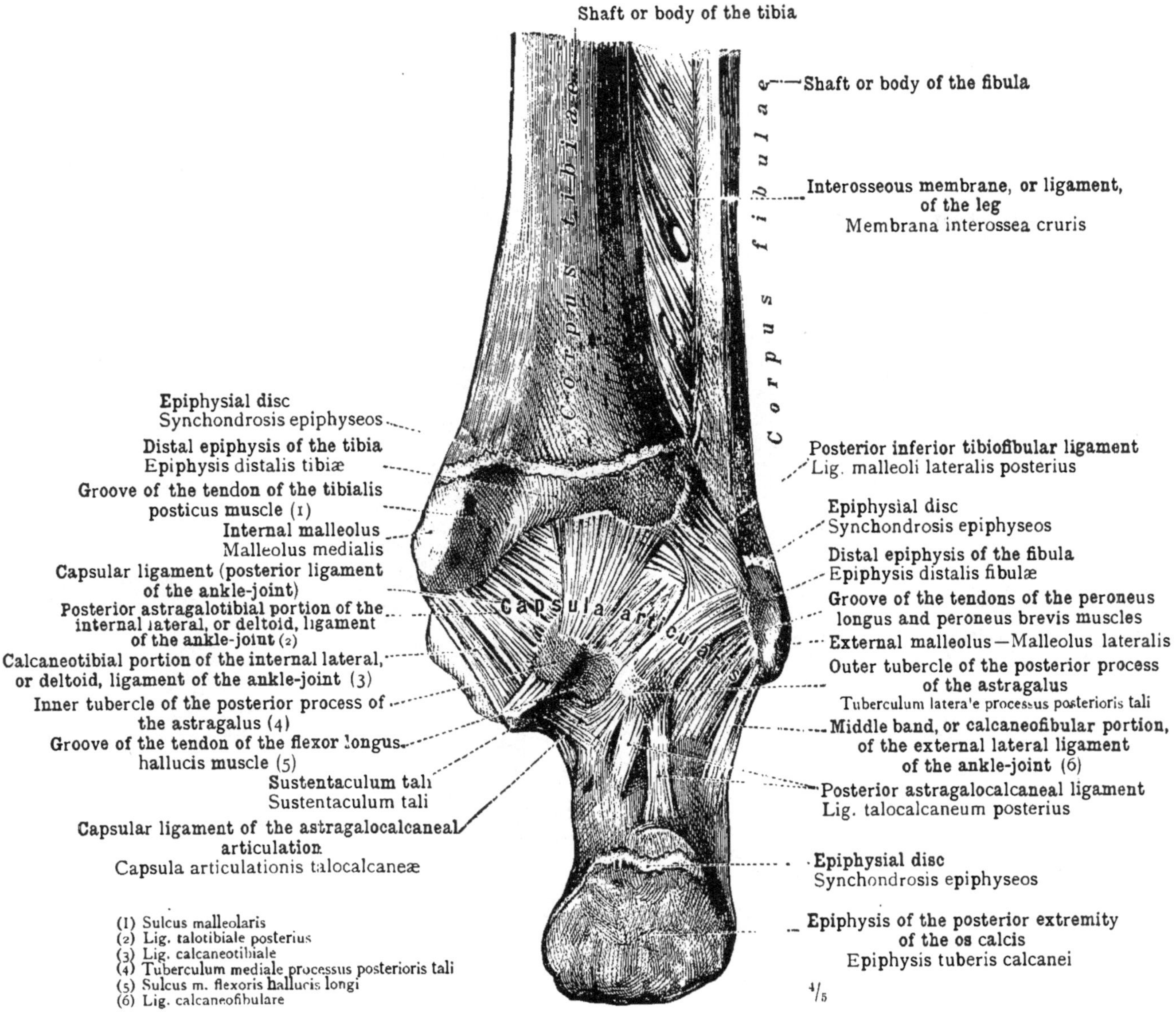

FIG. 479.—THE CAPSULAR LIGAMENTS AND THE SUPERFICIAL POSTERIOR LIGAMENTS OF THE ANKLE-JOINT AND OF THE ASTRAGALOCALCANEAL ARTICULATION. THE RELATIONS OF THE DISTAL EPIPHYSIAL DISCS OF THE TIBIA AND FIBULA TO THE ANKLE-JOINT. THE POSTERIOR PORTIONS OF THE LATERAL LIGAMENTS OF THE ANKLE-JOINT: LIGAMENTUM TALOTIBIALE POSTERIUS, THE POSTERIOR ASTRAGALOTIBIAL PORTION OF THE INTERNAL LATERAL, OR DELTOID, LIGAMENT OF THE ANKLE-JOINT; LIGAMENTUM CALCANEOTIBIALE, THE CALCANEOTIBIAL PORTION OF THE INTERNAL LATERAL, OR DELTOID, LIGAMENT OF THE ANKLE-JOINT; LIGAMENTUM CALCANEOFIBULARE, THE MIDDLE BAND, OR CALCANEOFIBULAR PORTION, OF THE EXTERNAL LATERAL LIGAMENT OF THE ANKLE-JOINT. LIGAMENTUM TALOCALCANEUM POSTERIUS, THE POSTERIOR ASTRAGALOCALCANEAL LIGAMENT.—SYNDESMOSIS TIBIOFIBULARIS: LIGAMENTUM MALLEOLI LATERALIS POSTERIUS, THE POSTERIOR INFERIOR TIBIOFIBULAR LIGAMENT. (THE ANKLE-JOINT AND THE ASTRAGALOCALCANEAL ARTICULATION OF THE RIGHT LEG, SEEN FROM BEHIND.)

Articulationes pedis The articulations of the foot.

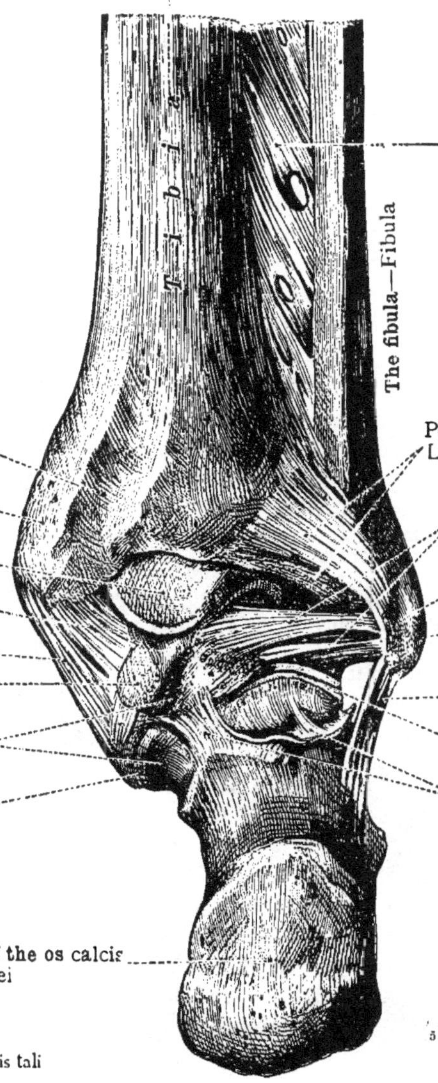

FIG. 480.—ARTICULATIONES TALOCRURALIS ET TALOCALCANEA, THE ANKLE-JOINT AND THE ASTRAGALOCALCANEAL ARTICULATION; SYNDESMOSIS TIBIOFIBULARIS, THE INFERIOR TIBIOFIBULAR ARTICULATION: LIGAMENTUM MALLEOLI LATERALIS POSTERIUS, THE POSTERIOR INFERIOR TIBIOFIBULAR LIGAMENT. THE POSTERIOR PORTIONS OF THE LATERAL LIGAMENTS: LIGAMENTUM TALOTIBIALE POSTERIUS, THE POSTERIOR ASTRAGALOTIBIAL PORTION OF THE INTERNAL LATERAL, OR DELTOID, LIGAMENT OF THE ANKLE-JOINT; LIGAMENTUM CALCANEOTIBIALE, THE CALCANEOTIBIAL PORTION OF THE INTERNAL LATERAL, OR DELTOID, LIGAMENT OF THE ANKLE-JOINT; LIGAMENTUM TALOFIBULARE POSTERIUS, THE POSTERIOR BAND, OR ASTRAGALOFIBULAR PORTION, OF THE EXTERNAL LATERAL LIGAMENT OF THE ANKLE-JOINT; LIGAMENTUM CALCANEOFIBULARE, THE MIDDLE BAND, OR CALCANEOFIBULAR PORTION, OF THE EXTERNAL LATERAL LIGAMENT OF THE ANKLE-JOINT. (THE ANKLE-JOINT AND THE ASTRAGALOCALCANEAL ARTICULATION OF THE RIGHT LEG, SEEN FROM BEHIND.)

The thin posterior portion of the capsule of the ankle-joint has been removed The posterior portion of the capsule of the astragalocalcaneal articulation has been separated from its attachment to the astragalus external to its attachment to the posterior process of that bone, and turned backwards on to the os calcis.

Articulationes pedis—The articulations of the foot.

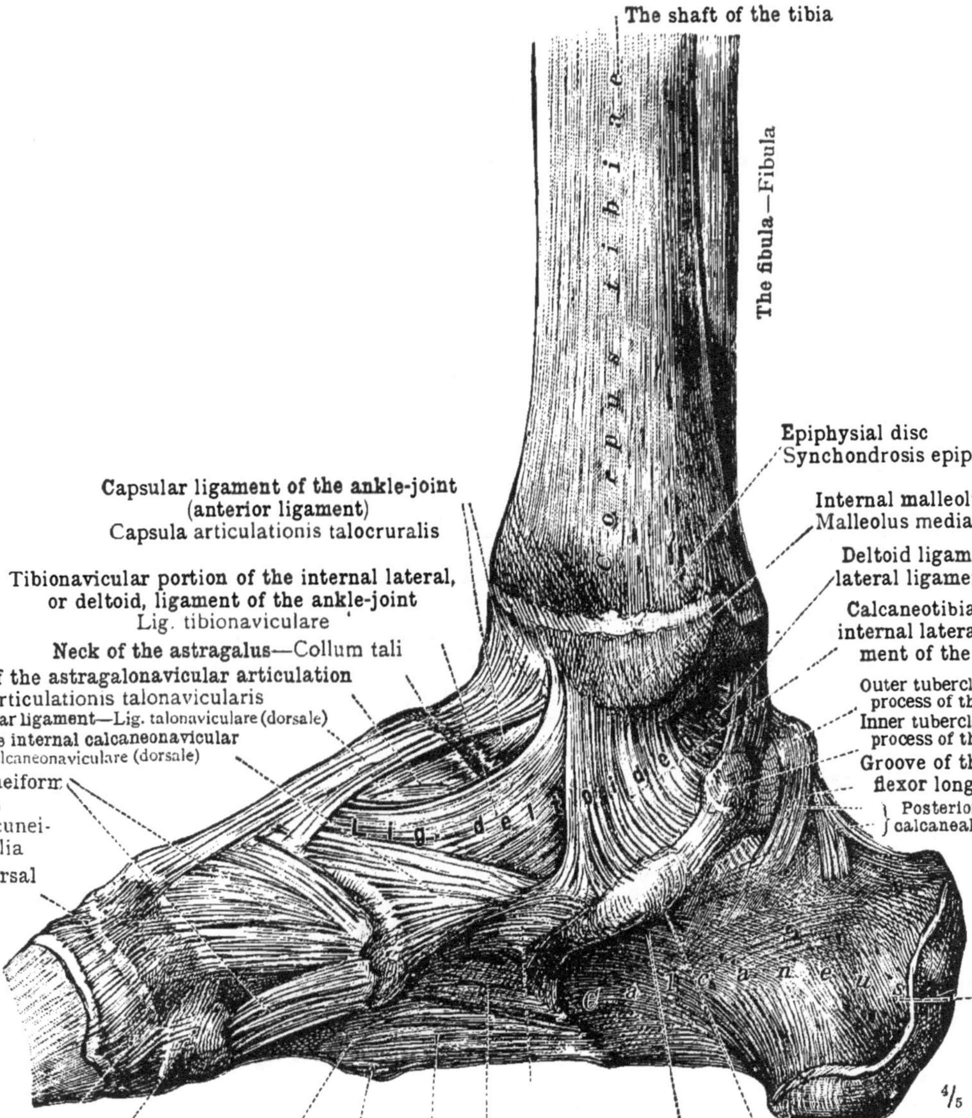

[1] See note [1] to p. 248.

Fig. 481.—The Superficial Internal Ligaments of the Ankle-Joint and of the Astragalocalcaneal Articulation, and the Relation of the Distal Epiphysial Disc of the Tibia to the Ankle-Joint. (The Right Tarsus, with the Adjoining Portions of the Tibia and Fibula and of the First Metatarsal Bone; seen from the Inner Side.)

Articulationes pedis—The articulations of the foot.

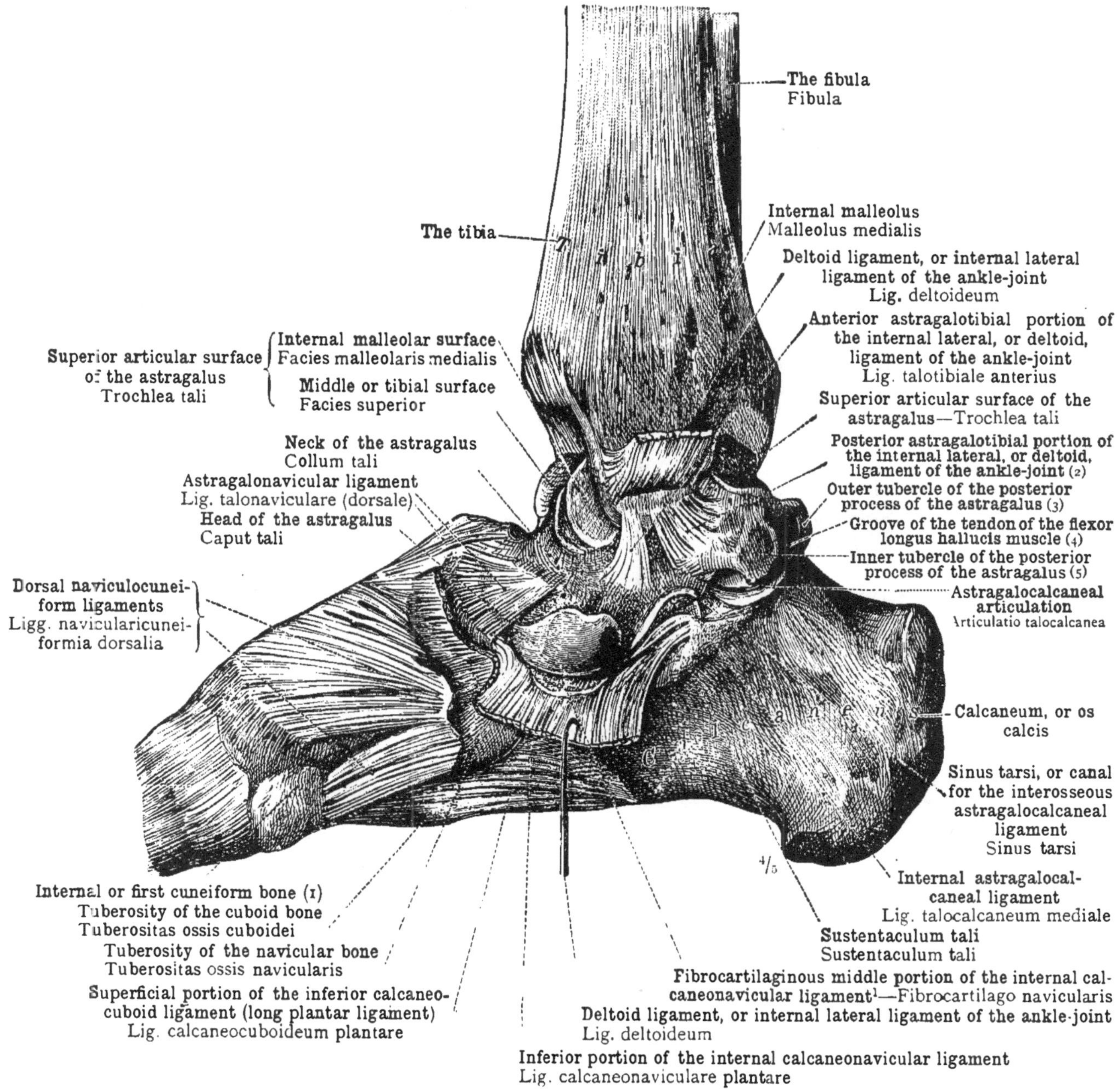

(1) Os cuneiforme I. (2) Lig. talotibiale posterius (3) Tuberculum laterale (4) Sulcus m. flexoris hallucis longi (5) Tuberculum mediale

[1] See note [1] to p. 248.

FIG. 482.—THE DEEP INTERNAL LIGAMENTS OF THE ANKLE-JOINT AND OF THE ASTRAGALOCALCANEAL ARTICULATION. (THE RIGHT TARSUS, WITH THE ADJOINING PORTIONS OF THE TIBIA AND FIBULA AND OF THE FIRST METATARSAL BONE; SEEN FROM THE INNER SIDE.)

The deltoid ligament (internal lateral ligament of the ankle-joint) has been cut across the middle, and the divided ends have been turned up and down. The capsular ligaments of the ankle-joint and of the astragalocalcaneal articulation have been removed, except for the deeper special bands.

Articulationes pedis—The articulations of the foot.

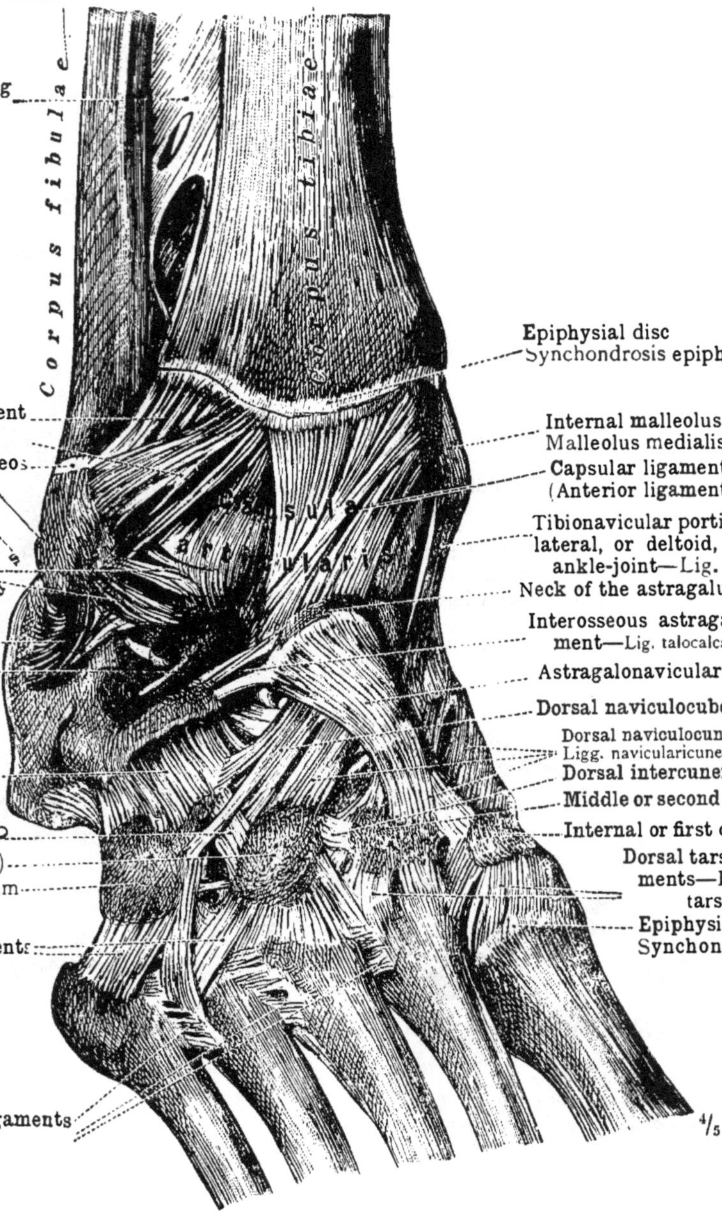

(1) Lig. talofibulare anterius
(2) Lig. calcaneofibulare
(3) Os cuneiforme III.
(4) Lig. talonaviculare (dorsale)
(5) Lig. cuboideonaviculare dorsale
(6) Lig. intercuneiforme dorsale
(7) Os cuneiforme II.
(8) Os cuneiforme I.

FIG. 483.—ARTICULATIO TALOCRURALIS, THE ANKLE-JOINT; SYNDESMOSIS TIBIOFIBULARIS, THE INFERIOR TIBIOFIBULAR ARTICULATION. THE RELATIONS OF THE DISTAL EPIPHYSIAL DISCS OF THE TIBIA AND FIBULA TO THE ANKLE-JOINT. ARTICULATIONES INTERTARSEÆ ET TARSOMETATARSEÆ, THE INTERTARSAL AND TARSOMETATARSAL ARTICULATIONS; ARTICULATIONES INTERMETATARSEÆ, THE INTERMETATARSAL ARTICULATIONS. LIGAMENTA TARSI DORSALIA ET TARSOMETATARSEA DORSALIA ET LIGAMENTA BASIUM DORSALIA; THE DORSAL LIGAMENTS OF THE TARSUS, THE DORSAL TARSOMETATARSAL LIGAMENTS, AND THE DORSAL PROXIMAL INTERMETATARSAL LIGAMENTS. (THE RIGHT TARSUS WITH THE ADJOINING PORTIONS OF THE TIBIA AND FIBULA AND OF THE METATARSUS; DORSO-EXTERNAL ASPECT.)

The joints are unopened except for the astragalocalcaneal, astragalonavicular, and naviculocuneiform articulations, which have been partly opened.

Articulationes pedis—The articulations of the foot.

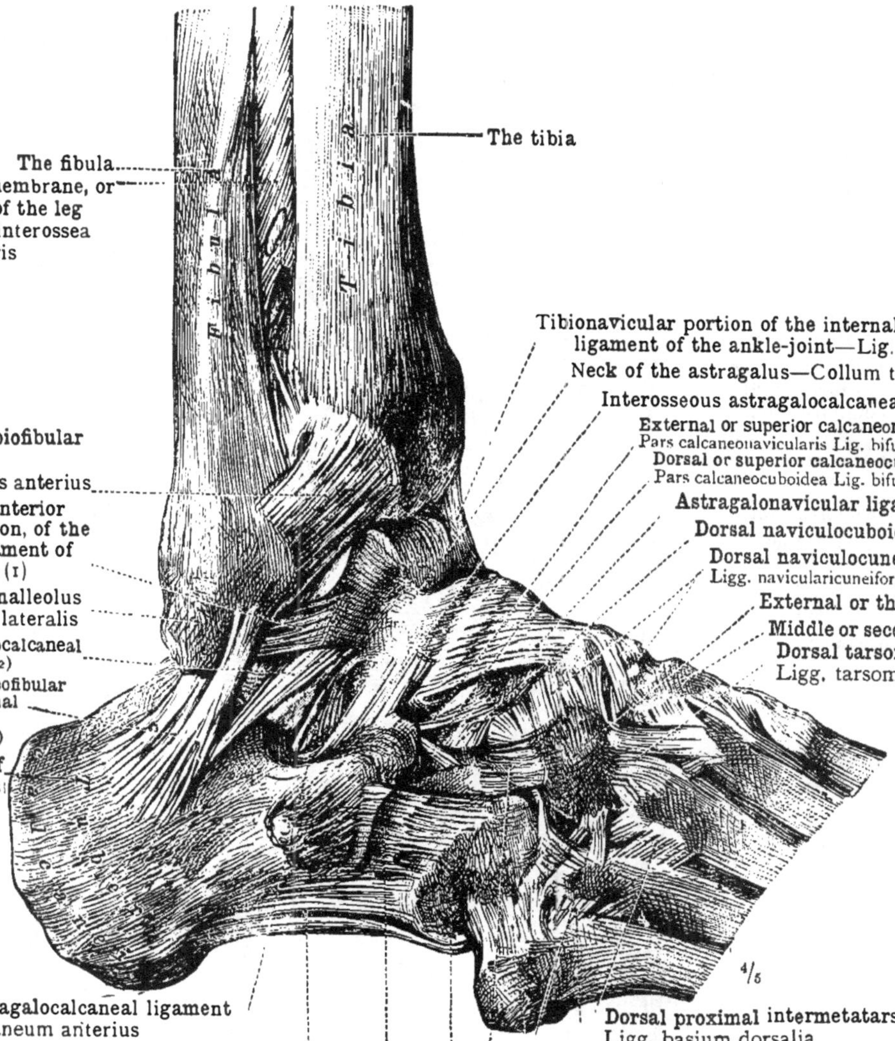

(1) Lig. talofibulare anterius
(2) Lig. talocalcaneum laterale
(3) Lig. calcaneofibulare
(4) Lig. talocalcaneum interosseum
(5) Lig. talonaviculare (dorsale)
(6) Lig. cuboideonaviculare dorsale
(7) Os cuneiforme III.
(8) Os cuneiforme II.

[1] The strongest part of this ligament is situate external, and not superior, to the calcaneocuboid articulation; it would therefore be more appropriately named the *external calcaneocuboid* ligament.—TR.
[2] In the English nomenclature these are regarded as two distinct ligaments, not, as by Toldt, as two parts of a single ligament.—TR.

FIG. 484.—ARTICULATIONES TALOCRURALIS ET TALOCALCANEA, THE ANKLE-JOINT AND THE ASTRAGALOCALCANEAL ARTICULATION; LIGAMENTUM MALLEOLI LATERALIS ANTERIUS, ANTERIOR INFERIOR TIBIOFIBULAR LIGAMENT. THE ANTERIOR AND MIDDLE BANDS OF THE EXTERNAL LATERAL LIGAMENT OF THE ANKLE-JOINT (LIGAMENTUM TALOFIBULARE ANTERIUS ET LIGAMENTUM CALCANEOFIBULARE): LIGAMENTA TALOCALCANEA, LATERALE. *ANTERIUS, ET INTEROSSEUM: THE EXTERNAL, *ANTERIOR, AND INTEROSSEOUS ASTRAGALOCALCANEAL LIGAMENTS.—ARTICULATIONES INTERTARSEÆ ET TARSOMETATARSEÆ, THE INTERTARSAL AND TARSOMETATARSAL ARTICULATIONS; ARTICULATIONES INTERMETATARSEÆ, THE INTERMETATARSAL ARTICULATIONS: LIGAMENTA TARSI DORSALIA, LIGAMENTA TARSOMETATARSEÆ DORSALIA, ET LIGAMENTA BASIUM DORSALIA, THE DEEPER DORSAL TARSAL AND TARSOMETATARSAL LIGAMENTS, AND THE DORSAL PROXIMAL INTERMETATARSAL LIGAMENTS. (THE RIGHT TARSUS, WITH THE ADJOINING PORTIONS OF THE TIBIA AND FIBULA AND OF THE METATARSAL BONES; DORSO-EXTERNAL ASPECT.)

The anterior ligament of the ankle-joint and the lateral portion of the capsule of the astragalocalcaneal articulation have been removed.

Articulationes pedis—The articulations of the foot.

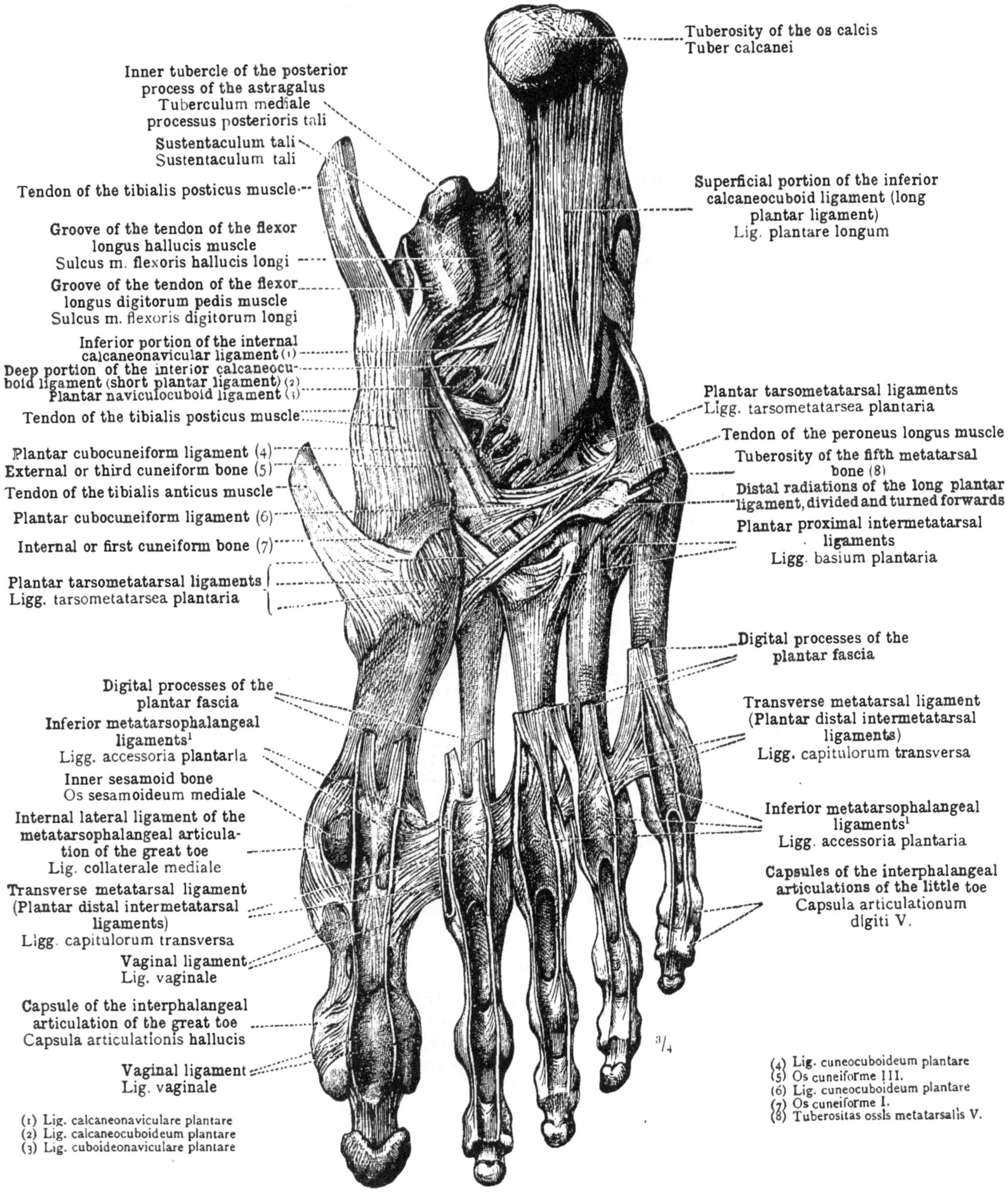

[1] *Fibrous* or *sesamoid plate* (Quain), or *glenoid plate* (Macalister).—TR.

FIG. 485.—THE SUPERFICIAL LIGAMENTS OF THE PLANTAR SURFACE OF THE RIGHT FOOT AND THE RELATIONS OF THE TENDONS OF THE TIBIALIS ANTICUS AND POSTICUS AND OF THE PERONEUS LONGUS MUSCLES TO THESE LIGAMENTS. LIGAMENTA TARSI ET TARSOMETATARSEÆ, THE TARSAL AND THE TARSOMETATARSAL LIGAMENTS: LIGAMENTA BASIUM PLANTARIA, LIGAMENTA CAPITULORUM TRANSVERSA, ET LIGAMENTA ACCESSORIA PLANTARIA; THE PLANTAR PROXIMAL INTERMETATARSAL LIGAMENTS, THE TRANSVERSE METATARSAL LIGAMENT, AND THE INFERIOR METATARSOPHALANGEAL LIGAMENTS (*see note above*); THE RELATIONS OF THESE LIGAMENTS TO THE DIGITAL PROCESSES OF THE PLANTAR FASCIA.

Articulationes pedis—The articulations of the foot.

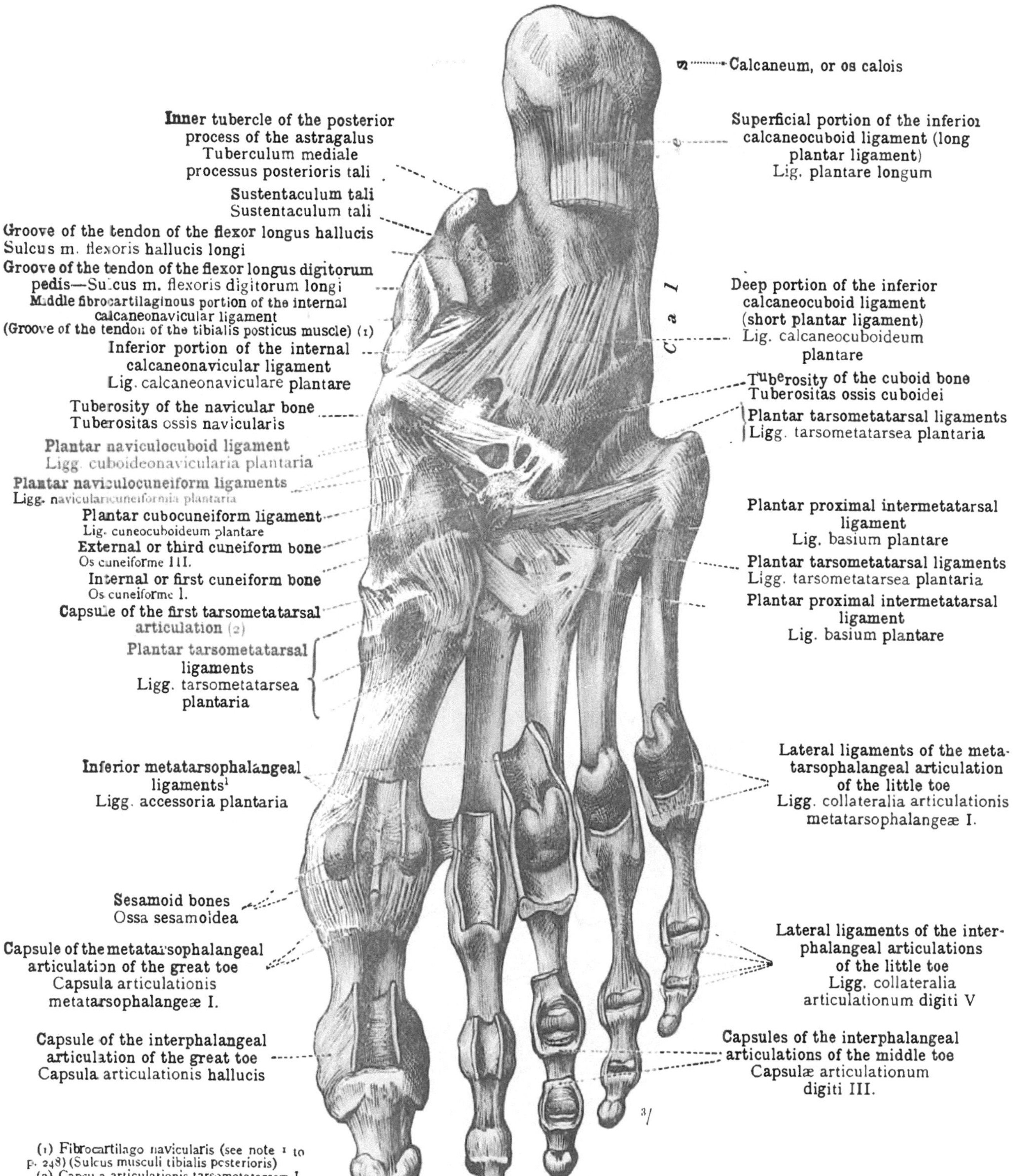

See note to p. 246.

FIG. 485.—THE DEEP LIGAMENTS OF THE SOLE OF THE FOOT AND THE SESAMOID BONES OF THE METATARSOPHALANGEAL ARTICULATION OF THE GREAT TOE.

In the preparation shown in Fig. 485 the tendons of the muscles were removed, also the long plantar ligament except for its posterior extremity, and the transverse metatarsal ligament and the digital processes of the plantar fascia were cut away. Some of the metatarsophalangeal and interphalangeal articulations have been opened ; others have been left intact.

Articulationes pedis—The articulations of the foot.

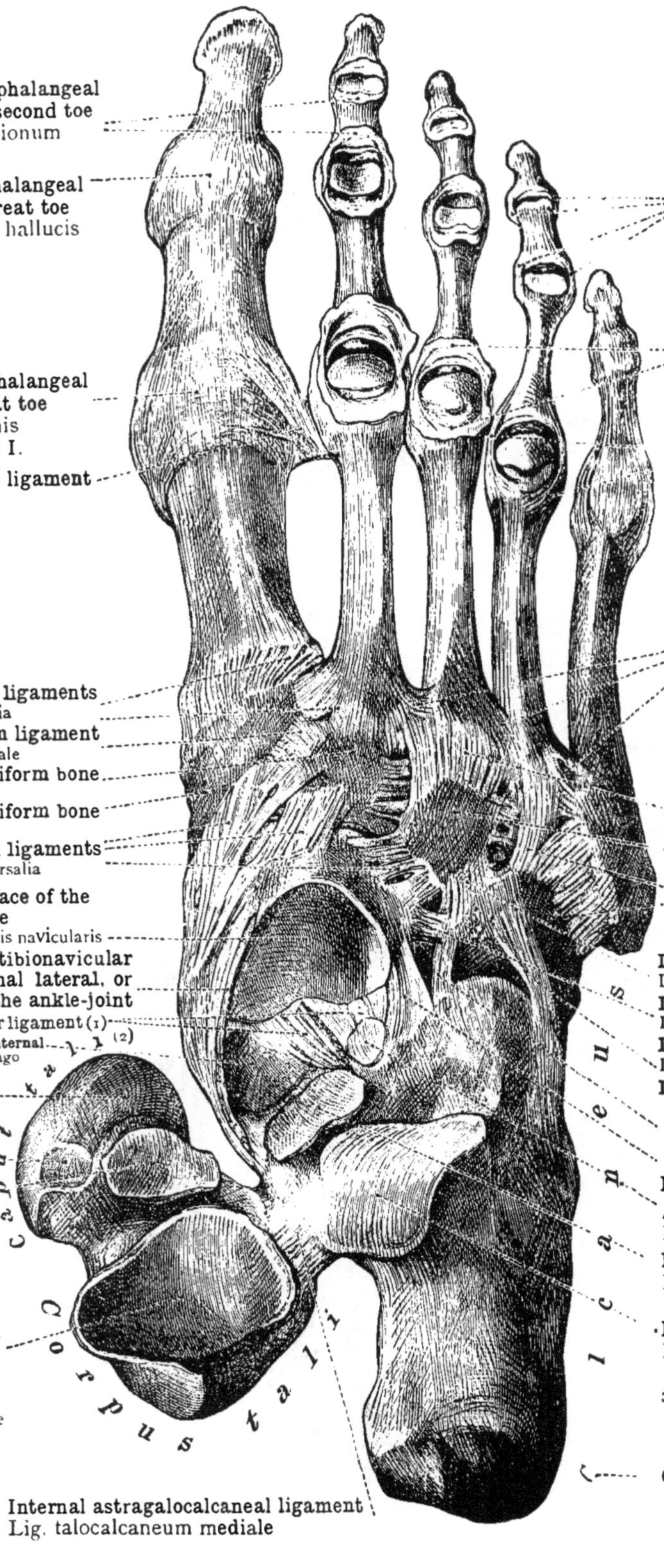

¹ *Fibrocartilago navicularis:* This term, though a most suitable one, is not employed by English anatomists. It is applied by the author to the middle fibrocartilaginous portion of the internal calcaneonavicular ligament, the *superior* surface of which articulates with a special facet on the head of the astragalus, between the internal of the three facets for the os calcis (posteriorly) and the facet for the navicular bone (anteriorly). The internal articular facet of the os calcis, the facet on the superior surface of the *fibrocartilago navicularis*, and the posterior articular facet of the navicular bone, thus form a continuous articular surface for the head of the astragalus. The *inferior* surface of the *cartilago navicularis*, likewise cartilaginous in texture, forms, as shown in Fig. 487, the groove for the tendon of the tibialis posticus muscle.—Tr.

² See note ¹ to p. 245.

FIG. 487.—THE ARTICULAR SURFACES OF THE ASTRAGALOCALCANEONAVICULAR ARTICULATION, THE DEEP LIGAMENTS OF THE DORSUM OF THE FOOT, THE METATARSOPHALANGEAL AND INTERPHALANGEAL ARTICULATIONS OF THE TOES. (THE RIGHT FOOT SEEN FROM THE DORSAL SIDE.)

The capsule of the astragalocalcaneal articulation was removed, with the exception of the internal astragalocalcaneal ligament; the capsule of the astragalonavicular articulation was also removed with the exception of its internal and plantar walls; and, after removing the interosseous astragalocalcaneal ligament, the astragalus was rotated inwards (on the internal astragalocalcaneal ligament as a hinge), until its inferior surface looked directly upwards.

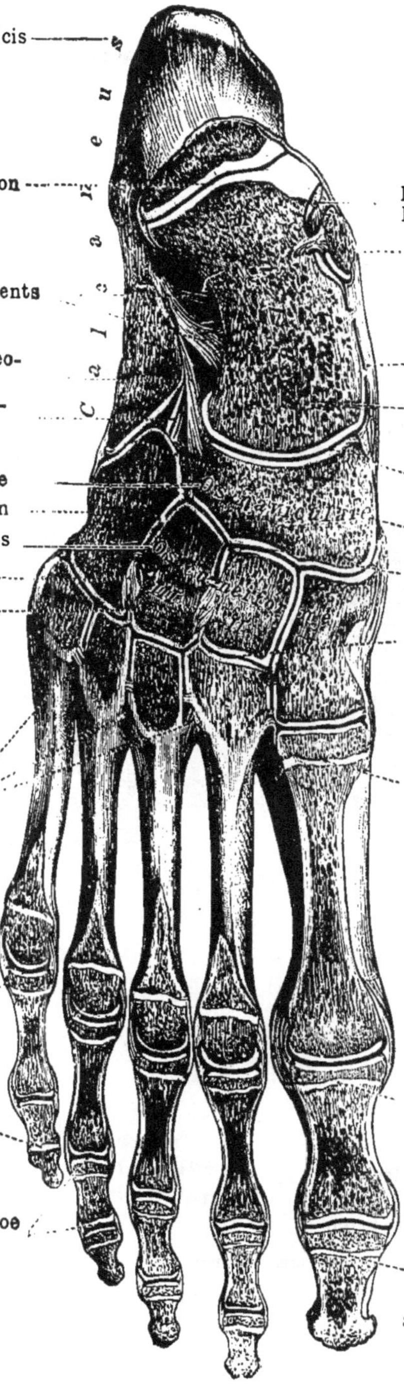

[1] See note [1] to p. 245.

[2] Known also as the *mediotarsal* or *mid-tarsal* joint. It is through this joint (the two parts of which are, however, entirely separate articulations) that the foot is divided in Chopart's amputation.

[3] It is through the tarsometatarsal articulations that the foot is divided in Lisfranc's amputation.

FIG. 488.—ARTICULATIONES INTERTARSEÆ ET TARSOMETATARSEÆ, THE INTERTARSAL AND TARSOMETATARSAL ARTICULATIONS, SHOWING CHOPART'S (MEDIOTARSAL) LINE, AND LISFRANC'S OR HEY'S TARSOMETATARSAL LINE: LIGAMENTA TARSI INTEROSSEA ET LIGAMENTA CUNEOMETATARSEA INTEROSSEA, THE INTEROSSEOUS LIGAMENTS OF THE TARSUS, AND THE INTEROSSEOUS METATARSOCUNEIFORM LIGAMENTS. ARTICULATIONES INTERMETATARSEÆ, THE INTERMETATARSAL ARTICULATIONS. ARTICULATIONES METATARSOPHALANGEÆ, THE METATARSOPHALANGEAL ARTICULATIONS. ARTICULATIONES DIGITORUM PEDIS, THE INTERPHALANGEAL ARTICULATIONS OF THE TOES. THE RELATIONS OF THE EPIPHYSIAL DISCS OF THE METATARSAL BONES AND OF THE PHALANGES OF THE TOES TO THE RESPECTIVE ARTICULATIONS. (HORIZONTAL SECTION THROUGH THE ARTICULATIONS OF THE RIGHT FOOT OF A YOUTH AGED SEVENTEEN YEARS. SUPERIOR SURFACE OF THE LOWER SEGMENT.)

Articulationes pedis—The articulations of the foot.

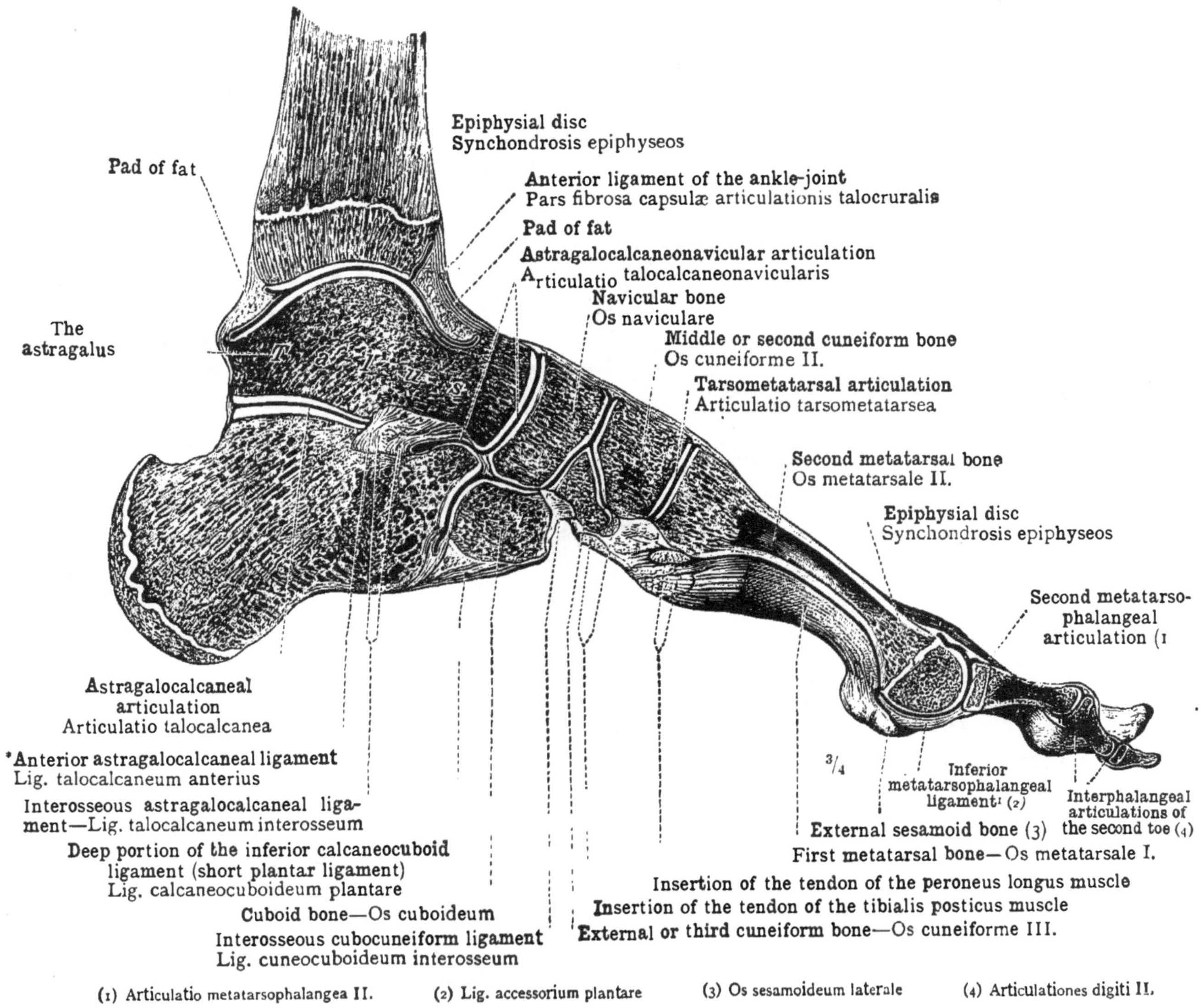

(1) Articulatio metatarsophalangea II. (2) Lig. accessorium plantare (3) Os sesamoideum laterale (4) Articulationes digiti II.

[1] See note to p. 246.

FIG. 489.—THE ARTICULATIONS OF THE RIGHT FOOT OF A YOUTH AGED SEVENTEEN YEARS, SEEN IN SAGITTAL SECTION, AND SHOWING THE RELATIONS OF THESE ARTICULATIONS TO THE EPIPHYSIAL DISCS.

The section passes through the distal extremity of the tibia, the astragalus, the os calcis, the middle cuneiform bone, the second metatarsal bone, and the phalanges of the second toe.

Articulationes pedis—The articulations of the foot.

INDEX
TO THE ARTHROLOGY

Certain names in this Index have an asterisk (*) prefixed; these, as more fully explained in the Translator's Preface, being terms that form part of the English nomenclature used in this work, but which are not commonly employed by English anatomists. To other names a dagger (†) is prefixed; these are Latin names used by the author in the original work, but not included in the official nomenclature of the "Anatomische Gesellschaft."

M.

N.

O.

P.

R.

S.

T.

V.

W.

Z.

This book has been produced in line with the EU GPSR guidelines about the safety of products.

The General Product Safety Regulation is the European Union's updated framework for ensuring that all consumer products, including books, are safe for consumers.

This book has been printed by CPI books GmbH. The printer has issued safety certificates for the materials - like ink, paper and glue - being used.

The product identifier is: 9786256629608

The author is responsible for the content of the book, is the publisher of the works and bears full responsibility for it.

The book has been published via Bookmundo. Bookmundo enables any author to share their stories with the rest of the world via printed books and ebooks and a broad distribution network.

Bookmundo will act as an intermediary in regard to questions about safety and will address them to the printer / author. Should there be any question in regard to the safety of the product, please contact us.

Bookmundo
Delftsestraat 33
3013AE Rotterdam
The Netherlands
info@bookmundo.com